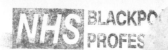
Breaking Down Barriers

Breaking Down Barriers

ACCESS TO FURTHER AND HIGHER EDUCATION
FOR VISUALLY IMPAIRED STUDENTS

Jane S. Owen Hutchinson
Manager Physiotherapy Support Service (RNIB), London

Karen Atkinson
Manager RNIB Resource Centre
Department of Health Sciences
University of East London

Jenny Orpwood
Former Member Physiotherapy Support Service (RNIB)
University of East London

Consultant Editor
Jo Campling

RNIB
challenging blindness

**Published in collaboration with the
Royal National Institute for the Blind**

Stanley Thornes (Publishers) Ltd

First printed in 1998 by:
Stanley Thornes (Publishers) Ltd
Ellenborough House
Wellington Street
CHELTENHAM
GL50 1YW
United Kingdom

98 99 00 01 02 / 10 9 8 7 6 5 4 3 2 1

A catalogue record for this book is available from the British Library

ISBN 0-7487-3344-2

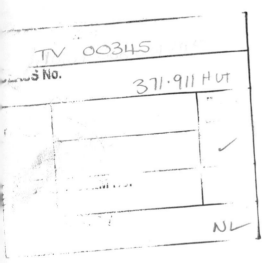

Typeset by WestKey Ltd., Falmouth, Cornwall
Printed and bound in Great Britain by T.J. International Ltd., Padstow, Cornwall

Contents

Foreword

This book will be of great value in removing barriers to further and higher education for blind and partially sighted students. It should be required reading for many educationalists and other staff who are responsible for teaching and assisting students.

Everyone should have the opportunities to reach his or her full educational potential, since learning through life is essential to the future success of our nation. We need the creativity and enterprise of *all* our people. But in the past, we have too often ignored or neglected opportunities for students who have some form of disability. The degree to which people with disabilities achieve their learning ambitions is, I believe, a measure of the effectiveness and the civilization of the educational system. This book should help many institutions to make progress, at least in respect of visual impairment.

One key concept, which the authors embrace, is the idea of inclusive learning. The idea is startlingly simple yet profound: we need to avoid the idea that the difficulty lies with the student. Instead, colleges and universities should understand and respond to the individual student's needs. We should concentrate on understanding how people learn, how they can gain greater access to information and have the practical support and technology to overcome obstacles to learning, and work on equal terms. The broader application of the idea is obvious if we are serious about widening participation and reaching out to those with a history of educational disadvantage.

It would certainly have been helpful to me if staff and students alike had had the opportunity to know a little about how best to be helpful, how to avoid being patronizing and how to offer practical help, before I went to university. I was lucky, those around me responded very positively and attitudes were remarkably open and inclusive. This is not always the case and anything which can smooth the way, or open up minds to how best to 'include me in', will make a very real difference.

I am, therefore, pleased to provide the Foreword to this book, and I urge its readers to put the good guidance it offers into practical effect.

David Blunkett
Secretary of State for Education and Employment
July 1998

Preface

Purpose

History, legend and literature have contributed much to the perpetuation of many popular myths and misconceptions about the effects of impaired vision on the lives of blind and partially sighted people. Although some of these myths are relatively innocuous, others are positively inimical, since they serve to license discriminatory practices founded on ignorance or prejudice. Lack of knowledge and understanding about visual impairment and its practical significance has frequently resulted in what we consider to be an unacceptable restriction in the range of life choices and opportunities presented to blind and partially sighted people.

Our concern in this book is with visual impairment alone, although we readily acknowledge that many blind and partially sighted people may have additional impairments. With a specific focus on post-school education, our principal objective is to replace fiction and conjecture with factual information and practical guidelines for both disabled students and the staff (at all levels) who work with them. Our wish is to contribute towards dismantling some of the numerous disabling barriers that many visually impaired people face when entering or participating in educational programmes within the further, higher and continuing education sectors. Our hope is that the information contained here will help colleges and universities to create accessible environments for visually impaired learners and that it will encourage blind and partially sighted people of all ages to assert their rights to receive full access to the goods, facilities and services offered by all post-school educational providers.

Philosophy

This book reflects our general commitment to the philosophy and language of the social model of disability. We believe that there is no intrinsic reason why blindness or partial sight should, *per se*, represent a barrier to full participation in society in general and education in particular. Rather, we contend that such barriers are – initially at least – erected by society: the attitudes of non-disabled people towards disability, reflected both in the construction of the external environment – including the creation of a culture of 'normality' – and in the language used to describe disabled people and their experiences. These features collectively characterize the individualistic model of disability, which depicts disability as an individual problem, placing all the responsibility for solving that problem on the victim. The disabled sufferer is expected to seek a cure for what is regarded as an illness so that conformity to what is considered to be a normal social role can occur. Feelings of guilt often drive disabled people to search, relentlessly, for medical treatment and to undergo rigorous forms of therapy and rehabilitation whose principal objective is independence at all costs. The secret of attaining this desirable state lies with the professional expert who will, in exchange for compliance with certain rules, impart the appropriate knowledge and skills to the patient. The relationship is one characterized by inequalities: all the power and control lie with professionals who often regard themselves as legitimate gatekeepers of disabled people's services. The concepts of choice and rights are meaningless and are subordinated to the needs of professional workers. The disabled person invariably becomes socialized into believing that this dependence is acceptable and that s/he must be grateful for any charity. That the goods, facilities and services offered to disabled people are invariably inferior to those available to non-disabled citizens should not be surprising, given the difference that exists between them. (See Chapter 3 for further discussion and analysis of the concept of barriers.)

Many writers on visual impairment and authors of texts that discuss access issues in education are not themselves disabled. We believe that a book that seeks to deal with disability issues in education can be credible only if it is written from considerable personal experience, both of disability itself and of providing teaching and support services to blind and partially sighted students in special and mainstream contexts. Two of us have disabilities. We have each received education in special and mainstream institutions and, as disabled learners, relate to all three of the possible educational experiences identified by Tomlinson (FEFC, 1996): 'total exclusion', 'isolation' and 'increasing integration' (Florian, 1997). We have been disadvantaged on many mainstream programmes in establishments where equal access to the academic curriculum and to the external environment was, for disabled students, rarely considered a priority. We want to contribute towards changing this situation by raising awareness of the barriers faced by disabled learners.

All of us have considerable experience as teachers in special and mainstream institutions, where we have been involved in the provision of both teaching and support services to disabled students. Whilst we acknowledge that there have been considerable improvements in post-school provision over the last decade, discriminatory practices within educational institutions continue, sometimes unchallenged. We believe that lack of effective legislation has contributed to this problem. In spite of the Further and Higher Education Acts (1992), the traditional approach to provision for disabled students in the post-school sectors is, in the UK, often crisis driven and piecemeal, standards varying dramatically from one institution to another. It is significant that colleges and universities are exempt under the terms of the Disability Discrimination Act (1995). This effectively licenses the college to abrogate responsibility for its disabled students. Curriculum access is denied for a variety of reasons. Those commonly identified are associated with lack of cross-college human, physical and financial resources and poor standards of teaching practice. We believe, however, that other, perhaps more complex (and controversial in relation to the social model of disability) reasons can be identified. These are related to personal history and experience of the world and the way in which each individual interacts with society and deals with the barriers presented to them. For example, assertiveness skills may not have been developed; some disabled students may never have had the opportunity to cultivate some of the personal strategies which help to reduce anxiety levels and facilitate learning (see Chapter 5). Knowledge is power and our wish is that this book will go some way to redressing the inherent inequalities that often characterize staff–student relationships. We hope that the inclusion of theoretical and practical information, whilst being useful to educational providers, will also be helpful to blind and partially sighted people in enabling them to take greater control of their educational choices, leading to increased participation in post-school educational experiences.

Many years' experience of working with disabled students – and numerous battles with 'the system' – have led us to espouse a philosophy that contends that education is, in itself, a basic human right to which everyone should have access. It should be inclusive and should value people as autonomous, interdependent social human beings whose individual choices deserve respect and whose potential for achievement is inextricably linked with the flourishing of society in general (see Chapter 4). We believe that institutions have a responsibility to facilitate the admission, education and transition of disabled students and that staff engaged in curriculum delivery have a duty to ensure that each person gains full access to all aspects of that experience, irrespective of individual differences. Consultation and dialogue between staff and disabled students through the establishment of both formal and informal mechanisms should help to ensure that services are meeting consumer needs. Our experiences suggest that there is a correlation between low standards of teaching practice and poor curriculum access by disabled students who are effectively excluded from learning; where standards are high, everyone is included in an enhanced educational experience.

For inclusive education to represent more than just an *ad hoc* response towards meeting the access requirements of disabled students, however, we believe that colleges and universities will necessarily have to become involved in a continual process of critical evaluation of policy and operational issues. This process will, we hope, result in the adoption of institution-wide strategic plans, which, in turn, will ensure that future practice takes account of everyone's rights (see Chapter 12). We would emphasize that this process must not be confined to the academic curriculum but must include the social and cultural aspects of student life (see Chapter 11). Whilst we acknowledge that some establishments are attempting to address these issues, we believe that a radical rethinking of an institution's philosophy is required if claims to offer equal access and opportunity to all learners are to be taken seriously.

Practice

As a consequence of providing support services to visually impaired students, we have, over the years, acquired considerable knowledge and insight into the practical implications of making the curriculum accessible to everyone. Our belief that attitude and cultural change will – albeit slowly – be facilitated partly by education has led us to organize and develop various training and awareness-raising programmes for college staff throughout the UK. Many of these programmes have been successful in altering approaches to disability and in initiating improvements in provision, but these have usually been in departments that have already admitted, or are about to admit, disabled students onto a course. In general, we remain concerned about the lack of interest and motivation by staff in attending training programmes that consider issues of equal opportunity and curriculum access. We can only speculate on the reasons for this response: no doubt the lack of human and financial resources are significant contributors. We do, however, receive numerous requests for what one higher education tutor described as a 'manual' and another as a 'bible' of visual impairment and every aspect of its cause, effect and management in the post-school educational context. Our response to such requests is to emphasize that the benefits to be gained from participating in an awareness-raising and training programme might be greater than those of perusing a textbook.

Over time, however, the potential usefulness of such a resource has become increasingly apparent. To the best of our knowledge, no such single volume is commercially available. Information is often in booklet or leaflet form and accessible only to those with a working knowledge of the specific voluntary organizations, agencies and institutions through which it is obtainable. A considerable amount of valuable material is also available in specialist journals and periodicals, as will be evident from the frequent references throughout this text. Literature on disability is increasing but the focus of many texts is general and writers rarely deal with blindness and partial sight in any significant depth. Those works that deal exclusively with visual impairment are either largely autobiographical or written primarily from a medical model perspective. The number of textbooks on eye physiology, pathology and treatment is considerable, but these are highly specialized and academic, using esoteric language. This apparent gap in the market, together with the constant exhortations we receive from students, staff, colleagues and friends to document our work, has finally galvanized us into action. We hope it has all been worth it!

Method

We attempt in the body of the text to draw together the disparate strands of the available theoretical and practical information on visual impairment from a wide range of sources and also provide relevant details from our own experiences. Our intention is that the book should be used as a one-stop, general reference for all staff and visually impaired students and we envisage that people will dip into it when faced with a particular issue. Because we perceive the book to be an initial resource manual, we have included medical information (with a glossary of terms, abbreviations and descriptions of practitioners' roles for quick reference). That we have chosen to place this information in appendices and a glossary reflects our fundamental wish to focus on the social as opposed to the medical aspects of disability, although we remain convinced that medical facts should not be omitted from a book of this nature, since they may, in some instances, serve to empower visually impaired people, for example, during consultations with medical and paramedical practitioners. Finally, and for convenience, we have included a list of names and addresses of organizations with whom readers might wish to make contact.

A note on terminology

During every staff training session in which we have participated, the issue of terminology inevitably arises. 'Do blind people like being referred to as visually impaired or blind or without sight? Should we describe people who have limited vision as partially sighted or as having a visual impairment?' The 'nomenclature' debate among blind and partially sighted people continues with little prospect of ever reaching a consensus. Our response to the above questions is that there are no rules – except perhaps that it is unacceptable, as has happened on numerous occasions, to describe someone as having 'bad' eyes. Each blind or partially sighted person has probably given the matter considerable thought and has developed personal preferences. We recommend, therefore, that all staff should raise this issue with individual students, whose wishes can then be ascertained and respected. As authors, we have tried to remain mindful of the debate whilst recognizing that no solution will be totally satisfactory. In the text, therefore, we strive to remain consistent. We use the terms 'blind' and 'partial sight' to refer, respectively, to people who have no sight and those whose sight is significantly limited. On some occasions when both groups are being discussed together, we use the term 'visually impaired' for convenience, although we acknowledge the underlying implications of doing so.

Aspirations

Although the numbers of visually impaired students entering post-school education is increasing, many blind and partially sighted people continue to express fears about undertaking educational programmes in mainstream institutions because they believe that they will be unable to participate fully in the curriculum. Will the staff understand the issues relating to disability? Will the college provide adequate and appropriate study facilities and other resources? As staff who work closely with visually impaired people, we are committed to realizing the ideal of equal access. One of the ways in which we believe this might be achieved is by publishing a resource manual that seeks to address, from a theoretical and practical perspective, the concerns of both disabled learners and personnel working at all levels in educational institutions. The Royal National Institute for the Blind's mission is to challenge blindness and the many barriers faced by blind and partially sighted people. We hope that everyone who reads any part of this work will also take up that challenge and that, as a consequence, some of society's most disabling barriers confronting visually impaired citizens will eventually be broken down.

References

FEFC (Further Education Funding Council) (1996) Inclusive Learning: Principles and Recommendations: A Summary of the Findings of the Learning Difficulties and/or Disabilities Committee FEFC, Coventry.

Florian, Lani (1997) 'Inclusive Learning': the reform initiative of the Tomlinson Committee. *British Journal of Special Education*, 24, 1, pp. 7–11.

Acknowledgements

As well as acknowledging our indebtedness to the wealth of literature on disability and the various aspects of visual impairment, we should like to express our sincere thanks to all those students, colleagues and friends with whom we have worked over the years and who have contributed significantly towards our own personal and professional development as lecturers and student advisers in post-school education and to the successful establishment of RNIB's Physiotherapy Support Service. In particular, we should like to thank our colleagues Shirley Garner, Cheryll McCandlish, Archie Roy and Richard Stowell, who have acted as informal reviewers of this text and whose constructive feedback has been invaluable. Frances Blackwell's considerable expertise in relation to counselling visually impared people has enriched the text and we are most grateful for her input. Our sincere appreciation goes to Andy Buchan and Julia Willis for all their administrative support in supplying information and documentation on request, often at very short notice. Our Technical Consultant, Paul Guyver, produced all the photographs and diagrams as well as contributing to Chapter 8 and we are indebted to him for all his hard work and commitment to this project over the past months. Maureen Crosby and John Milligan provided helpful advice in relation to some of the content of Chapter 11 for which we are most grateful. Thanks are also due to staff in RNIB's publications department for their cooperation in enabling us to reproduce the official logo, and to Tony Wayte of Stanley Thornes (Publishers) for his constant encouragement.

Jane S. Owen Hutchinson
March 1998

Introduction 1

As the title of this book reflects, our principal concern is with breaking down the barriers that blind and partially sighted people face when entering, and participating in, post-school education. Barriers of many kinds are encountered, which are primarily constructed not by the presence of a visual impairment but externally, by society. They are erected by people's preconceived attitudes and beliefs about disability and their consequent treatment of disabled people, by an often hostile physical environment whose negotiation relies heavily on visual ability; and by financial constraints (at both a national and an institutional level), resulting in the general lack of personal and college resources made available to facilitate study. Inevitably, each individual will react differently to these social experiences and secondary barriers may then be created. In its own way, however, each barrier represents a restriction of access: a denial of goods, facilities and services which non-disabled people often take for granted. Throughout this book, we seek to identify a number of these barriers, to suggest reasons for their existence and to explain some of the effects their presence has on visually impaired people. We then attempt to dismantle them and to reconstruct situations in which blind or partially sighted people can enjoy the same access rights to everything on offer as non-disabled people.

Chapters 2 and 3 are devoted to what we consider to be some of the most pernicious barriers: people's attitudes and beliefs about disability. With the focus on visual impairment, we begin by exposing the plethora of myths and misconceptions concerning blindness and partial sight and endeavour to replace fiction with factual information. Of course, other impairments are equally susceptible to such manipulation and the following chapter therefore considers disability in general, arguing for the adoption of a theoretical model that locates the 'problem' of disability firmly within society, rather than within each disabled person. This establishes the premise upon which we begin to examine the concept of barriers. We contend that people are disabled not by their impairment *per se*, but by the various primary barriers that have been systematically created by a society that is generally intolerant of difference. Inevitably, however, each individual will experience a unique set of reactions to such treatment and the ways in which s/he responds to it will depend upon a multiplicity of factors related to that person's particular personality and life history. We recognize that the social model of disability represents a controversial perspective. We believe, however, that to ignore personal reactions to social phenomena is to deny the existence of what might be termed secondary barriers, which, for many of us, are all too real and can, in themselves, be as disabling as those primarily created by society.

In view of our wish to confront such issues, Chapter 4 focuses on the individual and discusses some of the developmental, educational, psychological, socio-cultural and personal consequences and effects of blindness and partial sight. A chronological approach is taken and the discussion is related to the post-school educational setting, indicating some of the implications for teaching and learning. The emphasis on the significance of personal history in the context of disability should not lead to the conclusion that the individual is exempt from taking any responsibility for dealing with the disabling effects of society. Based on the premise that knowledge is power and that management of disability is a skill that can be improved with practice, Chapter 5 encourages the belief in self-efficacy and tackles the controversial subject of adopting an individual strategic approach to social challenges. Some definitions are proposed and the chapter examines the concept of a personal strategy. Personal strategies are identified as techniques and are grouped under different categories and we offer a list of suggestions under each heading. It is emphasized, however, that no panacea exists and that the choice whether or not to adopt a particular approach lies, ultimately, with each individual.

Continuing the theme of the personal management of visual impairment, Chapter 6 begins with an introduction to the topic of low vision. First, the principles and procedures of a low vision assessment are discussed and the process by which people with low vision might acquire a chosen piece of equipment is explained. Second, in order to facilitate future choice, many examples of low vision appliances and equipment are given. Because orientation and mobility issues play an important role in the personal management of visual impairment, the chapter also provides examples of appliances and equipment designed to facilitate moving around in the external environment, including some recent technological advances.

For any prospective student, decisions about which course of study to undertake are as much dictated by the geographical location of the institution, its architectural features and the characteristics of its external environment as by the specific contents of the programme on offer. For prospective blind and partially sighted students, however, orientation and mobility issues may take priority over other considerations. The availability of a fast and reliable public transport service, the layout of the campus and the design of buildings and other facilities are often of greater importance than course profile and, in many cases, dictate an applicant's choice of institution. Chapter 7, therefore, provides detailed and specific guidance on the underlying principles of improving environmental access for *all* students, including those with a visual impairment. Consistent with the principle of inclusivity, some examples of best practice are given, together with advice on obtaining more detailed information.

Chapter 8 is devoted to technology and explores solutions to the numerous barriers faced by visually impaired people when attempting both to access printed material and to communicate with others in written form. It focuses on the considerable range of equipment that is currently available, both commercially and through specialized manufacturers and outlets. With the educational environment in mind, the chapter provides a comprehensive overview of the increasing range of technological apparatus from which blind and partially sighted people can choose in order to facilitate study.

For education to be genuinely inclusive, entry to and participation in the institution's academic programmes is also of crucial importance to all students. Chapter 9 considers the general trends within further and higher education and focuses particularly on changes that have contributed towards increasing opportunities for all under-represented groups. With particular reference to visually impaired students the chapter then discusses some of the procedures that may be involved in ensuring that visually impaired people are given the same chances to compete for access to courses as their sighted peers. Chapter 9 also emphasizes the significance of transitional phases within the lives of disabled people and documents two of the phases that are deemed to be of particular importance within the post-school educational context.

Chapter 10 focuses on the more specific issues associated with accessing the academic curriculum. If the burgeoning advances in technology have increased the access possibilities for visually impaired learners, such developments have also proved invaluable to staff when faced with the task of making the different components of the course programme accessible to blind and partially sighted students. By frequent reference to such equipment as well as to other methods, this chapter provides a step-by step guide to many ways in which the various elements of the academic curriculum can be rendered accessible to blind and partially sighted learners.

Whilst full participation in the academic programme is often denied to visually impaired people through lack of equal access with their non-disabled peers, the hidden curriculum often presents even more significant barriers. Post-school education is not confined to the activities undertaken in a lecture or seminar room: it includes the social, cultural and recreational features and experiences of life at college. When considering access issues, this aspect of a disabled student's experience is often forgotten. For this reason, Chapter 11 gives a brief tour around the range of goods, facilities and services that are available and to which disabled students should have equal access.

In the final chapter, the various topics that have been considered in earlier chapters are drawn together by the suggestion that the most appropriate method of creating an accessible learning environment for visually impaired students is for the college to adopt a strategic approach to policy and planning. Only through the development of an agreed institutional philosophy can developments take place and the components of 'best practice' be transformed from an ideal into reality. A genuine commitment to inclusiveness will guarantee that, in colleges at least, the number of barriers to access encountered by disabled students will be significantly reduced.

The book is intended as a reference manual and, therefore, includes appendices containing factual medical information. The first of these gives an overview of the anatomy and physiology of the eye; the second provides brief notes on some common conditions that can cause visual impairment. The glossary should enable readers to retrieve information relatively quickly and the list of practitioners and their roles is intended to clarify any misconceptions concerning their specific remit in relation to the management of visual impairment.

Illusion or reality? Some myths and misconceptions about blindness and partial sight

Visual impairment is a complex phenomenon which has, over the centuries, been the subject of a wealth of myth and legend. This in turn has served to obscure many of the stark realities associated with blindness and partial sight. 'Sight loss is one of the commonest causes of disability in the UK. Almost a million people are blind or partially sighted. That's one in sixty of the population.' (Royal National Institute for the Blind, 1997.) 'Of these, 380,000 are blind and 579,000 are partially sighted. Only eight per cent were born with a visual impairment. Sixty-six percent of visually impaired people are over 75 years old and 72% are women.' (Royal National Institute for the Blind, 1994a.) (For statistics relating to numbers of visually impaired students in post-school education, see Chapter 12): Research conducted by Royal National Institute for the Blind (RNIB) in 1994 (RNIB, 1994a), however, indicates that many misconceptions continue to thrive unchallenged. If some practical understanding of visual impairment is to be gained, these myths – and the assumptions behind them – will need to be challenged.

Blindness

Contrary to popular belief, only about 18% of blind people in the UK are described as seeing nothing at all (Bruce, McKennell and Walker, 1991). More accurately, blindness may be described as 'severely distorted vision', many people being aware of some visual input and six out of ten being able to read large, clear print. (Royal National Institute for the Blind, 1994a). It is, however, important to dispel the myth that those blind people who see 'nothing' experience complete darkness: 'I feel quite clearly that, as a totally blind person, my life is not lived in darkness' (Wilson Goddard, 1995.) In his discussion on the concept of 'brightness', Gregory (1986) attempts to explain:

> The simplest of the visual sensations is brightness. It is impossible to describe the sensation. A blind man knows nothing of it, and yet to the rest of us reality is made up of brightness and of colour. The opposed sensation of blackness is as powerful – we speak of a 'solid wall of blackness pressing in on us' – but to the blind this also means nothing. The sensation given to us by absence of light is blackness; but to the blind, it, like light, is nothing. We come nearest to picturing the world of the blind, who have no brightness and no black, by thinking of the region behind our heads. We do not experience blackness behind us: we experience nothing, and this is very different from blackness. (Gregory, 1986)

Discussions with numerous blind people indicate that Gregory's description has some relevance, but a semantic problem exists. Whilst it is possible to understand the concept of 'nothingness' on an intellectual level, is it possible – or even appropriate – to try to unravel the subjective experience of 'nothingness'? What does it mean to say that a blind person experiences 'nothing'? Logical difficulties inevitably arise when attempts are made to describe an experience in terms of an absence of something, although this problem is not always recognized.

The question, however, may be posed differently: what is it like to experience sight loss? A detached retina has been identified as a 'dark curtain coming over', but not the descent of 'nothingness'. (Disabled Living Foundation, 1991). The adjective 'dark' may have been chosen because, for that person, it represented a more accurate depiction of the experience. Perhaps 'darkness' describes the short, transitional phase from sight to its absence but does not reflect the experience of 'blindness'.

People determined to pursue this quest for knowledge about blindness often resort to 'simulation' exercises. Blindfolds are eagerly donned and removed by enthusiastic participants on rehabilitation and other training programmes that purport to provide experiences of blindness. All these students experience, however, is what it is like to wear a blindfold for thirty minutes or so; they do not gain any genuine insight into the disabling experience of blindness. They do not even have the experience of sudden sight loss as some tutors claim. The problem is that these traditional teaching methods serve only to reinforce those misconceptions that they were presumably designed to dismantle. They encourage the 'tragic' view that blindness must equal 'darkness' – with all its connotations – and reinforce the misconceived belief that a non-disabled person can 'experience' disability. (See below for further discussion of simulation).

Indeed, the attempt to experience the experiences of others is, in itself, an ill-conceived enterprise. The notorious ambiguity of the language with which personal experiences are described often serves only to emphasize the difference between one person's experience and that of another. If disability issues are to be understood at all, this understanding is more likely to be gained through analysis of the objective: the political, economic and socio-cultural context in which disabled people operate.

Partial sight

If descriptions of blindness as 'nothingness' are fraught with difficulties, depictions of partial sight seem to be even more problematic. The frequent identification of partially sighted people as 'partially blind' testifies to a general failure to understand the phenomenon of impaired vision. The possible reasons for this are numerous. They include: the inherent ambiguity of the term itself; the disconcertingly infinite variety and essential uniqueness of each person's (often fluctuating) visual experience; the contrasting personal histories of those affected; and the general problem of semantics. Attempts to communicate something of the nature of partial sight do, however, seem worthwhile, in spite of the associated communication problems.

The following questions will be familiar to many partially sighted people: 'What can you actually see?', 'Can you see that tree over there'? and 'How much can you see?' These are questions that are destined to produce unsatisfactory answers. If the person responds to the first enquiry by cataloguing the objects seen, this gives little indication of functional vision: the ways in which residual sight can be used to best advantage. Furthermore, it communicates nothing about the nature of a visual loss, whether this is central or peripheral or both. If the answer to the second question is 'yes', this also represents an unsatisfactory response:

> . . . my intellect tells me that I do not see that tree as the person asking me does. I assume that the sighted person can see the individual leaves, maybe even the veins on those leaves. BUT I DO NOT KNOW. At 25 yards I can see the yellow number plate on the car in front of the one in which I am travelling, but I cannot read the figures.
> (Bradbury, 1996, original emphasis)

As with the third question, it is impossible to provide a coherent response without some reference to the visual experiences of the enquirer. To inform someone of how much you can see necessarily involves comparison with what that person can see, and, by definition, a partially sighted person does not possess such access. Even if the partially sighted person has experienced full vision, s/he can only respond to the questioner by referring to memories of that experience which may be unreliable. Although these questions may evoke feelings of frustration in the respondent, they are, nevertheless, often genuine attempts to gain an understanding and, as such, deserve serious attention and a considered response.

In an effort to formulate some answers, it might be helpful to consider a selection of cases of partial sight, beginning with peripheral field deficit. In general, the corollary of equating blindness with darkness seems to be the assumption that people whose visual field is restricted in some way necessarily experience a degree of darkness proportional to the field loss and the variety of restriction (Disabled Living Foundation, 1991). Such associations may underlie the popular choice in the medical literature of diagrammatic representations of different field defects in which a proportion of the field is represented as shaded or dark. (See Appendix A: Figure A.3. As with the correlation of blindness with darkness, the equation is inappropriate because it results in an over-simplification of the picture. It is unwise to assume that field loss will be experienced as darkness although some people affected by disorders of the retina at the back of the eye (for example, retinitis pigmentosa) describe feelings of 'standing at the exit of a tunnel whose walls are black, merging into a kind of grey' (sometimes described as 'tunnel vision'). Other individuals identify a cloudy haze surrounding relatively clear images. (Disabled Living Foundation, 1991). It is worth emphasizing, however, that two people with apparently the same impairment may recount different visual experiences. (See Appendix B for information on specific eye conditions).

Not everyone describes the 'tunnel vision' sensation: some people claim to be 'completely unaware of a field loss' (Disabled Living Foundation, 1991). This latter experience is identified by individuals affected by a variety of hemianopsia, where the appropriate part of the visual picture is merely 'absent': the individual perceives 'nothing' because the relevant cerebral component of the visual image is affected (Disabled Living Foundation, 1991). People with congenital impairments of the lens, such as cataract, describe a contrasting experience of having 'no side vision': a bilateral and generalized field restriction (Disabled Living Foundation, 1991). Again, it is not darkness but 'nothingness' that is perceived and the individual is unaware of the width of the unrestricted visual field. It is because they experience 'nothingness' and not darkness that most visually impaired people remain unconscious of their peripheral field restriction. There appear, however, to be two exceptions to this. First, in some cases of retinitis pigmentosa, a combination of peripheral and central visual loss is described. The pattern is haphazard and individuals state that they are intellectually aware of areas of 'nothingness' but, because of the brain's compensatory perceptual mechanisms, they perceive a coherent picture. Second, in progressive retinal diseases, a critical point is reached when the person is conscious of a disabling reduction in vision (Disabled Living Foundation, 1991).

In contrast to peripheral field restrictions, impairment of central vision caused by the typical 'floaters' of some varieties of retinal disorder, or the often large 'clouds' of some degenerative macular conditions, is more noticeable and easier to imagine. These 'floaters' or 'clouds' are often described as 'black' or 'dark', and by one person as 'mustard' (Disabled Living Foundation, 1991). Similarly, loss of visual acuity (clarity of distance vision), typically experienced by people with cataract or glaucoma, is quickly identified and it is this central visual deficit that prompts early visits to the GP or optometrist. (See Glossary for definition.) Reductions in visual acuity do not, as is often believed, necessarily result in a blurring or fragmentation of images, although these experiences are identified in glaucoma and corneal tears, respectively. Rather, it might be more accurate to suggest that those images are indistinct or unrecognizable – as they might appear to a sighted person who stands too far away for comfortable recognition. To many partially sighted people, everyday objects appear small and often flat if the myopia is associated with additional problems of depth perception (Disabled Living Foundation, 1991). (See Appendix B for information on specific eye conditions.)

A communication problem still, however, remains. It has been decided not to include diagrams/photographs in this text that purport to convey something of the subjective experience of visual impairment. (See, for example, Disabled Living Foundation, 1991; RNIB, 1994b; Ford and Heshel, 1995.) None of these is successful – they may even be inappropriate – partly because of the limitations of two-dimensional representation and partly because they are created by non-disabled (usually medical) personnel. 'Nothingness' cannot be represented on paper and both monochrome and colour representations of, for example, tunnel vision fail, as do slide photographs.

Many trainers believe that something of the nature of these experiences is captured by simulation exercises in which participants are asked to wear spectacles whose lenses have been adapted, supposedly to resemble various forms of residual vision. Others contend that such exercises are not designed to simulate the experience of visual impairment but rather to remove visual cues from the environment and thus to encourage course members, through personal experience, to consider how various practical issues can be approached without sight. Appreciation of the wide variety of visual impairments should lead to the conclusion that it is inappropriate to categorize all visually impaired people as 'partially sighted' and then claim to understand the implications of such a disability. This in turn should result in recognition of the condition-specific implications for the educational process and the considerable range of strategies that need to be developed by personnel who deliver services to visually impaired users. It is suggested that simulation exercises can provide personal experience of the extent to which people with unimpaired vision rely upon visual cues and, as such, represent a genuine challenge to their current methods of practice.

As indicated earlier, however, the true worth of simulation exercises is debatable. That they convey something of the experience of visual impairment remains questionable, since it is doubtful whether any form of simulation of disability is either possible or justified (see French, 1996). Participants in such exercises undertake simulation exercises with the prior knowledge that their duration is predetermined: the blindfold or spectacles will eventually be removed. Non-disabled participants remain so. Indeed, the same applies to disabled participants: they do not experience the disability of others. If simulation exercises have any value, perhaps this lies in the (essential) debriefing period afterwards. During such sessions, the group facilitator can encourage participants to identify and discuss

the intrinsic limitations of such activities and can encourage debate as
to whether simulation does, indeed, provide a genuine insight into
the practical significance of visual impairment. Is participants'
subsequent practice likely to undergo permanent change leading to
improved access to services for visually impaired people or are they
likely to focus on the somewhat depressing perspective held by R.D.
Laing:

> I cannot experience your experience. You cannot
> experience my experience. We are both invisible men. All
> men are invisible to one another. . . . I cannot avoid trying
> to understand your experience, because although I do not
> experience your experience, which is invisible to me . . . yet
> I experience you as experiencing. I do not experience your
> experience but I experience you as experiencing. I
> experience myself as experienced by you. And I experience
> you as experiencing yourself as experienced by me. And so
> on. (Laing, 1973)

Before the attempt to share the experiences of others is abandoned
as a pointless exercise, however, it may be helpful to consider an
alternative means by which some insight into the subjective
experience of partial sight may be gained. An understanding of
perceptual processes could be useful here.

It has been noted above that vision is associated with perceptual as
well as sensory processes. Perception is identified with active attempts
to organize sense data and interpret its significance in terms of
present context and past experience, thus involving memory. The
brain engages in information processing. Meaningful patterns are
created out of random stimuli, rendering the world intelligible. All
the senses are involved. These processes are as active in visually
impaired people as they are in sighted individuals. It is axiomatic that
if one sensory input is deficient in some way, the other senses will be
actively developed and utilized in an attempt to compensate for this
deficit. The part played by the remaining senses in the selection and
testing of hypotheses, therefore, tends to be considerable. What is
often unrecognized, however, is that residual visual input is also
exploited and put to its maximum use. An understanding of the

experience of visual impairment may be enhanced, therefore, if the complexities of visual as well as other perceptual processes are appreciated.

Further insights into visual impairment

The eye/camera analogy

Traditionally, the eye/camera analogy is used to explain some of the eye's functions. Its focusing mechanisms – involving changes in the focal length of the lens according to the distance of an object from the observer – are compared to those of a camera, the photo-sensitive film being compared to the retina. Although some similarities between the human eye and the camera may exist, there are limits beyond which it is inappropriate to draw such analogies.

How does a camera work? Not only must an object be brought into focus on the film by use of an appropriate lens, but the prevailing lighting conditions must be of adequate intensity for the subject of the potential photograph to be clearly 'seen' by the camera. The device possesses two systems for regulating the amount of light that passes through the lens: the shutter speed and the size of the aperture can both be altered as necessary. The shutter may be compared to the eyelid: when it is closed, no image is seen. The aperture is analogous to the pupil which constricts and dilates in automatic response to environmental lighting changes. The photo-sensitive film on to which the camera lens focuses the image of the outside world resembles – but does not replicate – the retina with its network of specialized photo-receptor cells. When stimulated, the retina relays messages along the optic nerve to the brain, which contains cells specialized for vision arranged in a sheet – the 'inner screen' (Frisby, 1979). The screen contains potentially active, moderately active and inactive cells that respond, respectively, to bright, grey and dark spots present in the environmental picture. The 'inner screen' cells replicate a pattern of light and dark that characterizes the shape of the retinal image of the external world. Thus, if a black cat on a white rug is seen, the activity pattern of the 'inner screen' cells mirrors the cat image; the establishment of this pattern on the 'inner screen' causes the observer to see a cat. In this respect, then, the observer represents the camera: when the camera 'sees' a cat, the resulting snapshot will be of that cat. The camera and the observer are thus depicted as passive recipients of a visual image.

But is this how a cat is 'seen'? The analogy disintegrates at the film/retina point. The retina has been described as an outgrowth of brain tissue. Gregory's comments on the practical significance of this are instructive:

> It [the retina] is a specialised part of the surface of the brain which has budded out and become sensitive to light, while it retains typical brain cells functionally between the receptors and the optic nerve (but situated in the front layers of the retina) which greatly modify the electrical activity from the receptors themselves. Some of the *data processing* for *perception* takes place in the eye, which is thus an integral part of the *brain*. (Gregory, 1986, emphasis added)

The 'homunculus' (little man) or 'picture view' of vision is described and dismissed by Dodds (1988), who dismisses it because it ignores these crucial components of seeing. Because it accepts the 'picture view' of vision, the eye/camera analogy – equating the camera with the observer – it misrepresents 'seeing' as a passive, non-analytical process. This is to ignore the perceptual component associated with cerebral information processing (Dodds, 1988, 1993; Humphreys and Riddoch 1987; Disabled Living Foundation, 1991). Meanwhile Ornstein (1988) describes the eye as 'the most important avenue of personal consciousness'. Contrary to Bradbury (1996) (see below) he estimates that 90% of incoming information is transmitted by sight but cautions that we do not perceive objective reality but that we are engaged in a process of continual construction of our world. Sensory information is gathered, modified, organized and interpreted by the brain in the light of memories, beliefs and expectations.

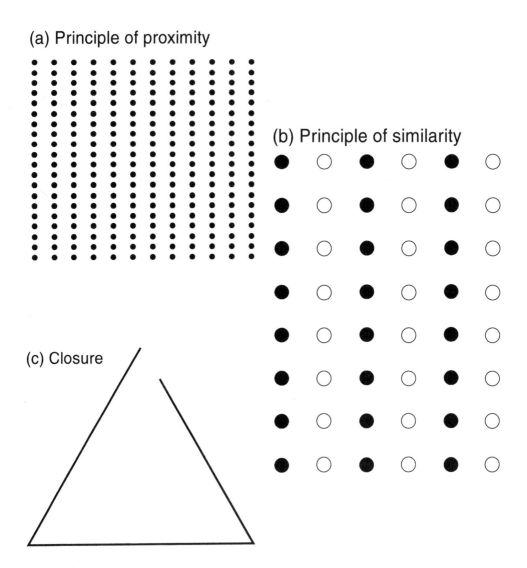

(a) Principle of proximity

(b) Principle of similarity

(c) Closure

Figure 2.1 Proximity, similarity and closure. (a) The dots are seen as forming columns as the vertical spacing is narrower than the horizontal spacing. (b) The dots group on the basis of having similar colours. (c) This diagram is seen as a triangle with part of one side missing. If shown this shape very briefly, subjects will report seeing a complete figure and are unaware of the interrupted outline. They 'close' the shape mentally.

Perception cannot, however, occur in the absence of sensory input but, as Gross (1992) also emphasizes:

> the sense data constitute only the 'raw material' from which our conscious awareness of objects is constructed. . . . to the extent that we perceive the world as it really is, we do this indirectly, through analysing, interpreting and trying to make sense of sensations. . . . the sense organs are part of the perceptual system as a whole.

Associated with perception are the principles of Gestalt (see Figure 2.1; Humphreys and Riddoch, 1987). Under normal circumstances, organization of in-coming visual stimuli into meaningful 'wholes' or images comprising 'figure' and 'background' is automatic. It becomes conscious only when such stimuli present problems to the brain's information-processing mechanism, for example, when objects are too distant to be identified, or when two alternative, but equally plausible, interpretations can be selected, as illustrated by two examples of 'ambiguous figures' (see Figures 2.2 and 2.3). Confusion and frustration are experienced by the observer who is required to select and retain a hypothesis about which element of the picture comprises 'figure' and which constitutes 'background' or on which surface the 'X' is placed: two possibilities can be 'seen'.

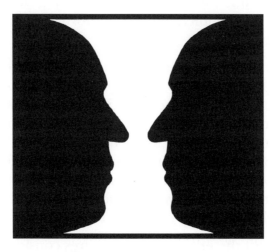

Figure 2.2 Faces or a vase?

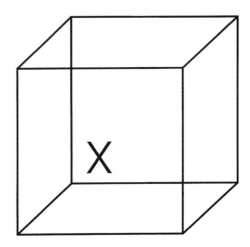

Figure 2.3 The Necker cube. Note that the cross can appear at either the front or rear of the transparent cube.

Consternation and even disorientation may be felt after prolonged periods of gazing at such figures.

Now imagine a world in which 'ambiguous figures' are regularly presented. This begins to approach something of the subjective experience of visual impairment: the conscious – and often continual – necessity to select and test hypotheses relating to impoverished or absent visual input. Because this input often proves to be inadequate and unreliable, additional information processing of other sensory stimuli is required to supplement visual information in order to make sense of the environment:

> Sight provides the brain with 80% of the information it receives. I suspect that the percentage of information derived from sight in those people with residual vision is considerably lower and that more comes through the other senses, particularly hearing. I know from my own experiences that my other senses guide my eyes to focus on the information that my brain requires and that my brain has learnt to interpret incomplete and often inaccurate information which my eyes convey to it. (Bradbury, 1996)

Manoeuvring about the environment requires considerable energy expenditure because, unlike sighted individuals, blind and partially sighted people cannot take their world for granted. Incoming sense data must be regularly tested against past experience and conjecture, utilizing cognitive skills to interpret sensory input. It will be appreciated that this process demands considerable mental effort. If this level of concentration is maintained for protracted periods of time, the effect can be exhausting. Many blind and partially sighted people are subjected to these kinds of stresses throughout much of their life.

Typical questions asked by people with residual vision are: 'Is that a red post box or is it a person wearing a red coat?'; 'Is that a street sign or merely a different coloured brick?'; 'Is that the entrance door or is it a window?' Look again at the ambiguous figure and now consider familiar instances of camouflage, a principle that relies on the normal ability to distinguish figure from background. There are many occasions on which partially sighted people experience the effects of (unintended) camouflage: they are unable to distinguish figure from background and consequently do not see some objects at all.

Perhaps some concrete examples might help. Many visually impaired people describe their external environment as 'disordered' or 'chaotic'; the bombardment of unrecognizable stimuli – visual, auditory, olfactory and tactual – is such that time is required to attempt to make sense of it. Imagine standing in the middle of a building site with all its open trenches, scattered debris and mounds of rubble. Consider the dexterity and skill required to negotiate this kind of hazardous environment. For a blind or partially sighted traveller, entering an unfamiliar, crowded building and trying to locate a designated area or negotiating the bustling streets of a large city can often represent similar chaos. Both skill and concentration are required.

Take a second, highly dramatized, example. During a country walk, a rambler perceives a small moving object several hundred feet away in front of some trees. The sighted person fleetingly questions the identity of the object and concludes that it is either a rabbit or a squirrel. The matter rests there. The identity of the object is of no material significance to the rambler, speculation merely represents a passing inquisitiveness and the entire incident is soon forgotten. If an understanding of the experience of visual impairment is to be gained, it is important first to note that speculations concerning the identity of objects within the environment often take place at a distance of only a few feet from the individual. Second, the perceptual process itself is at the forefront of consciousness precisely because of the problems presented by the abundance of ambiguous and possibly unintelligible visual stimuli.

Reconstructing the above example, imagine, this time, that during a country walk, the route takes you across a field. As you crest a small rise, you are aware of a large animal in fairly close proximity to you. What is it? You decide that it is either a docile cow or a ferocious bull. Your safety is thus in jeopardy. Because you are unable to identify the animal accurately, you cannot afford to take any risks. You certainly cannot afford the luxury of stopping to extricate the powerful monocular which you religiously keep in your pocket in order to gaze at its anatomy to determine its identity (if such equipment is of any use at all). You must move out of its way immediately in case it is, in fact, a bull. This places a further demand upon you: you must negotiate, accurately, the immediate territory if you are to escape from potential annihilation. Your concentration is rapidly diminishing. In panic you manage to select an appropriate escape route across the open space but, travelling at some considerable speed, you have no time in which to consider where you are going. When you eventually stop, you are completely disorientated and have no clue as to how you arrived at your present location. There is no one around to ask for assistance. You then employ all your remaining powers of logic and determination and, mentally exhausted, you eventually discover your original path. Phew!

The overdramatization is intentional. The considerable time and effort required by blind and partially sighted people to make sense of the plethora of incoming visual stimuli should not be underestimated. The necessity to be alert at all times has practical implications. Temporary lapses in attention and concentration may result in jeopardizing personal safety. The luxury of relaxation is often denied. Anxiety and stress can be reduced, however, by developing appropriate personal strategies that deliberately exploit the principles of Gestalt.

Depth and distance

The automatic utilization of monocular and binocular cues to depth and distance facilitates the interpretation of the environment and our negotiation of it (see Figure 2.4). Some partially sighted people have impaired depth perception. Imagine walking about in a world where everything appears to be flat, or one in which objects loom up at you as if out of nowhere. This is, potentially, an unsafe place. Under some environmental conditions, the danger can be increased for many visually impaired people, all of whom will have a personal preference for some conditions above others. There are two striking examples of situations in which the perception of depth cues is rendered particularly problematic.

First, walking down a tree-lined avenue in brilliant sunshine where the sudden and dramatic changes in the prevailing light conditions effectively prevent any useful visual adaptation. It is similar to the experience of being at a disco or fairground, where the rapidly changing lights produce an increased sensory stimulation designed, initially, to create pleasure and excitement but which, eventually, cause visual disorientation. The deep shadows cast by the trees are perceived as dark and appear virtually indistinguishable from any steps or holes that might be present in the path. Flights of steps may be mistaken for shadows because they appear to be dark and flat. The consequences of these misperceptions will be obvious. In passing, it is also important to note that, on dull days, curbs and flights of steps are often perceived as continuations of the flat pavement, again with predictable consequences.

Second, walking along a brightly lit busy street on a rainy night fails to provide the necessary frame of reference against which to judge the relative position of objects ahead. The experience can be compared to being in a cave surrounded by water in which the bright lights attached to the roof and walls are reflected. The sensation may also be compared to walking on reflecting glass, the dazzling effect of the bright street lights and car headlamps appearing to spring from below as well as from above. Because of these conditions, no colour contrasts are perceived, thus objects, people and steps are indistinguishable from the darkness.

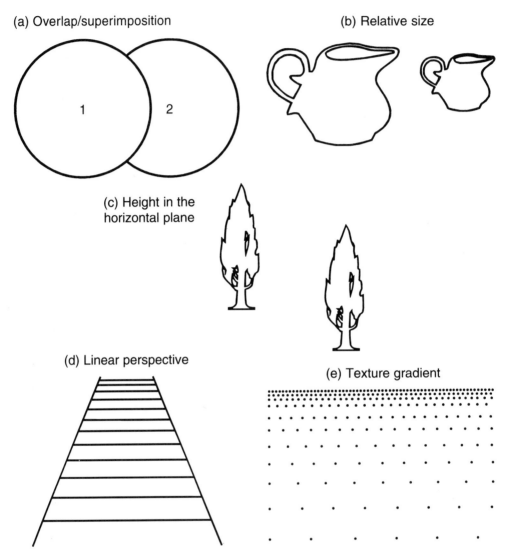

Figure 2.4 Effects of perspective obtained from two dimensions. (a) Object 1 overlaps and appears to cut off the view of object 2. Object 1 is presumed to be nearer. (b) With small objects (especially those known to have constant size, e.g. milk pots), the smallest one appears further away. (c) Objects placed higher in a picture appear further away. (d) Parallel lines (e.g. railway tracks) appear to converge and recede into the distance. (e) Grain or texture seems finer as the distance increases.

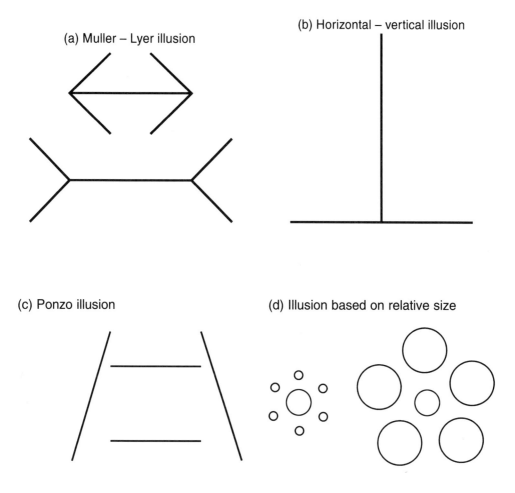

Figure 2.5 Geometric illusions. (a) The lines are the same length but the one with the outgoing fins always looks longer. (b) The vertical line appears longer even though they are both the same length. (c) The two horizontal lines are the same length but the upper line appears longest when they are set between two lines converging. (d) The two centre circles are the same size but the one on the left appears larger.

Illusions

Descriptions of the subjective experiences of visual impairment would be incomplete without mention of the concept of illusion (see Figure 2.5). Given the above, it is not surprising to learn that the part played by illusion in the lives of many blind and partially sighted people is often considerable. Illusion (see the diagrams) occurs because an incorrect perceptual hypothesis has been selected: the object appears to be something it is not. When a sighted person moves around the environment, hypotheses about the identity of objects are usually correct: reality is perceived as reality. With a lack of adequate sensory information, incorrect hypotheses are made about reality and it is experienced as illusion. To take examples from the street scene, a church spire might be perceived as a conifer tree; a low moon might be taken to be a street light.

The impossible object

Look at the diagram of 'the impossible figure' (Figure 2.6). Try to identify and define your feelings as you look at it. The reasons why this object is impossible to interpret are related to the problems of perceiving three-dimensional forms represented on a two-dimensional surface. In the search for a correct interpretation, first one and then another hypothesis is selected with the result that neither of them is satisfactory. The object is impossible. All efforts to

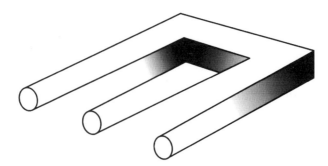

Figure 2.6 The impossible figure. This drawing looks like a 'U' at one end but has three prongs at the other!

solve the problem are defeated. For people with a visual impairment, many commonplace objects are perceived as 'impossible'. It is now not a matter of 'Is this a docile cow or is it a ferocious bull?', it is a question of 'What on earth is this?' It will be appreciated that, if encountered with monotonous and predictable regularity, such impossible objects cause visually impaired people to experience a variety of emotions ranging from mild irritation to extreme frustration and anger. Look again at the figure and try to imagine the experience of regularly encountering such impossible objects during the course of everyday living. This diagram has been used by our team in lectures and discussions on visual impairment because it expresses, for some of us, the often impossible task of making sense of the world.

Utilization of perception

It would be incorrect to conclude from the above that the perceptual world of visually impaired people is one in which the impossible always dominates the possible. The possible is approached via various routes: the development of personal strategies (see Chapter 5) represents one approach. It will be helpful to focus on one particular strategy in order to complete this attempt to describe some of the subjective experiences of visual impairment. The strategy concerns the utilization of the phenomenon of Gestalt.

Making sense of a range of apparently random stimuli associated with moving around in the external environment is not always easy, even with considerable effort. There may be many reasons for this, not the least important of which are related to the nature of the visual impairment and its onset. It takes time and practice to transform these initially meaningless visual and other sensory stimuli into an intelligible form, shape or pattern. It is on this process of pattern construction and interpretation that emphasis should be placed and not on the precise nature or specific identity of what is seen: as suggested above, many visually impaired people do not always perceive objects as they really are. A simplified description of the process will communicate something of what a visually impaired person might have experience of, for example, a street scene when stepping out from a building and onto the pavement.

For the first few seconds, the scene appears as a kaleidoscopic jumble of meaningless images. Any necessary adjustment to the light changes may take time. As the person actively tries to make sense of the picture, it begins to rearrange itself into a recognizable pattern. Certain objects can now be positively identified and may be seen clearly and distinctly against their background. Many objects will elude such positive identification and will be tentatively classified as either X or Y. Other objects will present more difficulty because they will appear, initially, as 'impossible'. Their identity may, however, be determined and this is done by matching the subjective visual image of the object against a memorized range of possible alternatives, each capable of producing a similar retinal image. For example, a red blur or speck in the distance is merely a red blur or speck. On closer scrutiny, it becomes either a person dressed in a red coat or a post-box. The process of elimination then begins and, as a result of learning and past experiences of similar visual images of red blurs or specks, it is decided that this particular blur or speck is in fact a post-box, because its shape and size conform to those of known post-boxes previously seen at approximately this distance. Of course, this represents a conjecture or an educated guess rather than a statement of fact. In the street scene, there will probably always be at least one 'impossible' object but, unless this is considered to be of some practical significance, little energy will be expended on scrutinizing it.

It may be helpful to illustrate one more instance of the utilization of Gestalt. Having made some sense of the street scene from the doorway of the building, the visually impaired traveller proceeds along the pavement in search of a particular street. Infuriatingly, but predictably, the street signs are often positioned at a height well above eye level, making the letters impossible to read. Unless the person can use a distance monocular, s/he would probably seek help in finding the street. In many instances, however, utilizing Gestalt can provide the necessary assistance. Individual words are perceived as unique patterns, according to their component letters. (Think of the way in which poor handwriting is read: the meaning of the words is interpreted by decoding their pattern which conforms to memories of what each word looks like.) Thus, as long as the pattern displayed on the wall of a street can be recognized, it is not necessary to be able, literally, to decipher the individual letters. The pattern of 'Water Lane' does not look like 'Manbey Park Road'. A similar strategy can be used to identify the destination of an approaching bus or tube train, which is often travelling far too fast for a partially sighted person to be able to read the letters.

The utilization of Gestalt is therefore a strategy that, because of its practical value, seems to be worth cultivating. It is also helpful in conveying the nature of the subjective experience of visual impairment because, by analysing the process, something of the arduousness of visual and other sensory interpretation and subsequent management is conveyed, skills that are all too easily taken for granted when eyesight is unimpaired. The active and conscious cultivation of the principles of Gestalt provides the visually impaired person with one of a valuable set of personal strategies (see Chapter 5).

Residual vision

Although the importance of vision in dealing with the activities of daily living is acknowledged, sight is often afforded undue reverence by people who are afraid of losing it (Royal National Institute for the Blind, 1994a). These fears may be associated with misconceptions about eye damage consequent upon certain practices and it is important to clarify the situation. Eye damage, generally speaking, cannot be caused by the following: (a) excessive reading; (b) reading in poor light or too close to text; (c) undertaking tasks that require fine visual acuity (e.g. sewing); (d) long periods of writing; (e) long periods of watching television; (f) sitting very close to a computer screen; (g) wearing glasses of the incorrect prescription (except in certain specified cases in children); (h) dim lighting conditions; (i) general overuse of the eyes. This is not to deny that protracted periods of reading, using a computer monitor or similar precision tasks may cause headache, severe eye symptoms and even migraine.

The eye itself cannot be damaged by overuse: fatigue is generally the most common result (Disabled Living Foundation, 1991; Small, 1994). Other common misconceptions are worth correcting: (a) cataracts do not have to be mature for surgery – they can be removed at any age; (b) contact lenses cannot cure myopia, which returns after the lenses have been removed; (c) people with hypermetropia do not have such good distance vision as people with full sight; (d) eye washes are not necessary and may cause irritation if used frequently; (e) removal of the eye causes blindness and it is never removed for eye surgery; (f) exercising the ocular muscles does not improve eye health, restore vision or correct refractive errors (Small, 1994). Finally, some visually impaired people experience reading and spelling difficulties. It is generally believed that reading problems are not usually due to visual impairment but may be associated with other difficulties such as dyslexia. It has, however, been suggested by some of our colleagues that there is a connection between a spelling difficulty and visual impairment (see Chapter 4).

Because of the general problems of understanding functional residual vision and its significance, confusion often arises when a partially sighted person is registered as 'blind' (see below). It is rarely appreciated that the way in which someone interacts with the environment is contingent upon a multiplicity of variables including: gender; ethnicity; race; social class; age and nature of onset of the impairment; eye condition (stable/fluctuating signs and symptoms); environmental factors; (the weather, internal lighting conditions); and personality. All human beings are unique. No two individuals will necessarily have the same, or even similar functional vision and it is a mistake to believe that knowledge gained from acquaintance with one partially sighted person automatically provides accurate information about another (Barnes, 1996). Although certain principles may act as guidelines, the term 'partial sight', itself, contra-indicates the learning of a rigid set of rules in relation to a person's abilities. For example, it is often assumed that the prescription and wearing of glasses represents a panacea. Whether lenses have been prescribed or not will depend not only upon the ophthalmologist's philosophy, but also upon diagnosis: some impairments are not correctable by the introduction of external or internal lenses. (See Appendix B and

Glossary for further information and definitions.) Indeed, both varieties of lenses may prove to be more of a hindrance than a benefit to some people. Spectacles tend to restrict the visual field and often bifocal lenses cause image distortion and visual disorientation; contact lenses may cause inflammation with excessive eye watering and periods of misty vision. Similarly other low vision equipment and adaptations do not solve all problems and are not statutorily provided, although many are obtainable in the UK under certain highly restricted government schemes (Disabled Students Allowance; Access to Work).

That sight is often afforded undue reverence leads to the contentious assumption that to possess some sight is necessarily preferable to being blind. A superficial analysis of partial sight might lead to this conclusion but personal, social and cultural factors require consideration (see Chapters 3 and 4).

Stereotyping

The visual system is, in human beings, the most highly developed of the senses: 'because the sense of which they make overwhelmingly the most use is sight, . . . sighted people just cannot imagine how blind people can manage without it' (Magee and Milligan, 1995). Typical responses to blind and partially sighted people include denial, disbelief, fear, horror, wonderment, confusion, pity, grief, indifference, hostility, rejection and even amusement. It is often assumed that blindness or partial sight either renders the 'victim' completely immobile and incapable of performing even the simplest of tasks; alternatively, the person suddenly acquires supernatural qualities, with the power to perform miracles. In the former case, there is believed to be a concomitant loss of all intellectual faculties rendering the person mentally as well as visually impaired. In the latter case, endowment with a compensatory 'sixth sense' occurs or else, at the very least, one (or more) of the remaining senses is enhanced out of all recognition: the person is unquestionably 'gifted' in recompense for impaired or absent sight (Disabled Living Foundation, 1991).

It was suggested earlier in this chapter that, whilst attempts to describe the experience of blindness caused difficulties, similar efforts to depict partial sight were even more fraught with problems. Perhaps these difficulties account for the fact that people's reactions to blindness appear to be less problematic than do those to partial sight, possibly because the concept of 'blindness' is, in itself, less ambiguous. Experience suggests that the behaviour of blind people evokes less confusion, because it displays fewer inconsistencies. The social unease that partial sight generates is perhaps reflected in the apparent reluctance among the public to respect the wishes of many individuals who describe themselves as 'partially sighted'. As already noted, it is with monotonous and irritating regularity that partially sighted people are referred to as 'partially blind' (Disabled Living Foundation, 1991) (see Chapter 4).

Irrespective of the level of visual impairment, there is, amongst the general public, a preoccupation with an individual's eye condition and its prognosis. Some people assume that, irrespective of circumstances, visual improvement is impossible; others are convinced that the impairment is merely temporary and eagerly await its reversal. These contrasting reactions reflect the overwhelming fear of sight loss noted earlier (Royal National Institute for the Blind, 1994a) and represent different methods of dealing with what is perceived as an essentially negative experience and a socially unacceptable phenomenon (see Chapter 3). It is important, however, to challenge such assumptions.

It would, of course, be incorrect to deny that these negative attitudes do not adversely affect visually impaired people. It is hardly surprising that many experience feelings of depression as a consequence of the way in which society treats people with impairments, but it important not to collude with the prevailing myth which has its origins in the individualistic model of disability and which claims that the presence of depression is due, entirely, to psychological reactions associated with sight loss. Research has demonstrated that the development of depression can result as a consequence of light deprivation (Rosenthal, Sack, Gillin et al., 1984). An example of the physiological cause of mild depression is the familiar condition known as seasonal affective disorder (SAD) which is experienced by significant numbers of the population during winter months and for which light replacement therapy has been shown to be an effective treatment (Wehr, Skwere, Jacobson *et al.*, 1987). The brain is affected by light in two ways: directly by impulses from the optic nerve, and by the secretion of melatonin, a hormone whose production occurs as a response to light. Melatonin plays a part in determining the sleep/wake cycle. Many blind people experience a disruption in sleep pattern which is successfully restored by melatonin replacement therapy. This has led to the speculation that, because the brain can no longer be affected by light, the depression sometimes observed could have a physiological cause (Dodds, 1993).

It is important to emphasize that visually impaired people experience the same range of emotions as non-disabled individuals. They enjoy a variety of social and cultural activities (Royal National Institute for the Blind, 1994a), full participation in which is often limited only by the existence of socially created barriers. There are, for example, visually impaired artists and photographers, some of whom are recognized for their talents, as David Henderson testifies:

> I've been told my photographs are exceptional not because
> I have a sight problem, but exceptional by anybody's
> standards. There's no reason why any visually impaired
> person should not take decent pictures. (Quoted in
> Hermeston, 1997)

Contrary to popular belief, the presence of attitudinal and environmental barriers in the employment context does not necessarily indicate that all visually impaired people consider themselves to be at a disadvantage. Research into the attitudes of a selected group of visually impaired professionals (French, 1990) reveals that many positive aspects to blindness and partial sight were identified in relation to working with ill and disabled people. These included: 'an increased knowledge of disability, the ability to empathise, the need to make physical contact with people who are often isolated and lonely, the breaking down of professional barriers, and the positive role models they, as disabled people, are able to provide.' (French, 1995).

It is worth emphasizing that visually impaired people are, like all human beings, complex individuals. They are to be found in all social strata and possess the same range of strengths and weaknesses as might be found in any identifiable group. They learn from their experiences in much the same way as do sighted people. The assumption is made that the person who knocks over a vase of flowers does so because of impaired vision, whereas this may be due to clumsiness. Many people display high levels of skill and manual dexterity which have developed through practice. Everyone's method of managing their visual impairment is unique.

Some blind and partially sighted people are also deaf and/or have a learning difficulty; some *are* musical. Although many are exceptionally talented in specific areas, however, it is untrue that visually impaired people have 'a sixth sense' which enables them to 'locate the right building or the right ingredients when cooking a meal' (Royal National Institute for the Blind, 1994a). In their attempt to emphasize this point, Magee and Milligan (1995) echo Bradbury's (1996) point made earlier:

> . . . nature (fortunately) makes available to human beings a great deal of redundant information through more senses than one; and because sight is in modern conditions so much more efficient than the other senses sighted people have got into the habit of disregarding a lot of the information the other senses provide, or can provide. However, blind people can learn to use this when they put their minds to it.

Any residual visual sense, together with the other available senses can thus be cultivated as a compensatory personal strategy to enable people to operate effectively within the environment. This may or may not be a deliberate, conscious process. With practice, the components of a skill often become automatic. (See Chapter 5.)

Registration and access to goods and services

Each local authority keeps a register of blind and partially sighted people living in its area. The register is held by the social services department, or by the local voluntary society

for visually impaired people, acting as agents for the local
authority. The register is confidential. The aim of the
register is to help local authorities provide the best service
they can for people with a visual impairment. To do this,
they need a record of all the people with a visual
impairment in their area, and what kind of services they
need. (Royal National Institute for the Blind, 1997. See also
Royal National Institute for the Blind, 1995)

In an attempt to dismantle current misconceptions, it is useful to
note some definitions and criteria with regard to registration in the
UK.

People who retain some sight can qualify for the blind
register, even when their remaining sight is not expected to
get worse. Registration as blind means that, according to
the National Assistance Act 1948, a person is 'so blind as to
be unable to perform any work for which sight is essential'.
(Ford and Heshel, 1995)

This introduces two concepts: visual acuity (measurable) and visual
ability (contingent upon a multiplicity of variables). (See Glossary.)
Ambiguities inherent in this latter term would seem to be largely
responsible for the prevailing misconceptions concerning both the
meaning and practical significance of blindness. Cullinan (1986)
notes that 'anyone with a visual acuity of less than 6/60 (that is, who
cannot read the top line of the standard optician's chart) may be
considered for registration as blind. (These figures refer to the visual
acuity in the better eye, after correction.)'

Ford and Heshel (1995) state that a person is considered to have
met the criteria of the 1948 Act 'if only the top letter on the test
chart (called a Snellen Chart) can be seen when the eye specialist
holds the chart just in front of him' (3/60 vision). Registration as
blind will be considered if a person has 6/60 central vision, but
whose field vision is considerably restricted (Ford and Heshel,
1995). Cullinan (1986) adds that 'Not more than 7 to 10 per cent of
people on the "blind" register . . . are there because of reduced
fields alone.'

Dodds (1988) identifies the cause of much confusion and highlights the general tendency to ignore a person's functional vision:

> . . . an individual registered as blind may nonetheless have sufficient residual sight to benefit from low-vision training. In the UK this means in practice that the low-vision client is likely to be a person who has between 3/60 and 6/60 of visual acuity; that is to say between one-twentieth and one-tenth of the acuity of a normal eye. However, what this figure might mean in practical terms is not at all obvious. This is because the acuity figure reflects the client's ability to read high-contrast, static letters whilst sitting in a chair. Whilst this may be vital information to the optician who may be able to prescribe a corrective lens to enable the client to read print again, it is of little use to those of us who may wish to ascertain how well he can get around and look after himself. (Dodds, 1988)

Dodds (1993) further contends that there is a 'contradiction between the social conception of blind as meaning "without sight" and the legal definition of blind which is based on criteria such as degree of acuity and integrity of the visual field'.

Cullinan (1986) suggests that it is the perceived objectivity of the concept of 'visual acuity' (introduced by the National Assistance Act, 1948) and the ambiguity inherent in the notion of 'visual ability' that are responsible for the arbitrary nature of registration in the UK. (Visual acuity is the only criterion of blindness in the USA (Kleinstein, 1984)).

Contrary to popular belief, 'there is no legal definition of partial sight. Some authorities place the limit at 6/24.' (Dodds, 1988). The term refers to people whose sight is impaired to the extent that it is considered to be disabling (see Ford and Heshel, 1995). Many people retain the misconception, however, that an apparently partially sighted person can – or should – be registered as blind. This may be because, in terms of measurements of visual acuity, the distinctions remain confusing. Ford and Heshel (1995) attempt to explain:

Partially sighted people may be able to distinguish objects no better than a 'blind' person, but their field of vision may not be so limited. Alternatively, they may be able to see more clearly than anyone registered blind, but only within a very limited area. When their eyesight is tested on the Snellen chart, they can read the top letter at the usual distance of six metres. If they can read the next three lines down, they will still qualify for registration if their field of vision is limited, perhaps because they suffer, for example, from a disease such as retinitis pigmentosa or glaucoma. People with one eye will not qualify for the partially sighted register unless the sight in their remaining eye is seriously affected. (Ford and Heshell, 1995)

(For further clarification of the above terms see Chapter 6.)

To be registered as blind or partially sighted, consultation with an ophthalmologist is necessary. A report of the person's vision is prepared, together with a recommendation for the individual's name to be entered in the appropriate register. In England and Wales, the BD8 form is used; the BP1 is used in Scotland and the A655 in Northern Ireland (Ford and Heshel, 1995).

Although registration acts as a gateway to many statutory and voluntary services, 77% of those eligible are not registered (Bruce, McKennell and Walker, 1991). The range of available services to which registration entitles visually impaired people is not, however, identical for those on both registers, nor are these services automatically received as rights by those who are entitled to them. (See Ford and Heshel (1995) for further information.)

That the criteria for registration as either blind or partially sighted are arbitrary and therefore unsatisfactory is reflected in the equally haphazard interpretation of the concept of need. It is a myth that all blind and partially sighted people receive appropriate or adequate support in the form of information and advice regarding their visual impairment, counselling services, financial assistance, mobility and independence training and help with securing employment. For example, only 5% of visually impaired people receive adequate mobility training, in spite of the fact that 52% require some assistance in getting about. Twenty-two percent of visually impaired people choose to use a white cane. Only a small number of white canes are issued free of charge, however, and relatively few people receive adequate instruction in how to use the cane. Contrary to general assumptions, most visually impaired people do not have the option to train for a guide dog. Only 1% are guide dog users, many being elderly and unwilling or unable to take responsibility for an animal's welfare (Bruce, McKennell and Walker, 1991). The general public has many illusions about the abilities of a guide dog, some believing that the dog has superhuman qualities which enable it to act as its owner's carer (Royal National Institute for the Blind, 1994a).

Access to information in an appropriate format represents a major concern for many blind and partially sighted people. It is often assumed that Braille is a widely used medium whereas only 19,000 visually impaired people in the UK are Braille readers. This is largely due to the fact that many lose their sight during later life, when it becomes more difficult to learn Braille. In general, most prefer to use large print or cassette tapes and many rely upon others to read to them (Bruce, McKennell and Walker, 1991). Because of the limited availability and range of books and other documents in Braille, audio cassette and large print, access to information for visually impaired people remains seriously restricted. Whilst production of such material is expanding and is increasingly available on CD-ROM and via electronic means, such high-tech, often complicated equipment is not available to everyone, with the consequence that blind and partially sighted people are denied the choices that non-disabled people take for granted.

Ford and Heshel (1995) note the benefits of registration in terms of access to goods and services, but acknowledge the inherent injustices in the system, especially in relation to elderly people. In the UK, registration is voluntary and, for those who choose to register, familiarity with 'the system' and methods of accessing services is crucial, negotiation with an ophthalmologist often being required before registration can be issued. Some visually impaired people choose not to register, believing that the cost in personal and social terms far outweighs the benefits offered. Any act of registration is a 'rite de passage . . . a social marker that one's role in life has changed . . . such as marriage or divorce, or "coming out" ' (Dodds, 1993). The fact that many visually impaired people do not, in Dodds' words 'go public' perhaps reflects their wish not to be identified as 'disabled' because of the stereotypes associated with this label. (See above and Chapter 3.)

The need to shatter illusions

An attempt has been made to explode some of the myths and misconceptions associated with blindness and partial sight. It is acknowledged that to press the point too far often succeeds only in reinforcing the perceptions of some individuals who, for various reasons, wish to cling steadfastly to their own illusions. It is hoped, however, that by engaging in dialogue with visually impaired people, the attitudes of non-disabled people towards those with disabilities will change over time as a consequence of the development of greater mutual understanding.

References

Barnes, C. (1996) Visual impairment and disability, in *Beyond Disability: Towards an Enabling Society*, (ed. G. Hales) Open University and Sage, pp. 36–44.

Bradbury, C. (1996) How much can you see? A view from a person with residual vision. *Viewpoint*, **50** (229), 15–17.

Bruce, I., McKennell, A. and Walker, E. (1991) *Blind and Partially Sighted Adults in Britain: The RNIB Survey*, Vol. 1, HMSO, London.

Cullinan, T. (1986) *Visual Disability in the Elderly*, Croom Helm, London and Sydney.

Disabled Living Foundation (1991) *Visual Handicap: A Distance Learning Pack for Physiotherapists, Occupational Therapists and Other Health Care Professionals*, DLF, London.

Dodds, A. (1988) *Mobility Training for Visually Handicapped People: A Person-Centred Approach*, Croom Helm, London and Sydney.

Dodds, A. (1993) *Rehabilitating Blind and Visually Impaired People: A Psychological Approach*, Chapman & Hall, London.

Ford, M. & Heshell, T. (1995) *BBC In Touch 1995/96 Handbook*, 12th edn, In Touch Publishing, Cardiff.

French, S. (1990) The advantages of visual impairment: some physiotherapists' views. *New Beacon*, **74** (872), 1–6.

French, S. (1995) Visually impaired physiotherapists: their struggle for acceptance and survival. *Disability & Society*, **10** (1), 3–20.

French, S. (1996) Simulation exercises in disability awareness training, in *Beyond Disability: Towards an Enabling Society* (ed. G. Hales), Sage, London.

Frisby, J. (1979) *Seeing*, Oxford University Press, Oxford.

Gregory, R.L. (1986) *Eye and Brain*, 3rd edn, Weidenfeld & Nicholson, London.

Gross, R.D. (1992) *Psychology: The Science of Mind and Behaviour*, 2nd edn, Hodder & Stoughton, London.

Hermeston, R. (1997) A man of vision. *Disability Now*, September, 12.

Humphreys, G.W. and Riddoch, J.M. (1987) *To See but Not to See: A Case Study of Visual Agnosia*, Lawrence Eribaum Association, London.

Kleinstein, R.N. (1984) Vision disorders in public health. *Annual Review of Public Health*, (5), 369–84.

Laing, R.D. (1973) *The Politics of Experience and the Bird of Paradise*, Penguin, Harmondsworth.

Magee, B. and Milligan, M. (1995) *On Blindness*, Oxford University Press, Oxford.

Ornstein, R. (1988) *Psychology: The Study of Human Experience*, Harcourt Brace Jovanovich, New York.

Rosenthal, N.E., Sack, D.A., Gillin, J.C. *et al.* (1984) Seasonal affective disorder: a description of the syndrome and preliminary findings with light therapy. *Archives of General Psychiatry*, 41, pp. 72–80.

Royal National Institute for the Blind (1994a) *Seeing It Our Way: Exploding the Myths about Blindness*, RNIB, London.

Royal National Institute for the Blind (1994b) *You and Your Sight: Living with a Sight Problem*, RNIB, London.

Royal National Institute for the Blind (1995) *All about Registering as Blind or Partially Sighted*, RNIB, London.

Royal National Institute for the Blind (1997) *Blindness: The Facts*, RNIB, London.

Small, R.G. (1994) *The Clinical Handbook of Ophthalmology*, Pantheon Pearl River, NY and Carnforth, UK.

Wehr, T.A., Skwere, R.G., Jacobson, F.M. *et al.* (1987) Eye versus skin phototherapy of seasonal affective disorder. *Psychiatry*, **144**, 753–7.

Wilson Goddard, J. (1995) Darkness invisible. *New Beacon*, **79** (933), 221–2.

Suggested reading

Allen, M. and Birse, E. (1991) *Journal of Ophthalmic Nursing and Technology*, **10** (4), 147–52.

Baker, M. and Winyard, S. (1998) *Lost Vision: Older Visually Impaired People in the UK*, RNIB, London.

Campling, J. (ed.) (1981) *Images of Ourselves: Women with Disabilities Talking*, Routledge & Kegan Paul, London, Boston and Henley.

French, S. (1988) Understanding partial sight. *Nursing Times*, **84** (3), 32–3.

Kiger, G. (1992) Disability simulations: logical, methodological and ethical issues, *Disability Handicap & Society*, **7** (1), 71–8.

Royal National Institute for the Blind (1996) Listening to Students: A Survey of the Views of Older Visually Impaired Students, RNIB, London.

Royal National Institute for the Blind (undated) *Future Vision: A Discussion Paper*, RNIB, London.

Tobin, M.J. (1995) Blindness in later life: myths, attitudes and reality. *British Journal of Visual Impairment*, **3** (2), 69–75.

3	**Disability**

What does the word 'disability' mean? What image comes into mind when you picture a disabled person? What language would you use to describe a disabled person? Your personal experiences (examples of which are given below, will all have an impact on your own attitude and response to disabled people:

- meeting or not meeting disabled people
- the newspapers and books you read
- the radio programmes you listen to
- the television you watch
- the advertisements you see
- your family's and friends' attitudes to disability.

Most people encounter barriers in their everyday lives that prevent them from doing what they might choose to do had their situation been different. People may experience barriers in the form of lack of wealth, education, housing or food. Disabled people will experience the same barriers as non-disabled people. Additionally, however, they encounter environmental, attitudinal and institutional barriers when trying to take a full part in society.

The aim of this chapter is to encourage readers to think more generally about the issue of disability as a broader concept that includes people with a visual impairment. It is hoped that the reader will gain some understanding of current issues around disability from a political/sociological perspective through a review of the social model of disability. This identifies the barriers disabled people experience in society. In view of the stance taken in this book, we have chosen to call these 'primary barriers'. Because the removal of primary barriers will not remove the person's impairment it is important to introduce the current debate concerning individual experience. Each disabled person will process and react to primary barriers in a unique way and therefore manage other people's attitudes, the environment and their own lives differently. Although we are committed to the principles and philosophy that underpin the social model of disability, we believe that there has been little reflection on how the individual disabled person reacts to primary barriers. We have chosen to call these personal reactions 'secondary barriers', because we consider them to be a direct consequence of an individual's experience of a disabling society. We hope that this will add an extra dimension to the disability debate that has not been considered previously. Finally, this chapter reviews parts of the Disability Discrimination Act 1995 within an educational context.

Models of disability

'Disability' is a term frequently used that has a number of meanings, depending on the user. It is a term that has been the subject of much debate among both professionals and disabled people. This book is attempting to approach disability – and therefore visual impairment – through an understanding of the social model of disability (Oliver, 1983). Generally speaking, the social model of disability seeks to empower the individual. It enables the individual to look at the 'perceived problems' and decide if they are that person's own responsibility or if in fact they are the responsibility of society. The social model of disability is relevant in a book of this nature because, as individual people, with or without impairments, we all function within a social context. Invariably the society in which disabled people find themselves is not ideal.

Definitions of disability

Traditionally, the limitations that disabled people experience have been perceived as a consequence of their physical, perceptual, intellectual or emotional impairment, as illustrated by the World Health Organisation's definitions of disability (World Health Organisation, 1980). The following definitions are the most commonly used when considering the provision of goods and services in the UK:

Impairment – any loss or abnormality of psychological, physiological or anatomical structure or function, for example loss of eyes.
Disability – any restriction or lack (resulting from an impairment) of ability to perform an activity in the manner or within the range considered normal for a human being, for example inability to see.
Handicap – a disadvantage for a given individual, resulting from an impairment or disability that limits or prevents the fulfilment of a role (depending on age, sex and social and cultural factors) of that individual, for example inability to read print.

The social model challenges these concepts and, to illustrate its different philosophy, the following definitions of disability are adapted from Disabled People's International (1981):

Impairment – the functional limitation within the individual caused by physical, mental or sensory impairment, for example, inability to see.
Disability – the loss or limitation of opportunities to take part in the normal life of the community on an equal level with others due to physical (environmental) and social barriers. For example due to the lack of Braille, large print or taped material, a person with a visual impairment is denied access to written information.

> In our view it is society which disables physically impaired people. Disability is something imposed on top of our impairments by the way we are unnecessarily isolated and excluded from full participation in society. Disabled people are therefore an oppressed group in society (Union of the Physically Impaired Against Segregation, 1976).

Oliver conceptualizes ideas behind disability in two models: the individual model and the social model (Finklestein, 1980; Oliver, 1983). The individual model of disability, sometimes referred to as the medical or charity model of disability (London Disability Resource Team Training Materials – undated) places responsibility on the individual with an impairment. The major thrust of this ideology has been to remove or cure the impairment. Oliver (1990) and Barnes (1991) would argue that, in western society, the dominant attitude towards disability is one of personal tragedy. This 'has served to individualize the problems of disability and hence leave social and economic structures untouched.' (Oliver, 1996)

Individual model of disability

The individual model of disability is seen every day and it is evident in the general attitudes that surround disabled people. Disability is usually perceived as an illness. If people are ill they should be in hospital where doctors will cure them. In fact, many disabled people are extremely healthy, but regardless of the state of an individual's health the impairment must be cured. Oliver (1983) describes this as the medicalization of disability. Most people's impairment, however, cannot be cured by medical intervention although some symptoms might be alleviated. Conversation with disabled people has revealed great doubt about many of the benefits derived from medical and particularly surgical intervention. Many disabled people feel that they are the subjects of medical experiments. Supporters of the social model would argue that 'the cure' is sought because society is so terrified by difference. It is deemed more socially responsible and acceptable to put part of the population through painful medical procedures with doubtful outcomes or keep them in large medical institutions (out of sight, out of mind), than to reflect upon attitudes towards difference and particularly those associated with disability. Although cure for an impairment is very rare, society has found it extremely difficult to examine itself, its values, its prejudices, how it constructs the physical environment, and how it organizes its institutions.

Doing disability all day long can be an exhausting process. I
don't mean the impairment . . . I mean having to spend a
significant part of each day dealing with a physical world
which is historically designed to exclude me and, even
more tiring, dealing with other people's preconceptions
and misconceptions about me. (Keith, 1996)

There is an ongoing issue within our culture regarding the need for
physical, intellectual and emotional wholeness and this is very much
reflected in Christian and other cultures. The notion of this ideal of
wholeness is perpetuated through the growth of some sects of
Christianity and due to the work of faith healers such as Morris
Cerullo, who believe that disability is a godly response to sin
(Shakespeare *et al.*, 1996, see also Hermeston, 1998).

The common notion which has been perpetuated is that sin and
disability are inextricably linked. Naude (1996) believes that, as a
disabled person, he is still created in the image of God. This radically
challenges paternalistic Christianity in a number of ways. It asks that
traditional thinking be updated and takes on board issues relating to
women, disabled people and gay and lesbian people within the
Church. Some disabled people feel positively rejected by the Church
at one level, whilst others are drawn into it as a means of hope and
salvation. Some disabled people not only have to deal with issues
relating directly to their impairment, but also carry a burden of guilt
because they believe they, or their families, must have sinned greatly
and hence God's wrath has brought about impairment.

A central feature within the 'individual model' of disability is the
concept of charity. The model depicts charity as exploiting the fate of
disabled people. Some people have argued that they are presented as
pathetic and dependent. This notion is further explored in Keith
(1996) who believes that 'The cultural message that you must be kind
to the "handicapped", is a very powerful one'.

In general, charity advertising tends to present disabled people in a
rather patronizing way. It presents an image of a disempowered
individual whose life is made possible only by the pity and
benevolence of the generous public, who are encouraged to dig deep
into their pockets. Some charities boast of the amount of money they

raise every year, especially the big television spectacles. In terms of the social model, charities are in themselves discriminatory. They are often set up to meet the needs of a group of people with a particular impairment, for example for people with epilepsy, spina bifida or a visual impairment. The money may not be allocated equally to all people who fulfil the charity's criteria. 'Rights' are not considered; no one has a right to the services offered by that charity. The charity will decide how it chooses to allocate its funds to 'worthy' individuals. Benefiting from access to the money, however, will often depend on whether the disabled individual or organization is aware that funds are available and can be applied for. Disabled people also need to possess the necessary skills and expertise to apply for funding, goods and services. Even then, applicants may still be unsuccessful and hence not receive any charity. The rallying cry of the supporters of the social model of disability is that there should be 'Rights not Charity'. The divide and rule principle that some charities operate must cease. Disabled people should have a right to goods and services and their quality of life should not be dependent upon what is, in effect, a lottery. The aims of the charities may be various but they usually include research into a cure as a major goal. For many disabled people, however, there are more pressing issues that are not related to the medical treatment of impairment, but are associated with overcoming the social barriers previously discussed. Charity's traditional response to this situation is to try to compensate disabled people by plugging the gap. This is evident in the direct funding of segregated transport, segregated schooling and so on, rather than addressing civil rights issues (Drake, 1996). Gradually, however, this paternalistic attitude is beginning to change. Charities such as RNIB and Scope are now addressing rights issues and looking at their management structures and strategies to include more disabled people. For example RNIB has reviewed its employment strategy and, as a priority, is committed to increasing the number of visually impaired and disabled people it employs (Royal National Institute for the Blind, 1994).

The charity image is continued throughout the popular media and in literature (Hevey, 1992). Tiny Tim in Dickens' *Christmas Carol*, is a character who is both tragic and brave. He is tragic because he has an impairment; he is brave because he tries to overcome his impairment and struggle on regardless. Reiser (1995) cites a number of stereotypical images of disabled people. Frequently, they are portrayed as the personification of evil especially in children's fairy tales such as 'Rumpelstiltskin' or the witch in 'Hansel and Gretel'. Similar images are seen in both classic and contemporary fiction. Examples of these are Mrs Rochester in *Jane Eyre*, Captain Hook in *Peter Pan* and blind Pugh in *Treasure Island*. Disabled people are rarely depicted as heroes of fiction unless they either overcome their impairment or it is cured, for example Heidi, or Mr Rochester in *Jane Eyre*. It is not uncommon for the British media to describe David Blunkett, the Labour MP and Minister for Education and Employment, in glowing terms in relation to the way in which he has overcome his disability and achieved such success – despite the fact that he is blind. He is depicted as a role model for other disabled people. No acknowledgement is made, however, of the primary barriers he had experienced while achieving his present position.

Language is a particularly strong weapon that has traditionally been used to serve specific ends. It can empower, but it may also disempower. It is interesting that many marginalized groups of people are not referred to as people at all, for example, the homeless, the unemployed and of course the disabled. The omission of the noun 'people' suggests that society may have difficulty in envisaging – and recognizing – people as having disabilities. Depersonalizing the issue of disability also legitimizes its relegation to a lower position on society's list of priorities. Disabled people are further dehumanized by referring to them by the name of their condition, for instance a paraplegic, a stroke and so forth. The effect of this is to reduce the person to an impairment. Medical labels say very little about an individual's impairment and say even less about the person themselves. A criticism made of orthodox medical and health professionals is the tendency to focus on only the part of the part of the body that is not functioning correctly. The person becomes a dismembered and eviscerated machine – the faulty part in need of repair. Parts of a person's body are referred to such as 'the cataract', 'the bad back' or 'the knee'. This conjures up an image of separate limbs and organs, rather than a person who is in need of appropriate healing or support (Owen Hutchinson, 1997). Human beings are further divided by the practice of having different professionals to deal with different parts of the body or impairments. It might, however, be suggested that by dehumanizing people into bodily parts, medical professionals can carry out their work more effectively. Frequently, medical interventions are painful and the ability to undertake these procedures is made possible by depersonalizing the process, for example likening it to carrying out carpentry or fixing a machine. This also serves to legitimize the dominance of professionals over their patients.

Traditionally, language regarding disability has been used to insult and abuse, for example 'spaz' or 'spastic', 'dummy', or the retort 'Are you blind?' should someone bump into something. This may reflect a deeply held belief that, in fact, disabled people are not full human beings and therefore do not have the right to full citizenship. Language also uses physical abilities and prowess to judge capabilities. For example the verb 'to see', is frequently used to mean 'to understand'. Oliver (1996) considers the use of walking as a metaphor for being 'manly'. Keith's (1994) poem 'Tomorrow I'm going to rewrite the English Language' addresses issues relating to walking/standing metaphors as well as sexist language, the implication being that if one is unable to see or walk then it is not possible to understand or to be successful. Language is used by many people in an imprecise way to describe everyday concepts and experiences. Through regular use of words these ideas and concepts are subliminally transferred into our belief system. We often fail to question why we use a certain word to describe a particular image, for example, 'she is confined to a wheelchair'. It is instructive to reflect upon these words in relation to perceptions and attitudes towards disability.

The social model of disability

The most important issue within Oliver's social model of disability is that of power which lies with everyone other than with the disabled person. Disabled people are not considered to be capable of taking

control over their own lives so someone else must take that
responsibility and consequently assume the power. Power, therefore,
lies with those who have received recognized 'training' – the medical
profession, social services, traditional charities and carers.

As Barnes (1996) states 'the majority of services for people with
visual impairments, as with provision for disabled people generally, is
dominated by non-disabled professionals steeped in the traditional
individualistic medical approach to disability'.

The social model of disability seeks to redress this balance of
power, reflected in the moves by some disabled people to establish
and manage their own organizations. These are known as
organizations 'of' disabled people. The control and power lies with
disabled people themselves as opposed to organizations 'for' disabled
people, where non-disabled workers hold the power.

Most people take for granted access to the environment, goods and
services. The assumption is that they will be able to go down the
street, get into their homes, use public transport, take up leisure
activities and be employed. Access to such facilities is considered to
be a common 'right'. These basic rights do not, however, necessarily
exist for many disabled people. Many are dependent upon charity for
the appropriate electric wheelchair to enable them to travel around
outdoors or to provide the necessary adaptations to their homes to
enable them to use the toilet, bathroom and kitchen.

Within the ideology of the social model, the following are required:

- the removal of physical and environmental barriers
- the changing of attitudes
- the absence of institutional barriers.

This would mean, for instance, that buildings and the built
environment would be physically accessible for all people; that
schools, colleges and universities should deliver the curriculum in an
accessible format; that transport systems should be redesigned to
allow impaired people to use them with ease. In terms of attitude
change, there would be recognition of the importance of difference,
and the experiences of disabled people would be valued.

The social model of disability recognizes that individuals may have
an impairment but that many of the problems experienced are

located within society itself and the way it is organized. The primary barriers are diverse. Some significant barriers are physical, such as steps, poor lighting and information in standard print; and attitudinal, such as prejudice. People are often entrenched in their preconceptions of what disabled people can and cannot do, especially concerning work, leisure and parenting. Society has devised systems that exclude disabled people from everyday life and experience, such as the educational system, which traditionally has legitimized the education of disabled people separately from their peers or, at best, offers inadequate support and resources in mainstream institutions. Where integration into the mainstream is offered, it often represents only a token gesture and does not reflect the philosophy of inclusivity.

Individual experience

The social model of disability has proved to be extremely important in the lives of many disabled people. It has taken away much of the individual burden of disability and has provided a rationale in which to interpret society's reactions to impaired individuals. It has been a liberating experience, giving disabled people strength and enabling them to work together to try to bring about change in society.

It has been argued, however, that by considering the individual disabled person only within the context of the social model of disability, a false impression of the nature of disability and impairment is given. The politicization of disability and impairment seems to imply that if all the primary physical, attitudinal and organizational barriers were removed disability would cease to exist. This is clearly not the case.

Some writers within the disability movement have challenged the social model of disability because it has ignored personal experience of impairment (Morris, 1991; French, 1993; Crow, 1996). For example, they contend that even if all the primary social barriers are removed, the individual will still be living a life with an impairment. For instance, some people will still experience pain even though they can get into buildings and a visually impaired person will still be unable to react to non-verbal cues in social situations. Crow (1996) believes that embracing the social model as a means of dealing with the oppression of disablement has effectively silenced individuals and their experience of impairment. The difficulty that some disabled individuals may experience, not only with their condition but also in dealing with the oppression encountered as a disabled person, has not been differentiated.

Oliver (1996) counters this attack and defends the social model because he believes that 'there is a thin line between writing subjectively and exposing things which are and should remain private'. He also states 'There is a danger in emphasizing the personal at the expense of the political because most of the world still thinks of disability as an individual, intensely personal problem'.

This stance has persuaded some disabled people to deny their personal experience of disability in their struggle to be accepted as 'normal' human beings who are capable of living, working and loving as any other person. This attitude has been reinforced by the role played by medical professionals and others. An example might be when disabled individuals are positively encouraged to spend many hours carrying out exhausting daily tasks like dressing, when perhaps that time and energy could be used in far more rewarding ways, not only for the individual concerned but also for society. 'Coping wonderfully' often hides a great deal of pain and exhaustion (see Chapters 4 and 5). Crow (1996) and French (1993) argue that there is something that lies between the concepts of impairment and disability as defined by the social model of disability that takes account of the individual's personal experience of impairment within society.

French (1993) states that:

Giving adapted computers, taped materials and large print books to visually impaired people does not have the effect of eliminating impairment. It may enable them to do a job which otherwise they could not do, but it will not transform them into sighted people: their working speeds will still be slower than average, they will not be able to scan print and

the act of reading and writing will still take more effort.
French (1993)

This debate is important in terms of beginning to understand the situation of the visually impaired student in undertaking a course of study. Visually impaired students often have to work much harder than their peers to achieve the same end result. The socialization of disabled people may be a factor in how they function as students. People with disabilities at any age frequently receive very mixed messages about themselves as disabled individuals. As mentioned earlier, there is the on-going bombardment of negative imagery concerning disability that all disabled people will experience. For some disabled people there are overriding messages from parents and teachers that 'you are as good as everyone else despite your disability'. This process of treating the person as 'normal' can have two opposing effects. On the one hand it can give the disabled person the same aspirations as everyone else, which is positive, in that the individual has an assumption that s/he will have access to all that society has to offer for non-disabled people. On the other hand however, it will be necessary to be better and work harder than non-disabled people even to get a chance of having an equivalent life. The student may experience some or all of the primary and secondary barriers mentioned earlier when trying to gain access to society. A negative outcome of this situation is that the disabled person may experience high levels of stress in trying to be 'normal', working long hours to achieve the same results as non-disabled peers.

Although disabled people are socialized to believe that they are as good as everyone else, this socialization also teaches them to be dependent. This has been described as 'taught helplessness' (Swain, 1993). Disabled children's lives differ greatly from their non-disabled peers', especially with regard to interactions with significant others. The prevailing relationships encountered may be with doctors, nurses, physiotherapists and other health care professionals rather than with peers and family (Leach, 1996; Mason, undated). A significant aspect of these relationships is that they are with 'experts': professionals, who supposedly know what is best for the child whilst providing no real choice or opportunity to make informed decisions.

This leaves the child with little or no control over his or her own life. 'While medical interventions may be appropriate for minimizing and monitoring the negative effects of impairment they are inappropriate for dealing with disability.' (Barnes, 1996.)

As Leach (1996) suggests, the phenomenon of taught helplessness is particularly seen in special schools: 'The system itself denied young people opportunities and circumstances in which they could have control over their own lives and education. The system is seen as creating dependency in that young people were passed from the hands of one professional to another . . . their needs determined by others.'

The only way for the individual to cope is to be passive, accepting the situation and the decisions made by professionals. Any child who questions this loss of control may become labelled as 'difficult' or even as exhibiting 'challenging behaviour'. Consequently, on reaching adulthood the individual has not had the necessary experiences and opportunities to practise making choices and taking decisions. The way in which young disabled people are socialized may have a great effect on their ability to take up full rights as citizens and, as part of this, to operate within the educational system.

Disabled people adopt a range of personal strategies to deal with the mixed messages received about themselves as individuals and about the position of disabled people in society in general. On the one hand they are expected to achieve as much as the next person, while on the other they are encouraged to be passive recipients of services, who are expected to be grateful for everything that is provided. Additionally, disabled people have to function with their impairment in an environment and society that is at worst hostile and at best patronizing.

Although the work of a number of writers (for example, French, 1993; Crow, 1996; Morris, 1991) has moved the disability debate forward, the complexities of the disabled person's individual response have not been fully explored. It should be possible to examine issues of psychological response to disability within the framework of the social model. The individual disabled person lives and develops within a society that presents barriers. Largely these primary barriers could be removed by:

- changes in the environment
- the way in which information is produced
- changes in practice
- individuals acknowledging their feelings about impairment.

The person will, nevertheless, still have an impairment. The primary barriers experienced by disabled people will initiate an individual response and may produce secondary, psychological barriers. Many will argue that this is an individual's responsibility and, therefore, the disabled person's problem. Disabled people have, however, been socialized within a disabling society and have, as a consequence, internalized the individual model of disability. The extent to which this socialization has an impact on the individual is variable and dictates the way in which that person deals with the world. It is this disabling society that has created an ongoing tension between the social context of disability, the individual experience of impairment and the personal reaction to disabling barriers.

Civil rights and the Disability Discrimination Act

The redefinition of disability, the development of the social model of disability and the growth of the disability movement have led to disabled people demanding change. The disability movement has evolved as a consequence of disabled people choosing to be together and setting up organizations that are controlled by themselves. Usually, these organizations of disabled people have evolved in response to common concerns (the removal of barriers) rather than having developed as a result of the needs of a particular impairment group, for example as demonstrated within the voluntary sector. Disabled people have compared their struggle for civil rights with that of other oppressed groups such as the women's movement, the black and minority ethnic movement and the gay movement (Leach, 1996). The adoption of equal opportunities policies by local authorities, the voluntary sector and some private companies during the 1980s raised issues of discrimination experienced by disabled people. For many, however, this has been nothing but a token gesture. It is only those employers who have designed and implemented well-planned strategies who have managed to increase the total number of disabled people in the work force (Leach, 1996). The reality of the position of disabled people is that they are still more likely to be unemployed than their non-disabled peers and to be employed in jobs below their capabilities (Barnes, 1991; Royal National Institute for the Blind, 1996). Barnes (1991) describes the level of discrimination experienced by disabled people in the UK throughout the social structure, including the educational system. He also highlights how past disability legislation has not been fully implemented and how attempts to secure even partial civil rights have not succeeded. In fact much of the UK legislation and regulations concerning disability include imprecise phrases such as 'reasonable and practical'. This makes it very easy for employers and service providers to avoid any obligation to ensure that disabled people have equal access.

Barnes (1991) identifies reasons why legislation is required to ensure that disabled people have equality with their non-disabled peers. On December 2 1995 the Disability Discrimination Act (DDA) 1995 passed through Parliament. The Act defines disability as 'A physical or mental impairment which has substantial and long-term adverse effects on a person's ability to carry out normal day-to-day activities.' (Disability on the Agenda, 1996.) It will, however, be years before much of it is fully implemented. The legislation was written as a response to the repeated and unsuccessful attempts to outlaw discrimination. It has been greeted with mixed feelings by people concerned with disability rights issues. The various groups that lobbied Parliament to ensure that the resulting Act was meaningful was perhaps the greatest achievement in terms of working towards common issues affecting all disabled people. This lobby included different disability groups working together in the Rights Now campaign, including voluntary agencies such as RNIB, Scope, SIA (Spinal Injuries Association) and BCODP (British Council of Disabled People). The Rights Now campaign members have, however, had their differences of opinion. On the whole, the organizations of disabled people believed that the legislation was insufficient and would not ensure that disabled people would have the same rights as their non-disabled peers. As noted above, the legislation couches provision and obligation in terms of what is 'reasonable' rather than what is 'rightful'. For this reason, some would say that it is the first piece of UK legislation that endorses discrimination against disabled people in certain circumstances. The Act, nevertheless, should help to dismantle many of the barriers that visually impaired people experience when carrying out everyday activities. It is a useful tool that will support the developments made by many institutions and it will be vital that organizations continue to develop their good practice to ensure that all barriers – physical and environmental, attitudinal and organizational – are removed to guarantee the full citizenship of disabled people.

Some people would argue that the legislation has been written using the individual and medical models of disability and therefore cannot address the discrimination that disabled people experience within society. The traditional charities, on the whole, have accepted that this is all that can be expected at present. They contend that something is better than nothing and encourage people to make full use of the legislation. Both the disability organizations and the traditional charities agree, however, that the fight for full civil rights must continue.

The Act itself has little to say about education. The most relevant components relate to the provision of goods and services. Ancillary services that are provided by institutions, however, such as student unions, catering services, contracted-out retail outlets or banking services will be included (Skill, 1997). Education is not considered to be a service under the Act. It places a duty upon the Funding Councils for Further Education (England and Wales) and the Funding Councils for Higher Education (Wales and Scotland) to require institutions funded by them to publish statements about their provision for disabled students (see Chapter 9).

Educational establishments should operate a complaints and appeals procedure in the event of colleges and universities not meeting the requirements stated. Further and higher education establishments, including teacher training colleges, should state their provision for access arrangements and any specialist equipment provided. In cases of non-compliance, the funding councils would be expected to act as the regulating body, and may decide to penalize institutions by withdrawal of funding. Colleges and universities are required to review their policies and continued funding will be contingent upon their implementation.

It is hoped that the Act will bring about a general cultural change. Not only will service providers acknowledge that they have an obligation to consider the needs and wishes of disabled people, but they will also recognize the economic sense of widening their customer base. Although education is not covered by the Act as a service, the change in culture may have repercussions, as disabled customers will demand a better service.

In relation to transition issues (see Chapter 9) it will be helpful to note that the Act also covers employment, although it places new responsibilities only on employers with 20 or more employees. With reference to the discussion above, it remains a matter for conjecture as to whether disabled people will have increased employment opportunities. In the event of suspected discrimination it falls to the employee to prove that discrimination has occurred. Cases would be taken to an industrial tribunal.

This chapter has given a brief overview of the social model of disability and has considered some of the ways in which disabled people are denied access to goods, facilities and services as a consequence of primary, socially constructed barriers. It has been suggested, however, that disabled people experience a unique reaction to these barriers, which may, in itself, be disabling and which needs, therefore, to be acknowledged and addressed. In order to provide a political context for these discussions, an introduction to the main features of the DDA has been provided, although readers are recommended to contact relevant government information departments to obtain current information on its implementation.

References

Barnes, C. (1991) *Disabled People in Britain and Discrimination*, Hurst & Co., London.

Barnes, C. (1996) Visual impairment and disability, in *Beyond Disability: Towards an Enabling Society* (ed. G. Hales), Open University and Sage, London, pp. 36–44.

Crow, L. (1996) Including all of our lives: renewing the social model of disability, in *Encounters with Strangers: Feminism and Disability*, (ed. J. Morris), Women's Press, London. pp. 206–26.

Disability on the Agenda (1996) *The Disability Discrimination Act: Education*, DL100, Disability on the Agenda, Stratford-upon-Avon.

Disabled People's International (1981) *Proceedings of the First World Congress*, Disabled People's International, Singapore.

Drake, R.F. (1996) A critique of the role of the traditional charities, in *Disability and Society: Emerging Issues and Insights*, (ed. L. Barton), Addison Wesley Longman, London, pp. 147–66.

Finklestein, V. (1980) *Attitudes and Disabled People: Issues for Discussion*, World Rehabilitation Fund, New York.

French, S. (1993) Disability, impairment or something in between, in *Disabling Barriers: Enabling Environments*, (eds. J. Swain, V. Finklestein, S. French and M. Oliver), Sage, London, pp. 17–25.

Hermeston, R. (1998) A very spirited debate, *Disability Now*, February, pp. 12.

Hevey, D. (1992) *The Creatures Time Forgot. Photography and Disability Imagery*, Routledge, London.

Keith, L. (1994) Tomorrow I'm going to rewrite the English Language, in *Mustn't Grumble*, (ed. L. Keith), Women's Press, London, p. 57.

Keith, L. (1996) Encounters with strangers: the public's responses to disabled women and how this affects our sense of self, in *Encounters with Strangers: Feminism and Disability*, (ed. J. Morris), Women's Press, London, p. 69–88.

Leach, B. (1996) Disabled people and the equal opportunities movement, in *Beyond Disability: Towards an Enabling Society*, (ed. G. Hales), Open University and Sage, London, pp. 88–95.

Mason, M. (Undated) *Parents in Partnership*, training materials, London.

Naude, J. (1996) Personal communication.

Morris, J. (1991) *Pride Against Prejudice: Transforming Attitudes to Disability*, Women's Press, London.

Oliver, M. (1983) *Social Work with Disabled People*, Macmillan. London.

Oliver, M. (1996) *Understanding Disability: From Theory to Practice*, Macmillan, London.

Owen Hutchinson, J.S. (1997) Health, health education and physiotherapy practice, in *Physiotherapy: A Psychosocial Approach*, 2nd edn (ed. S. French), Butterworth-Heinemann, Oxford, pp. 396–420.

Reiser, R. (1995) Stereotypes of disabled people, in *Invisible Children — Report on the Joint Conference on Children, Image and Disability* (ed. R. Reiser), Save the Children and the Integration Alliance, London, pp. 44–51.

Royal National Institute for the Blind (1994) *RNIB Strategy: 1994–2000*, RNIB, London.

Royal National Institute for the Blind (1996) *Out of Sight, Out of Work* RNIB, London.

Shakespeare, T., Gillespie-Sells, K. and Davies, D. (1996) *The Sexual Politics of Disability: Untold Desires*, Cassell, London.

Skill (1997) *The Coordinator's Handbook*, Skill, London.

Swain, J. (1993) Taught helplessness? Or a say for disabled students in schools, in *Disabling Barriers: Enabling Environments*, (eds. J. Swain, V. Finklestein, S. French and M. Oliver), Sage, London, pp. 155–62.

Union of the Physically Impaired Against Segregation (1976) *Fundamental Principles of Disability*, UPIAS, London.

World Health Organisation (1980) *International Classification of Impairments, Disabilities and Handicaps*, WHO, Geneva.

Suggested Reading

Garner, K., Dale, M. and Garner, S. (1997) *Education, Employment and Rehabilitation for Visually Impaired Adults: A Survey of Recent Research*, RNIB, London.

Visual impairment: some consequences and effects

4

Any book that attempts to consider some consequences and effects of blindness and partial sight must, we believe, address personal as well as social concerns. As has been suggested in Chapters 1 and 3, the barriers encountered by visually impaired people fall into two categories: primary (social) and secondary (individual reactions and responses to that impairment, and the ways in which the outside world treats people with impairments). It is, therefore, important to focus on the concept of impairment as well as on disability and to identify some of the medical and psychological issues which, for many blind and partially sighted people, represent significant obstacles to full participation in society. To disregard these secondary barriers is to deny their reality and, possibly, to trivialize their importance in the lives of disabled people. (See French, 1993; Keith, 1994; Morris, 1996.) Indeed, it could be argued that to acknowledge – rather than ignore – the physical, emotional and psychological effects of an impairment is, in itself, liberating and empowering. Based on the premise that all knowledge is power, enhanced self-awareness together with the possession of a range of information sources (including medical facts) will enable blind and partially sighted people to take a greater control over their lives, especially when dealing with professional personnel.

Perception and cognition: implications for learning

Visually impaired people employ the same perceptual and cognitive processes as sighted individuals but, 'for much of the information that regulates their interaction with their physical and social environment, they must consult different sources of information and acquire different sense data'. Thus 'there are important differences in the learning by which they become able to interpret the world around them accurately and respond to it appropriately.' (Foulke and Hatlen, 1992b). What is learnt from present experiences is coloured by past experiences which, in turn, will have been affected by earlier ones (Murphy and O'Driscoll, 1989). When attempting to understand the cognitive and perceptual abilities, styles and needs of visually impaired students and the implications for teaching, it will, therefore, be important to consider some of those experiences that provided the individual's earliest learning opportunities. (Foulke and Hatlen, 1992a; Millar, 1995).

Although the visual system is often regarded as the spatial system *par excellence*, supplying a rich source of spatial and temporal information, vision is not, of course, the only modality that provides the reference cues that coding of spatial information requires. The other sensory systems can play a vital role in interpreting incoming stimuli and almost all these systems contribute to the information upon which different forms of spatial organization depend (Dodds, 1988, 1993; Millar, 1995). Two important points, however, should be noted. First, the different sensory systems are specialized to analyse different complementary aspects of information from a variety of internal (body-centred) and external sources. Second, under normal conditions, the information from these sources typically converges and partially overlaps. Both this specialization and the redundancy of reference cues that results from the partial overlap are extremely important for the development of spatial coding, with and without sight (Millar, 1995).

The auditory system, for example, is specialized for the acquisition and analysis of time-varying stimuli and represents an impoverished source of spatial information. The identity, distances and directions of sounds can, of course, be estimated, a skill that can be developed with practice. Although the visual characteristics of objects are not conveyed via the auditory system, simultaneous sensory input can usefully supplement auditory information, for example, proprioception (the body's awareness of its position in space).

Working in consort, these other systems provide similar spatial information to that conveyed by the visual system, although this 'conglomerate' mechanism has some disadvantages:

(1) Poor capacity for pattern resolution: the abundance of detail that can be appreciated visually is not fully accessible through touch.

(2) Reduced volume of space that can be observed at one time and from one position: objects must be touched or handled individually and serially, a process that is not only time consuming but is a poor substitute for the simultaneous presentation of visual stimuli. Serial perception by touch is not, in any case, identical to visual perception: according to Gestalt principles, the whole is always greater than the sum of its constituent parts.

(3) In order to touch people and objects and to discover their relative positions beyond arm's length, a child may be required to travel to them. Exploration – and significant learning – cannot, therefore, occur before the development of locomotion, which may itself be delayed. The process of moving through space is time consuming. Information that is acquired serially may be incomplete and several attempts to acquire it may be necessary. The practical implications are significant. Blind infants are confronted with the task of combining small fragments of spatial information, acquired at many different times, to create memories of experience that subsequently lead to their conceptions of structured space. Spatial conceptions achieved in this way are less detailed and accurate than those possible from the kind of spatial observation of which a child with an unimpaired visual system is capable (Foulke and Hatlen, 1992a).

Millar's research (1995) suggests that, rather than utilizing external cues to give feedback on movement during the performance of spatial tasks, blind children tend to rely on frames of reference that are body centred, supplemented by memory. This is, she contends, 'not a question of inability, nor of developmental delay. It is not a question of waiting until they are older.' Rather, it is due to the specific conditions associated with lack of visual information. First, there is little direct and reliable information about the relationship between external surfaces which can provide spatial frame cues. Second, the redundancy of reference cues provided by the overlap of vision with other sensory input is lost. Without sight, therefore, 'cues from body-centred sources and from movements are more constant and reliable than external cues and therefore tend to predominate' (Millar, 1995).

Echoing Sheridan (1975), Murphy and O'Driscoll (1989) note that 'Vision plays a very important role in early development of skill. Sensory integration also involves past experience and long-term memory.' They argue that 'The link between movement and sensory information is a pre-requisite for normal anti-gravity mobility' and identify some of the consequences of blindness in childhood:

> Blind children develop along the same developmental sequence as sighted children (Adelson and Fraiberg, 1976) but are not motivated to explore and practise their motor skills and, of course, they will not practise any of the visual-motor skills in learning object permanence, object manipulation and spatial awareness, owing to their lack of vision. . . . Visually impaired children have difficulty in acquiring spatial orientation concepts necessary for proficient locomotion and independent mobility (Cratty, 1979). . . . Blind children have a tendency to immobility and passivity. (Murphy and O'Driscoll, 1989)

Due to the factors noted above, visually impaired children are often less inquisitive and tend not to explore other sensory inputs in the environment, such as sources of sound.

Millar (1995) points out, however, that the child's ability depends upon a number of variables, including individuality, the nature of the task to be completed, the available information sources and 'the ingenuity of parents and teachers in providing information.' One aspect of this is the degree to which visual information is transposed into non-visual information, although the substituted information needs to be made to converge and overlap with the child's existing reference cues and means of coding.

Millar's research suggests that blind students and those whose functional vision is seriously limited may require assistance to understand the relationship between external planes and surfaces, and that interest in solving spatial problems may well be lost if the material presented is inadequate or poorly integrated. Even though such students will, over the years, have learnt to attend to the information contained in the environment, to differentiate between relevant and irrelevant stimuli and to memorize appropriate details relating to the future performance of various tasks (Foulke and Hatlen, 1992b), staff will need to create a rich, structured learning environment which capitalizes on these abilities and facilitates them. Such strategies might, for example, include converting diagrammatic information into auditory or tactile media. Referring to undergraduate science programmes 'with a high visual content', Wild and Hinton (1993) argue that 'tactile methods of access to the high visual component can make a significant contribution to comprehension and understanding of the course work'.

This does not necessarily mean, however, that everything that can be seen by sighted learners, such as diagrams, maps and graphs, should automatically be converted to a tactile format. Not all blind and partially sighted people find this kind of representation easy to understand. Some prior learning is often necessary even though these representations may have some similarity to the features of the world that they are intended to symbolize. It will be important for the visually impaired learner to be familiar with the symbol system before it can be interpreted easily. Millar (1995) also contends that it is much more difficult to recognize two-dimensional configurations by touch than it is to produce them. This is particularly the case if the learner has no prior knowledge of the likely symbol systems that will be encountered.

If staff propose to issue raised diagrams to blind and/or partially sighted students, therefore, prior discussions with each individual will reveal the extent to which each particular learner feels comfortable with certain symbol systems, whether they are deemed likely to facilitate learning, and to what extent additional tuition of a symbol system may be required. For example, it is possible that some partially sighted learners may not have been introduced to diagrams in human biology classes at school because it was assumed that these would not be accessible. Whilst this might have been partly true, the reason for a student's declared dislike of diagrammatic representations is because of inadequate practice in their use. Such a student, having been given additional instruction in how to read a diagram, may come to appreciate the value of such a study method and may conclude that s/he have a particularly good visual memory which, until that time, had never been exploited.

Some other developmental issues

Reynell (1978) compared the abilities of blind, partially sighted and sighted children in the following five developmental areas: social adaptation; sensorio-motor understanding; exploration of environment; verbal comprehension; and expressive language. She concludes:

> . . . 10 to 12 months was the age at which the sighted group began to outstrip the visually handicapped children in most of the developmental areas. This divergence increased until towards the upper end of the scale (4 to 5 years for the visually handicapped) when more abstract thought processes began to develop. The effect on the visually handicapped group was also seen in the greater advantage of the partially sighted over the blind children. (Reynell, 1978)

She supports Foulke and Hatlen's (1992a) contention that 'nearly all the early stages of learning are visually dominated, and lay the foundations for higher intellectual processes' and argues that, although visually impaired children can compensate for their sensory deficit, they are, by this time, 1–2 years behind their sighted peers in most aspects of learning. Reynell believes that 'The early co-ordinating function of vision is such an enormous learning asset that it is unlikely any teaching can completely make up for its loss' (Reynell, 1978). She emphasizes, however, that 'appropriate and intensive early teaching' is crucial in laying the foundations for success in later life, a view echoed by Murphy and O'Driscoll (1989), Morsley, Spencer and Baybutt (1991), Foulke and Hatlen (1992b) and Millar (1995).

Of course, learning takes place in both formal and informal contexts and children's early psychological and social experiences play an equally vital role in determining their subsequent attitude towards themselves, their impairment, and society in general. Dorn (1993) catalogues a variety of parents' emotional responses to their visually impaired child and Pugh (1980) notes the 'profound effects' that blindness and 'even less severe visual impairment' can have on the 'physical, emotional and social development of a child and his family' (see also Kleinstein, 1984; Erin and Corn, 1994; Royal National Institute for the Blind, 1996). An example of one of these 'profound effects' might be due to a child's inability to focus on significant people and objects. Lack of eye contact, late or infrequent smiling or other communication difficulties may impair maternal and/or other forms of bonding (Dorn, 1993). Morse (1989) believes that 'vision must inevitably contribute to attachment.' If a visually impaired child looks different, this may elicit negative feelings and attitudes in relatives and friends which may lead, subsequently, to a damaging reduction in the amount of care giving (Thomas, 1982). Parents may experience a range of negative emotions about their visually impaired child (Dorn, 1993) which are inevitably picked up by the child and could lead to feelings of rejection and low self-esteem.

If protracted periods of separation from family and home environment are enforced at a critical point in the child's development (for example, due to hospitalization for eye surgery, or attendance at boarding school), this can represent an additional trauma, from which subsequent recovery might never be total. Childhood feelings of fear, desolation, guilt, eccentricity, inadequacy and rejection are often carried into adolescence and adulthood and can impair the quality of future social interactions. Limited opportunities to practise physical and social skills – including play –

will have important implications for the way in which subsequent life situations are managed. Enforced early self-reliance may lead to difficulties in establishing and maintaining intimate relationships in later years. Early experiences of witnessing other disabled children in pain or the death of a close friend can be devastating. It is not uncommon for the loss of a loved one to be trivialized by adults who encourage the child to adopt a stoical approach to the event. If the process of grieving is denied, this can have untold psychological repercussions for later life.

Some educational issues

Education: early years

Introduction to any variety of formal learning environment may prove stressful. Parental sensitivity to the child's visual impairment may produce certain compensatory attitudes and behaviour in both parent and child. If unrealistically high demands are made, the child may believe that only success will bring rewards of affection and approval: 'failure' will be punished. If expectations are unreasonably low, feelings of disempowerment may compound other issues:

> Children who do poorly as a result of vision disorders may be considered by their teachers to be poor students or have learning disabilities. Teachers and parents may subsequently lower their expectations for the child's performance. (M. Wesson, personal communication.) Unless the child complains, or the school provides a comprehensive vision screening, or the parents elect to have the child's eyes examined, the child will be at a disadvantage compared to classmates. This impaired ability may also negatively affect the child's behaviour. (Kleinstein, 1984)

The education of a visually impaired child is an issue to which parents give considerable thought. Following an assessment in which the child, her or his parents and a variety of professional personnel participate, all visually impaired children are issued with a statement of special educational need which makes recommendations regarding the most appropriate educational provision for each individual. The Local Education Authority (LEA) is required to respect the recommendations of the statement and to comply with the choices made by the child and her or his family. Making the choice between special and mainstream education is not easy and many parents agonize over such decisions, recognizing advantages and disadvantages in both approaches. These will be outlined.

Special education

It is not difficult to appreciate the reasons why special schools and institutions came into existence and still retain their appeal for some people. Their supporters argue that concept formation, psycho-motor skill acquisition and social skills learning are undertaken in a psychologically safe environment in which the visual problems of all children are identified and catered for. As well as holding the recognized teacher's certificate, academic staff are usually required to complete a supplementary programme which qualifies them to teach visually impaired learners. Designated resources guarantee a high staff–pupil ratio, staff being concerned with the identification and development of personal and social skills as well as academic abilities. A plentiful supply of specialized equipment and facilities permit full curriculum access for everyone.

Special schools, however, often require their pupils to be completely or partially residential. Separation from family and home environment may result in psychological damage associated with deprivation of family support and mainstream socio-cultural experiences. Opportunities for socializing with non-disabled children are often limited and role modelling is therefore restricted to other visually impaired individuals. Upon returning home for vacations, the child may feel isolated and excluded: there are no friends with whom to enjoy social activities. No practice in communicating the specific requirements of a visually impaired learner is provided because special needs are theoretically addressed. The ethos of the institution may be authoritarian and/or paternalistic. Pupils may develop distorted beliefs about reality. Because they have not been required to negotiate in respect of their special needs this skill may be underdeveloped, leading to potential difficulties at the tertiary level. Appropriate personal strategies may not be cultivated and personal autonomy may never be achieved. The remainder of life may be spent in sheltered or protected accommodation or depending upon the services and support of another person (see French, 1988; French, 1996).

Integrated education

Since the Education Act of 1981, children with special educational needs have received increased attention from educationalists in the UK. The Education Reform Act (1988) and the Children Act (1989) have guaranteed the maintenance of this profile. The general philosophy now purports to be one of inclusion, and the customary policy is to integrate such children into mainstream provision. The impetus for such practice came 'largely from a concern for the rights of children and young people with special educational needs (SENs)' (Wedell, 1995). Disability does not diminish rights to equal access and each LEA is statutorily required to ensure that the school makes adequate provision for the child's particular educational needs as identified in the Statement. Theoretically, this offers the visually impaired learner educational and social opportunities not available in a segregated educational context.

Learning is undertaken in a standard classroom environment. The visually impaired pupil may receive assistance from a full-time support worker whose role is to facilitate communication and learning. This situation provides more appropriate role models for academic, psycho-motor and social skill development. Both staff and non-disabled pupils benefit educationally and socially insofar as they too have a role model of a visually impaired person: learning about the concept of disability becomes a familiar part of their lives and they are less likely to regard other blind and partially sighted people as 'different'. Morse (1989) refers to educational studies conducted by McGuiness (1970) which concluded that 'students in itinerant programs develop a stronger self-image than do students in special schools owing to the number of friendships they develop with sighted peers.'

The success of integrated education, however, depends upon the realization of many ideals: adequate human, physical and financial resource provision, appropriate physical environment, abundance of specialized equipment, continual and effective support teaching services and the constant cooperation of other staff and pupils. It will also depend upon LEA general policies and provision that are subject to wide local variation.

It is not always the case that staff possess appropriate educational qualifications to be of practical help to the pupil within each of the variety of specific learning contexts. Some support staff are lay members of the public whose desire is to 'help'. Reports from some teachers of visually impaired students in UK further and higher education institutions suggest that the development of effective communication skills and personal strategies is inadequate in those children whose support staff have 'carried' them through primary and secondary school. The well-intentioned support may have been too intrusive for the appropriate development of personal autonomy and served only further to disable the learner (Wedell, 1995).

Where effective support does exist, it is often provided in specialized units, separated from the main classroom areas and regarded by many as segregation disguised as integration (Barnes, 1996). It is extremely cost intensive and, whilst it may facilitate the achievement of the numerous academic qualifications required by institutions of further and higher education, it may not, in the wider psychological and socio-cultural sense, guarantee adequate preparation of all visually impaired students for entry into the environment of tertiary education. Here the individual may have to take some personal responsibility for communicating with staff and negotiating appropriate learning environments. As in special schools, the perseverance, tenacity and assertiveness required may not be developed.

Stockley (1987) contends that:

> . . . successful integration depends on a number of factors coming together at the right time. The criteria of success

include appropriate attitudes, skills and preparation in the
child, the parents, the teachers and the administrators.

But it is perhaps the educational philosophy behind the concept of
integration which is the root cause of the problem: 'the stress in
integration is on the physical movement of the child from one place
to another without a concomitant expectation of necessary change by
the mainstream school' (Thomas, 1997). Integration is founded upon
a 'readiness model' (Lipsky and Gartner, 1996) which requires
learners to prove their readiness for inclusion into an integrated
setting rather than placing the onus on the school to demonstrate its
readiness to include them within its standard classes. Integration
describes the assimilation by the mainstream of identifiable categories
of children – those with sensory impairments, for example – whose
learning needs are assumed to be identical by virtue of their
disability. The establishment of separate teaching units is an example
of segregation disguised as integration, a practice that is predicated
upon the further misconceived assumption that it is legitimate to
exclude learners with different educational needs – and disabled
people in general – from the mainstream school environment.
Indeed, the entire concept of integration fails to recognize the
diversity of *everyone's* learning requirements:

> Teaching is focused on some concept of the aggregate
> learning needs of the pupils in a group which, in turn,
> leads to an assumed homogeneity of those pupils' learning
> needs. (Wedell, 1995)

Inclusive education

Although the terms are often used synonymously, integrated
education is not inclusive education. Ideologically, inclusive
education is founded upon a philosophy that values the individual
and acknowledges human diversity. Everyone is included in the
socio-cultural as well as the learning experience.

> The notion of inclusion . . . does not set parameters . . .
> around particular kinds of putative disability. Rather, it is

> about a philosophy of acceptance and about providing a
> framework within which all children (regardless of the
> provenance of their difficulty at school) can be valued
> equally, treated with respect and provided with equal
> opportunities at school. (Thomas, 1997)

In short, inclusion means moving from a preoccupation with
individual learning difficulties and disabilities to an agenda of human
rights. Attempts are therefore made to create a learning environment
that is accessible to all pupils: no one should be excluded.

Reality, however, often falls short of the ideal. For learning to be
genuinely inclusive, both school and post-school provision must be
redesigned 'where the needs of students with learning difficulties
and/or disabilities are seen as "cognate with those of all other
learners"' (Tomlinson Committee Reports, FEFC, 1996, cited in
Florian, 1997). Referring to tertiary education, Florian (1997) points
out that:

> Use of the term does not imply integrated provision but
> refers to the match between the needs of the learner and
> the demands of the course. As used in the Tomlinson
> Committee Report, 'inclusive learning' refers to how
> colleges effect this match and not necessarily to whether or
> not a course is integrated.

For inclusive education to represent more than just an *ad hoc*
response towards meeting the access requirements of visually
impaired learners, however, all educational establishments must
become involved in a regular and continual review process, to include
pupil/student input. This should stimulate reflection on policy and
operational issues, leading to the adoption of institution-wide
strategic plans which, in turn, will ensure that future practice takes
account of everyone's needs. This process must not be confined to
the academic curriculum but must include the socio-cultural aspects
of school and college life (see Chapter 12).

Inclusive education attempts to represent a 'unified system' that is
capable of responding to people as individuals rather than to follow
the 'tradition of parallel systems whereby some people receive

separate forms of education' (Ainscow, 1997). (See also Florian, 1997; and FEFC, 1996, 1997.) An inclusive philosophy is consistent with a pluralist culture that celebrates diversity and equality of opportunity.

> Even if schools and administrators are not convinced by the ethical arguments or empirical evidence in its favour, it seems likely that they will have to respond to an increasingly anti-discriminatory legislative environment backed by vigorous rights across the world.   (Thomas, 1997)

Ultimately, however, everyone's fundamental right to choose must be respected. The choice of educational institution lies with the visually impaired individual and his or her family. The young person's opinions and feelings should be taken into account by everyone involved in the decision making process.

Tertiary education

As will be evident from the previous discussion, the ethical and educational issues outlined above are as relevant to tertiary education as they are to the primary and secondary sectors. The advantages and disadvantages of special and mainstream provision continue to be vigorously debated, not least among visually impaired learners. The 1992 Further and Higher Education Acts and the Disability Discrimination Act (1995) require colleges to have concern for the access needs of disabled students and to implement appropriate support structures to meet those needs (see Chapters 3 and 12).

Between 1993 and 1996, staff from RNIB's Employment and Student Support Network (ESSN) were in contact with a peak figure of 2500 visually impaired students who were enrolled on some form of full-time or part-time post-school educational programme (RNIB ESSN Student Records). Such programmes include undergraduate, postgraduate, certificated, diploma and other vocational courses. Research has indicated that, within the context of higher education, many perform better than their sighted peers (Patton, 1993). Experience also suggests, however, that under-achievement – and the fear of it – is not uncommon. Some visually impaired students have enrolled on programmes that they know to be well below their capabilities; some have chosen courses that they would not have entertained had their sight been unimpaired. This inevitably affects their attitudes towards study and college life and restricts future career choice and opportunities.

Irrespective of their selection of course, all visually impaired students constantly make compromises. Processing written information takes longer than for sighted students and many additional hours are spent in keeping pace with course work (Lorimer, 1978; Tobin, 1985; Barnes, 1996). Postural positions that are often adopted in an attempt to access print material can result in other physical problems such as back or neck ache and gastro-intestinal disturbances (Francis and Brown, 1982). High-tech equipment designed to facilitate curriculum access is often prohibitively expensive and sometimes complicated to learn and use. Long battles to gain full participation on course programmes often contribute to the general stress experienced at college. Although some barriers to accessing and retrieving information can be overcome, the process is time consuming and the average library can present difficulties if, for example, catalogues are inaccessible and staff are not available to provide assistance.

Some psychological and social issues

All the above stresses may be compounded by many others both physical and personal. Examples might include adaptation to changes and/or deterioration in vision, or even loss of sight. Many people might identify with Dodds' (1993) contention that:

> Sudden and severe loss of sight can be an overwhelmingly distressing experience for the sufferer and, equally, those close at hand. This is particularly true when the individual has enjoyed normal or near normal vision for most of their life and as a result has taken their sight completely for granted.

If such an event occurs at any time during a student's educational programme it can cause a significant disruption; if it happens immediately prior to, or during, important examinations or practical, work-related placement, the consequences and effects can be devastating for an already anxious learner. Pain may or may not accompany deterioration in vision, which can be particularly disabling. Fears of being asked to leave the course or to repeat parts of it may drive some students to deny or mask the symptoms and may discourage them from seeking appropriate medical and academic help and advice.

Other stresses are associated with life-cycle and the social and cultural aspects of college life. All students are, of course, susceptible to life-cycle stresses but, with reference to 'adolescent turmoil', there is some evidence to suggest that 'in cases of visual impairment these difficulties may be more pronounced' (Stockley and Brooks, 1995). Pressures include: the need to be attractive, to make friends, to gain respect and to participate in cultural and recreational activities. For many blind or partially sighted students, a corridor full of bustling people, a crowded cafeteria or union bar can be an extremely frightening experience, especially during the initial weeks of the course. Moving around in such environments, recognizing people and making eye contact is difficult if not impossible. This can prevent a visually impaired student from being able to join a group of other students, who may, through lack of understanding, conclude that the student is anti-social. A sensitive student may become depressed and prefer solitude above participating in social events. Of course, such behaviour only serves to confirm other students' beliefs. Some colleges have recognized this potential problem and have addressed the issue by providing all new, visually impaired students with personal assistants whose role is to help with orientation and mobility. Such a practice can, however, have negative as well as positive consequences in that many visually impaired people experience embarrassment at being escorted around by a (sometimes) older person who reminds them of their parents.

Feelings of being different and social alienation may lead to an identification with other minority groups; conversely, negative socialization and the memories of painful personal experiences relating to disability can drive a visually impaired person to avoid any association with disabled people, or with organizations established to represent their interests. Clearly, each individual's response to the ways in which society treats him or her will be different but typical responses to visual impairment – congenital or acquired – include: general feelings of worthlessness and a decrease in self-esteem and self-confidence; fear; loneliness; depression; inadequacy; disbelief; denial; shame; guilt; anger; anxiety; grief; helplessness; isolation; defensiveness; resentment; envy; rejection; frustration.

Morse (1989) suggests that blind and partially sighted people may experience difficulties 'in establishing an adequate body image when deprived of accurate visual feedback regarding the functioning of their body or of the feedback of significant others. Obviously, if visual efficiency fluctuates or visual status suddenly deteriorates or improves dramatically these changes have an impact on the self-concept.' Feelings of inferiority are experienced and the person may seek to eliminate the anxiety-provoking discrepancy between how they perceive themselves and how others perceive them by evolving various defence mechanisms. They may or may not be 'aided' in this process by 'the overprotection of sighted people.' He identifies three methods designed to avoid anxiety frequently used by people with low vision:

> First, they obtain information about their performance (selective perception) and thus shun certain new or unpredictable situations. Second, they rationalize their inadequacies, project them onto others, or displace them onto the 'handicap' ('But I can't do that, I'm visually handicapped'). Third, they collapse or expand their perceptual field; that is, they become an expert in and devote their whole lives to a single endeavour or become involved in a multitude of activities or responsibilities.
> (Morse, 1989)

Other reactions will have equally significant implications and can, in themselves, be disabling, for example, feelings of inadequacy and worthlessness may engender doubts about the ability to form platonic and sexual relationships. A poor self-concept is more likely to develop (Morse, 1989). Denial may be reflected in tendencies to conform to expected social norms and strenuous attempts to behave normally at all costs (Barnes, 1996). For example, some people who describe themselves as blind but with some useful residual vision openly refuse to carry or use a white cane even though they admit to experiencing difficulty in getting around at night. With reference to student life, this might include an unwillingness to use low vision – or other specialized – equipment in public and difficulty in asking for assistance when this would be helpful.

It is important to emphasize, however, that it is the social situations created by the presence of a visual impairment, and not the visual impairment *per se*, which determine these reactions and the quality of life experiences (Hudson, 1994). Nevertheless, as a consequence of socialization, negative personal attitudes about disability may have developed which will further influence self-perception and the perception of other disabled people. Research conducted by Dodds, *et al.* (1991) suggests that there is a significant relationship between a visually impaired person's attitude towards visually impaired people in general and 'the degree to which they accept their own lack of sight' (Dodds, 1993).

As noted earlier, individual reactions to visual impairment vary considerably but have traditionally been compared to those of bereavement (Murray Parkes, 1980; see Dodds, 1989). The 'loss' model, however, may be unhelpful, as it originates from an individualistic perspective on disability as revealed in Dodds' analysis (Dodds, 1993). Not everyone is sad or despondent, although one significant cause of depression is the many negative attitudes towards impairment reflected in the numerous social and environmental barriers encountered.

Partial sight: some specific issues

It has been suggested (Chapter 2) that to possess some sight does not necessarily place the individual at an advantage. In certain contexts – negotiating the environment – even poor residual vision can be useful. Some partially sighted people believe, however, that their impairment creates more psychological and social barriers than blindness and is, therefore, more disabling. Referring to research by Bateman (1962), Morse (1989) contends that partially sighted people are inclined to be more self-pitying and less able to 'accept' their visual impairment than those who are blind. Further, parents of partially sighted children tend to show less understanding than do those of blind children (Morse, 1989). Because their abilities are determined by so many variables, some partially sighted people become ambivalent about their identity. That they perceive themselves as neither blind nor sighted can lead to a constant tension between the need for dependence and the wish for independence and normality.

Bowley and Gardiner (1980) believe that it is easier to communicate and empathize with blind people because of the many 'favourable images' associated with blindness. Experience confirms that the concept of blindness is less ambiguous than partial sight and therefore lends itself more easily to public education. This is not, of course, to deny that blind people are often the subjects of insensitive treatment: they are often ignored, patronized, frequently addressed indirectly (the 'does he take sugar?' syndrome), spoken 'at' and not 'to' and manoeuvred about as objects. Blind people – and those whose level of residual vision requires them to adopt non-sighted strategies – are frequently the target of what can only be described as verbal abuse. They are often the subject of undisguised public fascination and voyeurism, total strangers asking intrusive, personal questions relating to the impairment without doubting their right to receive information (see Morris, 1996).

Discussions with many partially sighted people reveal that, having witnessed such treatment, some consider that to have what is often described as an 'invisible' impairment is advantageous in that it enables them to appear non-disabled and thus to be treated as a non-disabled person. This, however, creates misunderstanding in terms of the person's (often incomprehensible) behaviour, which in turn causes confusion and ambivalence among the general public and testifies to the complex issues surrounding partial sight.

Partially sighted people may display, albeit unintentionally, ambiguous messages. Some may appear to be able to see much more than they actually can, while others seem to be more dependent than their degree of sight would warrant. Focusing on specific people and/or objects is sometimes achieved by squinting, looking above, below or beyond them. Peering, apparent staring, glaring or scowling are not uncommon signs displayed by people trying to utilize their residual vision to good effect. Further, since visual ability is often fluctuating and/or context dependent, the same partially sighted person might be able to dodge nimbly between shoppers in daylight but be rendered almost immobile at night. The reverse is also true: some people who prefer twilight conditions also experience disabling pain when in bright sunlight. Additionally, the person whose visual acuity enables him or her to read standard size print may, because of a field restriction, collide with objects and/or people while moving about. For these reasons, assistance is not always forthcoming and, even when it is actively sought, it may be denied or, if offered, may be inappropriate. That a partially sighted person displays unremarkable behaviour communicates very little: it does not necessarily signify that needs are being met but neither does it necessarily indicate that they are not (Disabled Living Foundation, 1991).

The implications of a marginal impairment are documented by Morse (1989), who notes that 'normal' appearance of the eyes leads others to expect 'normal' behaviour. He describes a familiar dilemma faced by partially sighted people:

> it is difficult for the low vision person to explain all the conditions of his or her loss. To say nothing invites false perceptions, yet, to offer a detailed account of what he or she cannot be expected to perform may be interpreted by meaningful others as offering excuses. (Morse, 1989)

As noted above, inability to recognize familiar people at a distance may lead some – especially those who are unaware of the person's visual impairment – to dismiss the partially sighted person as snobbish or anti-social. Eye contact may be difficult. Poor or inappropriate responses to non-verbal cues may result in the unwitting transmission of ambiguous messages, leading to misunderstandings. This problem is often intensified in group situations. The partially sighted person is denied valuable social/psychological information relating to other group participants, which may result in an inability to gain social acceptance and establish bonds with other members. The rational exhortation to declare an 'invisible' impairment is often easier to recommend than to execute, especially in new social gatherings. In spite of this, however, revealing the existence of an impairment is considered to be the most effective way of dealing with disability (Barnes, 1996). Sustained attempts at concealment only result in unnecessary energy expenditure and create considerable stress. Because some partially sighted people may experience ambivalence and even bewilderment about their impairment, they remain unable to decide the best course of action in social contexts. Feelings of alienation may, as indicated above, lead to the preference for lone pursuits.

Negotiating the environment

Most visually impaired people agree that successful negotiation of the environment requires considerable concentration and effort. Thus travelling around often increases general physical and mental tension and can be stressful. Such high stress levels are generally not experienced by sighted people, who take for granted an environment that is rich with informative visual cues. Blind people have access to no such cues; partially sighted people, as outlined in Chapter 2 will be required to interpret what are often perceived as ambiguous cues. It will be necessary to rely on other sensory input from which to obtain useful information, in particular, on the relatively impoverished auditory environment. Utilization of ambient and self-generated sound can, however, be effective and visually impaired people learn to attend to auditory input although it is generally more sequential than visual stimuli (Dodds, 1988; Dodds, 1993). That sound is a less reliable form of information than visual input is demonstrated by the fact that it can be time dependent. For example, a blind traveller can identify the destination of a particular train because of having learnt that a group of animated school children use this train to travel to school. Other means of identification would therefore need to be considered at times such as school holidays.

Many visual and perceptual disorders can affect mobility. There are numerous potential hazards associated with travelling around and it is regarded by many blind and partially sighted people as a major difficulty (Ford and Heshel, 1995; Royal National Institute for the Blind, 1997). Depending upon its nature, colour blindness could reduce the time taken to interpret signals that rely on colour for their significance. Logan (1982), referring to red/green blindness, identifies difficulties of 'scanning a background for a red object', adding that 'The subject may have an equal difficulty with green objects, but that matters less, because one is rarely scanning anywhere for a green object.' Logan states that the ability to discriminate red colours 'matters in road safety' (see also Wilson, 1989). Map reading may be difficult if colour vision is impaired, and may be impossible if the person has had no opportunities to develop and practise this skill or is unable to perceive fine detail. Impaired central vision may result in collision with other pedestrians or objects. Restrictions of peripheral vision (further reduced by the wearing of spectacles) may prevent a pedestrian from detecting a vehicle approaching from the side when looking straight across the road. Poor dark adaptation may render a person temporarily blind when entering or leaving buildings or subways. Perceptual disorders and/or poor contrast sensitivity may lead to accidents caused by an inability to identify outlines of doors, panes of glass, or flights of stairs (see Chapter 7). Reduced visual acuity has many repercussions. Difficulties experienced in attempting to read street signs, house and bus numbers, train and bus destinations and general noticeboards may precipitate headache which detracts further from concentration. Of the 500 visually impaired people who participated in a telephone survey, 44% did not use public transport on their own because of inaccessible timetable information, complicated operation of automatic ticket machines and lack of announcements at bus, tube and train station stops (Royal National Institute for the Blind, 1997).

Generalized disorientation may affect some visually impaired people. This can occur in situations such as: crowds; intense noise produced by roadworks or high winds; buildings with identical landmarks on each floor; and fog (where visual and auditory input is reduced). Psychological factors such as apprehension may affect a visually impaired person's willingness to travel around alone and may lead to the decision to use an escort.

Some personal issues

Barriers to access become particularly significant when they relate
specifically to personal issues such as self-image. For many visually
impaired people, the opportunity to make effective use of such
equipment as mirrors is unavailable, a frustration whose
repercussions can only be speculated upon. Although not everyone is
preoccupied with appearance, personal experience suggests that most
visually impaired people are to some degree concerned about how
they look. Access to relevant magazines is seriously restricted and,
although good colour memory can be developed, many people prefer
to ask family and friends or purchase the services of professional
consultants – at considerable cost – for information and assistance in
the selection of clothes and the application of some image-enhancing
techniques. Discussion with others increases confidence and goes
some way to improving this kind of access which non-disabled people
take for granted.

Loss of privacy represents an equally important consequence of
reduced access. Considerable information is received in the form of
written communication: personal mail, medical information, hospital
appointment details, benefit claim forms, financial statements and
bills. Forty per cent of those questioned in RNIB's telephone survey
stated that, in particular, financial information should be accessible
(Royal National Institute for the Blind, 1997). Unless appropriate
equipment is available – and scanners cannot read handwriting or red
ink – the visually impaired person must recruit the services of a
reader. The predominantly visual output of such machines as
cash-point dispensers can represent a further barrier and a
consequent invasion of privacy.

For many visually impaired people, the choice of where to live
is dictated to a great extent by the general accessibility of the
environment and by the level of local service provision, including
shops and other recreational and transport facilities. Some
students in higher education may choose to live in halls of
residence because they offer a high standard of accommodation
including on-site catering and laundry facilities. They are often
situated within easy reach of the main university campus, which

facilitates travelling to and from college. This is particularly significant for students who experience additional difficulties when travelling around at night because it provides them with the option to participate in social and recreational activities that take place on campus. The decision to live in a hall of residence may, however, represent a compromise. Mature students, for example, may have sacrificed living in a house with friends of a similar age because of its location and the potential access problems envisaged.

For visually impaired people living in private accommodation, other issues need to be considered, especially for those living alone. To assist with the management of general house maintenance, some choose to purchase cleaning, gardening and related maintenance services. The prospect of specific property improvements, however, may be daunting. Limited access to appropriate literature and the inability to undertake many DIY jobs such as painting and decorating is inconvenient and may be expensive if the services of professional personnel are recruited.

For 35% of visually impaired people polled, shopping was ranked as one of the top three frustrations (Royal National Institute for the Blind, 1997). Indeed, shopping can prove to be an interesting experience. The inexorable trend towards the impersonal hypermarket, often situated in places accessible only by private transport, has contributed to the increasing number of barriers faced by blind and partially sighted people. Even standard size supermarkets and department stores can prove difficult to negotiate. The constantly changing layout of goods often makes it impossible to find a particular item; food labels and price tags are invariably in minute print. Some visually impaired shoppers choose to take advantage of the telephone shopping and home delivery service offered by a few retailers. Others prefer to visit the store and obtain assistance from staff. Personal experience confirms, however, that this is by no means a guarantee that the person's shopping trolley will necessarily contain the items that appear on the prepared shopping list. Places such as markets are often avoided unless an escort is available.

The older learner: some issues

Any discussion on visual impairment and the implications for learning must not neglect the specific issues related to older learners, who are, by virtue of their age, likely to be affected by visual impairment. According to RNIB's (1997) student records, trends indicate that the number of older learners is increasing, with the highest percentage being in the age range of 26–40 years and a significant proportion aged 40–60 years. In 1996, RNIB launched a Life Long Learning Project, which is currently investigating the service needs of older visually impaired people interested in participating in an educational programme. For those over 55 years of age, learning has been defined as 'any activity which serves to maintain or enhance existing skills, as well as that which facilitates new learning' (Royal National Institute for the Blind, 1998). The project's findings suggest that many older visually impaired people are likely to seek new learning opportunities outside the further and higher education sectors and that local and national voluntary organizations, as well as residential establishments, are increasingly involved in the provision of educational activities. An initial mapping exercise reveals a low take-up of traditional courses by older learners, due, partly, to a perceived lack of appropriate college provision to meet their access requirements. The dearth of learning assessment mechanisms in part-time adult education is also a major issue and, to some extent, accounts for the limited take-up of formal learning opportunities by visually impaired older people. For adult returners – especially those who have become visually impaired since their most recent period of learning – the identification of learning support needs is critical to retention and motivation. The shortage of pre-course and on-programme study skills training that targets visually impaired people in general represents a further barrier for older people (Royal National Institute for the Blind, 1998).

Where institutions actively target older visually impaired learners, evidence suggests that those who have gained confidence through personal experience of one-to-one tuition and small group participation are most likely to show interest (Royal National Institute for the Blind, 1998). There are, however, many establishments that do not consider this group of students to rank high on the priority list of customers, as reflected in the poor quality of their current service provision. Many staff involved in delivering adult education programmes are operating in far from ideal circumstances. They may be teaching off site and/or out of hours and have limited or no access to such services as photocopying and technical support. Opportunities to take advantage of the college's general staff training and development initiatives may be limited or, if these are available, staff are expected to undertake courses in their own time and without receiving reimbursement. Being marginalized in this way is demoralizing and affects the quality of teaching practice and the relationship with learners. Although staff may be committed to the education of older visually impaired students, feelings of isolation and frustration at being unable to offer a quality service may persuade them, eventually, to withdraw from such activities.

In addition to visual impairment, other medical and social factors may affect an older person's learning abilities. For example, feedback from older learners indicates that there is an increased number of older people learning Moon in preference to Braille, in spite of the dearth of material available in this medium (Royal National Institute for the Blind, 1998). The system is, however, appealing for many older people, who may perceive Braille to be a complicated system beyond their capabilities and, if they have reduced tactile sensitivity, this may render Braille inaccessible. Trends indicate that Moon is also attractive to deafblind people, of whom there are a substantial number participating in a user group (Royal National Institute for the Blind, 1998). Older visually impaired people, however, demonstrate a general willingness to engage with new technology, although opportunities for doing so are more limited than those available to younger age groups. This has an impact on the training needs of older people which differ, in general terms, from those of younger learners (Royal National Institute for the Blind, 1998).

In common with non-disabled older people, those with a visual impairment may generally lack confidence in both their learning capabilities and social skills which may affect their performance in even medium size groups. Anticipation of receiving inadequate support and lack of familiarity with high-tech equipment may represent additional barriers to learning. Mobility difficulties and financial considerations may deter some from attending an institution unless transport is provided.

In conclusion, it is important for staff to take all of these consequences and effects into account when planning services for visually impaired students.

References

Adelson, E. and Fraiberg, S. (1976) Sensory deficit and motor development in infants blind from birth, in *The Effects of Blindness and Other Implications on Early Development* (ed. Z. Jastrazembska), American Foundation for the Blind, New York, pp. 1–15.

Ainscow, M. (1997) Towards inclusive schooling. *British Journal of Special Education*, **24** (1), 3–6.

Barnes, C. (1996) Visual impairment and disability, in *Beyond Disability: Towards an Enabling Society*, (ed. G. Hales). Sage, Thousand Oaks, CA, pp. 36–44.

Bateman, B. (1962) Sighted children's perceptions of blind children's abilities. *Exceptional Children*, **29**, 42–6.

Bowley, A.H. and Gardner, L. (1980) *The Handicapped Child: Educational and Psychological Guidance for the Organically Handicapped*, 4th edn, Churchill Livingstone, London and New York.

Cratty, B.J. (1979) *Perceptual and Motor Development in Infants and Children*, 2nd edn, Prentice Hall, NJ.

Disabled Living Foundation (1991) *Visual Handicap: A Distance Learning Pack for Physiotherapists, Occupational Therapists and Other Health Care Professionals*, DLF, London.

Dodds, A.G. (1988) *Mobility Training for Visually Handicapped People: A Person-Centered Approach*, Croom Helm, London and Sydney.

Dodds, A.G. (1989) Motivation reconsidered: the importance of self-efficacy in rehabilitation. *The British Journal of Visual Impairment*, **7** (1), 11–15.

Dodds, A.G. (1993) *Rehabilitating Blind and Visually Impaired People: A Psychological Approach*, Chapman & Hall, London.

Dodds, A.G., Bailey, P., Pearson, A. and Yates, L. (1991) Psychological factors in acquired visual impairment: the development of a scale of adjustment. *Journal of Visual Impairment and Blindness*, **85** (7), 306–10.

Dorn, L. (1993) The mother/blind infant relationship: a research programme. *British Journal of Visual Impairment*, **11** (1), 13–16.

Erin, J.N. and Corn, A.L. (1994) A survey of children's first understanding of being visually impaired. *Journal of Visual Impairment and Blindness*, March/April, 132–9.

FEFC (1996) *Inclusive Learning: Report of the Learning Difficulties and/or Disabilities Committee*, FEFC, Coventry.

FEFC (1997) *Mapping Provision: The Provision of and Participation in Further Education by Students with Learning Difficulties and/or Disabilities*, FEFC, Coventry.

Florian, L. (1997) 'Inclusive learning': the reform initiative of the Tomlinson Committee, *British Journal of Special Education*, **24** (1), 7–11.

Ford, M. and Heshel, T. (1995) *BBC In Touch 1995–96 Handbook: The BBC Radio 4 Guide to Services for People with a Visual Impairment*, In Touch Publishing, Cardiff, in association with BBC network radio.

Foulke, E. and Hatlen, P. (1992a) A collaboration of two technologies: part 1: perceptual and cognitive processes: their implications for visually impaired persons. *British Journal of Visual Impairment*, **10** (2), 43–6.

Foulke, E. and Hatlen, P. (1992b) A collaboration of two technologies: part 2: perceptual and cognitive training: its nature and importance. *British Journal of Visual Impairment*, **10** (2), 47–9.

Francis, I.C. and Brown, S.A. (1982) Abnormal head postures: a review of 116 patients. *Australian Orthoptic Journal*, **19**, 35–40.

French, S. (1988) Memories of the first day. *New Beacon*, **72** (856), 261–3.

French, S. (1993) Disability, impairment or something in between, in *Disabling Barriers: Enabling Environments*, (eds. J. Swain, V. Finkelstein, S. French, and M. Oliver), Sage, London, pp. 17–25.

French, S. (1996) Out of sight, out of mind: the experience and effects of a 'special' residential school, in *Encounters with Strangers:*

Feminism and Disability, (ed. J. Morris), Womens' Press, London, pp. 17–47.

Hudson, D. (1994) Causes of emotional and psychological reactions to adventitious blindness. *Journal of Visual Impairment and Blindness*, November/December, 498–503.

Keith, L. (ed.) (1994) *Mustn't Grumble: Writings by Disabled Women*, Womens' Press, London.

Kleinstein, R.N. (1984) Vision disorders in public health. *Annual Review of Public Health*, (5), 369–84.

Lipsky, D.K. and Gartner, A. (1996) Inclusion, school restructuring and the re-making of American society. *Harvard Educational Review*, **66** (4), 762–96.

Logan, J.S. (1982) The red-green blind eye. *Practitioner*, **226**, May, 879–82.

Lorimer, J. (1978) The limitations of Braille as a medium for communication and the possibility of improving reading standards. Division of Education and Child Psychology, British Psychological Society, *Occasional Papers*, **2** (2), 60–7.

McGuiness, R. (1970) A descriptive study of blind children educated in the itinerant, resource room and special school settings. *American Foundation for the Blind Research Bulletin*, **20**, 1–57.

Millar, S. (1995) Understanding and representing spatial information. *British Journal of Visual Impairment*, **13** (1), 8–11.

Morris, J. (ed.) (1996) *Encounters with Strangers: Feminism and Disability*, Womens' Press, London.

Morse, J.L. (1989) Psychosocial aspects of low vision, in *Understanding Low Vision*, 2nd edn (ed. R. T. Jose), American Foundation for the Blind, New York, pp. 43–54.

Morsley, K., Spencer, C. and Baybutt, K. (1991) Two techniques for encouraging movement and exploration in the visually impaired child. *British Journal of Visual Impairment*, **9** (3), 75–8.

Murphy, F.M. and O'Driscoll, M. (1989) Observations on the motor development of visually impaired children: interpretations from video recordings. *Physiotherapy*, **75** (9), 505–8.

Murray Parkes, C. (1980) *Bereavement: Studies of Grief in Adult Life*, Penguin, Harmondsworth, UK.

Patton, B. (1993) *RNIB Student Support Service: Provision in Higher Education*, RNIB, London.

Pugh, R. (1980) Development in sight. *Nursing Mirror*, 3 July, 30–2.

Reynell, J. (1978) Developmental patterns of visually handicapped children. *Child: Care, Health and Development*, (4), 291–303.

Reynolds, R. (1988) A psychological definition of illusion. *Philosophical Psychology*, **1** (2), 217–23.

Royal National Institute for the Blind (1996) *Taking the Time: Telling Parents Their Child is Blind or Partially Sighted*, RNIB, London.

Royal National Institute for the Blind (1997) *Blindness: The Daily Challenge*, RNIB, London.

Royal National Institute for the Blind (1998) *Report to the Life Long Learning Project Steering Group*, RNIB, London.

Sheridan, M.D. (1973) *Children's Developmental Progress: From Birth to Five Years the Stycar Sequences*, NFER Publishing, Windsor, UK.

Stockley, J. (1987) *Vision in the Classroom: A Study of the Integration of Visually Handicapped Children*, RNIB, London.

Stockley, J. and Brooks, B. (1995) Perception and adjustment: self and social. *British Journal of Visual Impairment*, **13** (1), 15–18.

Thomas, D. (1982) *The Experience of Handicap*, Methuen & Co., London and New York.

Thomas, G. (1997) Inclusive schools for an inclusive society. *British Journal of Special Education*, **24** (3), 103–7.

Tobin, M.J. (1985) The reading skills of the partially sighted: their implications for integrated education. *International Journal of Rehabilitation Research*, **8** (4), 467–72.

Wedell, K. (1995) Making inclusive education ordinary. *British Journal of Special Education*, **22** (3), 100–4.

Wild, G. and Hinton, R. (1993) Visual information and the blind student: the problem of access. *British Journal of Visual Impairment*, **1** (3), 99–102.

Wilson, R. (1989) Colour and the visually impaired rail traveller. *New Beacon*, **73** (861), 41–4.

Suggested reading

Allen, M. and Birse, E. (1991) Stigma and blindness. *Journal of Ophthalmic Nursing and Technology*, **10** (4), 147–52.

Beggs, W.D.A. (1990) The feelings associated with visually impaired travel – 1. *New Beacon*, **74** (882), 433–7.

Beggs, W.D.A. (1991) The feelings associated with visually impaired travel – 2. *New Beacon*, **75** (883), 1–6.

Blunkett, D. (1997) Editorial. *British Journal of Special Education*, **24** (4), 150–1.

Dodds, A.G., Howarth, C.I. and Carter, D.C. (1982) The mental maps of the blind: the role of previous visual experience. *The Journal of Visual Impairment and Blindness*, **76** (1), 5–12.

Dote-Kwan, J. and Hughes, M. (1994) The home environments of young blind children. *Journal of Visual Impairment and Blindness*, **88** (1), 31–68.

Dyson, A. (1997) Social and educational disadvantage: reconnecting special needs education. *British Journal of Special Education*, **24** (4), 152–7.

French, S. (1989) Mind your language. *Nursing Times*, **85** (2), 29–31.

French, S. (1991) What's so great about independence? *New Beacon*, **75** (886), 153–6.

French, S. (ed.) (1994) *On Equal Terms: Working With Disabled People*, Butterworth-Heinemann, Oxford.

Garner, K., Dale, M. and Garner, S. (1997) *Education, Employment and Rehabilitation for Visually Impaired Adults: A Survey of Recent Research*, RNIB, London.

Goffman, E. (1979) *Stigma: Notes on the Management of Spoiled Identity*, Penguin, Harmondsworth, UK.

Hill, E.W., Reiser, J.J., Hill, M.M. *et al.* (1993) How persons with visual impairments explore novel spaces: strategies of good and poor performers. *Journal of Visual Impairment and Blindness*, **87** (10), 295–301.

Jackson, R. and Lawson, G. (1995) Family environment and psychological distress in persons who are visually impaired. *Journal of Visual Impairment and Blindness*, **89** (2), 157–60.

Klatzky, R.L., Golledge, R.G., Loomis, J.M. *et al.* (1995) Performance of blind and sighted persons on spatial tasks. *Journal of Visual Impairment and Blindness*, **89** (1), 70–82.

Leicester, M. and Lovell, T. (1997) Disability voice: educational experience and disability. *Disability and Society*, **12** (1), 111–18.

Levitt, S. (ed.) (1984) *Paediatric Developmental Therapy*, Blackwell Scientific Publications, Oxford, London and Edinburgh.

Mason, H.L. and Tobin, M.J. (1986) Speed of information processing and the visually handicapped child. *British Journal of Special Education* (Research Supplement), **13** (2), 69–70.

Morris, J. (1995) Pride against prejudice: 'lives not worth living'. in *Health and Disease: A Reader*, 2nd edn, (eds. B. Davey, A. Gray and C. Seale), Open University Press, Buckingham and Philadelphia, 107–10.

Morris, N. and Parker, P. (1997) Reviewing the teaching and learning of children with special educational needs: enabling whole school responsibility. *British Journal of Special Education*, **24** (4), 163–6.

Oliver, M. (1983) *Social Work with Disabled People*, Macmillan, London.

Oliver, M. (1990) *The Politics of Disablement*, Macmillan, Basingstoke and London.

Oliver, M. (1996) *Understanding Disability: From Theory to Practice*, Macmillan, Basingstoke and London.

Preece, J. (1995) Disability and adult education – the consumer view. *Disability and Society*, **10** (1), 87–102.

Pring, L. (1982) Phonological and tactual coding of Braille by blind children. *British Journal of Psychology*, (73), 351–9.

Pring, L. (1983) Imagery and concreteness in the reading of blind and sighted children. *British Journal of Developmental Psychology*, (1), 365–74.

Roy, A. (1996) Access to education for visually impaired students – 1: 1656–1995. *New Beacon*, **80** (938), 4–7.

Roy, A. (1996) Access to education for visually impaired students – 2: 1884–1995. *New Beacon*, **80** (939), 4–7.

Roy, A., Dimigen, G. and Taylor, M. (1998) The relationship between social networks and the employment of visually impaired college graduates. *Journal of Visual Impairment and Blindness*, **92** (7), pp. 423–32.

Royal National Institute for the Blind (1996) *Listening to Students: A Survey of the Views of Older Visually Impaired Students*, RNIB, London.

Scullion, P.A. (1995) Oliver asks for more: rejecting illness, neglecting impairment, explaining disability and controlling rehabilitation. *British Journal of Therapy and Rehabilitation*, **2** (10), 521–2.

Seedhouse, D. (1988) *Ethics: The Heart of Health Care*, John Wiley, Chichester, UK.

Stewart, W.F.R. (1981) An education for friendship and love . . . Social/personal relationships and the sight-impaired child. *Inter-Regional Review*, (69), Summer, 29–37.

Shakespeare, T. (1994) Cultural representations of disabled people: dustbins for disavowal? *Disability and Society*, **9** (3), 283–99.

Slee, R. (1993) The politics of integration – new sites for old practises? *Disability, Handicap and Society*, **8** (4), 351–60.

Swain, J., Finkelstein, V., French, S. and Oliver, M. (1993) *Disabling Barriers – Enabling Environments*, Sage, London.

Thomas, A. (1998) *Within Reason: Access to Services for Blind and Partially Sighted People*, RNIB, London.

Tobin, M.J. (1981) Psychological development in blind infants. Paper presented at the Meeting on the Problems of Visually Handicapped Infants, Milan, 22–23 February 1980, published in *Cecita Infantile*, Prevenzione, Terepia, Recupero e Inserimento, Provincia di Milano.

Tobin, M.J. (1983) Do blind children need special perceptual and cognitive training? *LBMRC Research Newsletter*, **8** (3), 5–11.

Tobin, M.J. (1987) Special and mainstream schooling: some teenagers' views. *New Beacon*, **71** (837), 3–6.

Tobin, M.J. (1988) Visually impaired teenagers: ambitions, attitudes and interests. *Journal of Visual Impairment and Blindness*, **82** (12), 414–6.

Tobin, M.J. and Hunter, B. (1974) Assessing the manual dexterity of the visually handicapped. *New Beacon*, **58** (687), 169–72.

Tobin, M.J. and Hill, E.W. (1989) The present and the future: concerns of visually impaired teenagers. *British Journal of Visual Impairment*, **7** (2), 55–7.

Tooze, D. (1978) Mobility education for totally blind children.

Division of Educational and Child Psychology, British Psychological Society, Leicester, UK, *Occasional Papers*, **2**, (2), 53–4.

Tooze, D. (1981) *Independence Training for Visually Handicapped Children*, Croom Helm, London.

Urwin, C. (1978) Early language development in blind children. Division of Educational and Child Psychology, British Psychological Society, Leicester, UK, *Occasional Papers*, **2** (2), 73–87.

Varma, V.P. (ed.) (1973) *Stresses in Children*, University of London Press, London.

Vaughan, E. (1991) The social basis of conflict between blind people and agents of rehabilitation. *Disability, Handicap and Society*, **6** (3), 203–217.

Verplanken, B., Meijnders, A. and van de Wege, A. (1994) Emotion and cognition: attitudes toward persons who are visually impaired. *Journal of Visual Impairment and Blindness*, **88** (11), 504–11.

Walker, E., Tobin, M.J. and McKennell, A.C. (1992) *Blind and Partially Sighted Children in Britain: the RNIB Survey*, **2**, Stationary Office, London.

Wesson, M.E. (1964) The ocular significance of abnormal head postures. *British Orthoptic Journal*, **21** (14), 14–28.

Wills, D.M. (1968) Problems of play and mastery in the blind child. *British Journal of Medical Psychology*, **41**, 213–22.

Wills, D.M. (1978) Entry into boarding school and after. Division of Educational and Child Psychology, British Psychological Society, Leicester, UK, *Occasional Papers*, **2** (2), 39–44.

Wills, D.M. (1978) Work with mothers of young blind children. Division of Educational and Child Psychology, British Psychological Society, Leicester, UK, *Occasional Papers*, **2** (2), 32–8.

Workers Educational Association (1997) *Visually Impaired Students and the Workers' Educational Association: A Survey Report*, RNIB, London.

5

Personal strategies

Definitions and preliminary remarks

Previous chapters have discussed some of the social and
environmental (primary) barriers that disable visually impaired
people, and have suggested ways in which society might begin to
dismantle some of those barriers. Consideration has also been given
to what have been described as secondary barriers: an individual's
unique reaction to those primary barriers (see Chapters 3 and 4).
Although the aim of this chapter is to consider some of the ways in
which each individual can best manage his or her own reactions and
increase personal empowerment by adopting techniques to
manipulate the external environment, such strategies must not be
regarded as the principal means by which problems associated with
environmental or curriculum access should be overcome. They are
not substitutes for inappropriate building design, inadequate strategic
planning or poor teaching practice and it is crucial that visually
impaired people are not made to feel responsible for what are,
incontrovertibly, the institution's duties. It is not uncommon for
disabled people to experience this kind of guilt and for this reaction
to be exploited by unscrupulous service providers and by society in
general. Such responses are an example of the secondary barriers
mentioned above.

Guilt is only one reaction to impairment. Many blind and partially
sighted people describe various psychological responses to specific

situations which can be classified as secondary barriers and which can, in themselves, be debilitating (see Chapter 4 and also Barnes, 1996). Experience suggests, however, that to acknowledge these issues is, in itself, empowering and enabling and represents a positive strategic approach to managing life situations. Since this book seeks to address some of the important issues relating to visual impairment in the context of post-school education, we believe that it is important to include a chapter that discusses some techniques that disabled people can use to enhance empowerment, even though the emphasis is, necessarily, on the individual. Traditionally – and interestingly – the term 'coping strategies' is often used to describe the entire range of such techniques (see for example, Dodds, 1993).

By way of introduction it is important to consider the implications of the term 'coping strategy'. Citing Filip, Aymanns and Braukmann (1986), Dodds (1993) identifies the problem that 'The term "coping" is one of whose use is unfortunately inversely related to its precision . . . and it has been used in a multiplicity of ways to refer to a wide range of phenomena.' Dodds considers that 'Psychologists have not contributed much to the practicalities of coping' since they have tended to focus on abstract processes. He believes that 'coping' must encompass a practical element:

> In essence, coping refers to the ability of the person to reduce the mismatch between the resources at his disposal and the demands made upon him. Coping with sight loss has to take place on the perceptual, the behavioural, the cognitive and the emotional levels, and these are closely inter-related to one another. (Dodds, 1993)

This definition, however, still retains a very 'medical' flavour since, whilst it seeks to identify the various levels on which 'coping' takes place, all the responsibility for 'adjustment' seems to fall to the individual, without mention of society's obligations. (See Dodds' (1993) analysis of the concepts of 'self-esteem', 'self-efficacy', 'locus of control', 'learned helplessness' and 'attributional style'.) Within the medical model it is axiomatic that an individual is expected to 'cope' with disability regardless of the cost to that person. Success is judged by criteria that presuppose that 'normality' is a desirable state:

everyone would, if they could, wish to attain it. Those who do not, therefore, must be irrational. Society's approval is granted to those disabled people who are considered to be rational and who demonstrate compliance with its established norms. Such people, as a consequence of socialization, may have never questioned the legitimacy of these tenets. Their wish for social acceptance leads them to develop a range of sophisticated 'coping strategies' that are judged to be most likely to achieve this objective.

The term 'strategy' is identified as the 'art of conducting a campaign and manoeuvring an army' (*Chambers English Dictionary*, 1988) and the 'skilful management of getting the better of an adversary or attaining an end' and 'the method of conducting operations especially by the aid of manoeuvring' (*Hamlyn Encyclopaedic World Dictionary*, 1976). The definition is illuminating when considered in the context of disability. Society may be perceived as the 'adversary'. As noted above, some disabled people choose a compliant approach with which to counter 'enemy' attacks whereas others engage in defensive manoeuvres which are often dismissed as 'aggressive'. Whatever the preferred approach, the personal consequences of this continual – and apparently endless – warfare can only be speculated upon and the rational choice, surely, would be to seek an end to the conflict. By acknowledging that, in certain situations and at variable personal cost, some of the effects of society's disabling barriers can be reduced, conditions conducive to 'peace talks' with the adversary may be created. This is a positive tactic and one that is most likely to effect significant change through mutual dialogue, negotiation and education. It is an assertive approach, demonstrating strength and flexibility: a willingness to consider matters from a variety of perspectives.

It is in this latter sense that the term 'strategy' is used here. Because the emphasis is on personal choice and initiation and not on the reactive need to 'cope', the term 'personal' replaces the term 'coping'. The fundamental premise is that everyone has the capacity to effect change and that it is helpful to cultivate a positive attitude towards one's ability to affect the environment and thus initiate and promote change within it. Belief in oneself necessarily predisposes towards a motivation to develop the problem-solving skills that are crucial in the devising of effective personal strategies.

A personal strategy may therefore be defined as the means by which a disabled person seeks to take some control over a given situation in order to be able to manage the environment, negative attitudes, and poor practice. It is a means of compensating for the lack of equal access to society. It is also, however, a means by which a person's own resources are utilized to make the most of any given situation.

Although the following personal strategies have been found to be useful, some may be considered to be inappropriate, ineffective or unacceptable to certain people and in some specific cases. That such strategies cannot be implemented without considerable personal cost to the individual should never be forgotten. The 'luxuries' that non-disabled people take for granted are invariably denied to visually impaired people. The time and energy spent in (often repeatedly) explaining the practical significance of a visual impairment or in negotiating improvements in curriculum access is time and energy that non-disabled students are able to devote to other things: undertaking academic course work or engaging in social activities, for example (see French, 1992; Barnes, 1996). It should not be assumed, either, that for each perceived issue there necessarily exists a personal strategy: a panacea waiting to be discovered and utilized. An exhaustive list does not exist. Most visually impaired people believe that the development of such mechanisms is an ongoing process, with familiar strategies being modified and replaced by new ones designed to meet the demands of changing personal and environmental circumstances. Predictably, a healthy debate concerning the choice of a particular strategy to meet a specific perceived need testifies to the range of choices available. There are, however, some strategies that have consistently proved to be effective in given situations and an analysis of the reasons for their success reveals the presence of common characteristics. This in turn suggests the existence of a set of underlying principles which need to be considered when devising personal strategies. The emphasis is, however, on flexibility. Experience suggests that to regard these underlying principles as 'golden rules' is unhelpful, since this approach ignores the individuality of each particular person and circumstance. Discussion with others is always to be recommended, especially when considering service provision. Visually impaired students are encouraged to engage in dialogue with college personnel who need to take account of such variables as history, age and learning style when considering personal strategies. For example, older people whose vision is deteriorating may lack self-confidence and ingenuity; adolescents whose vision has always been impaired may approach new situations with unguarded enthusiasm and naivety. Development and utilization of personal strategies become easier with practice: they are skills that improve with regular self-monitoring.

Maximum use of residual vision

It was suggested in Chapter 2 that the value of eyesight may be overestimated. Many routine tasks are performed without continual reliance upon vision, for example, ascending/descending familiar flights of stairs. Arguably, some procedures – such as cleaning kitchen surfaces – might be more successfully executed if a concern with touch supplemented visual input. This is not, however, to deny the importance of vision in the management of everyday situations, including the learning environment. In general, people whose sight is limited want to employ their residual vision to maximum effect and are keen to adopt techniques that are designed to enhance the visual input.

Strategies to maximize residual vision

(1) Understanding the nature of the visual impairment helps to identify specific visual difficulties associated with it. For example, the use of eye movements often helps people with restricted fields of vision by enabling them to ascertain where the field is clear.
(2) Photophobia can be counteracted by using a shield, visor or wearing a baseball-type (peaked) cap. Glasses with dark or tinted lenses, or prescription (often ultraviolet) filters can reduce glare. An alternative is to half close the eyes to reduce the amount of light entering them.

(3) If binocular focusing is impaired, closing one eye sometimes clears the image.

(4) Object fixation is improved if attempts are made to replace or supplement head movements with eye movements. Practising eye control and regular exercise of the ocular muscles is useful and is rarely taught specifically, or formally. It is helpful to remember that staring causes the image to go out of focus.

(5) If nystagmus is problematic, prisms may be used to improve comfort and visual acuity.

(6) Eccentric viewing: if a central visual loss causes reading difficulties, moving the eye below or perhaps to the right of the image may help to project the image on to an active part of the retina.

(7) Steady eye strategy: associated with the above strategy, it is helpful to keep the eye steady while moving the reading material across the newly established line of (eccentric) vision. This technique may be difficult, especially if the target is large, heavy or fixed in position (Royal National Institute for the Blind, undated). Considerable practice is required.

(8) Practising visual activities such as scanning, blinking and focusing on different objects is useful. As with the above, such exercises may not have been taught formally.

(9) Familiarization with the range of visual appliances and equipment, how they are used and the methods by which they can be obtained may dramatically enhance access to goods and services.

(10) Familiarization with specific reading techniques has been demonstrated to improve reading speed and information processing (Backman and Inde, 1979; Ighe, 1993).

(11) Being aware of postural issues and adopting a comfortable position before commencing a task that is visually demanding facilitates more effective and efficient use of residual vision.

(12) Utilizing lighting, colour, size, shape and contrast to meet personal preferences facilitates control over the environment.

(13) Utilizing Gestalt principles (see Chapter 2) improves identification of words, people and objects and enhances the speed of information processing.

Environmental strategies

(1) Experience suggests that most visually impaired people choose to use some form of appliance to facilitate the process of getting from one place to another. Familiarization with the range of equipment and services that enhance environmental access, and the means by which they may be obtained, facilitates an informed choice.

(2) Preparation for any event is recommended. For example, verbal, written and tactile information about a proposed journey enhances control and often improves efficiency.

(3) Reconnoitring unfamiliar places and noting landmarks well before requiring their use are techniques designed to reduce the stress levels associated with travel.

(4) The point at which visually impaired people seek assistance from friends, colleagues or members of the general public varies considerably. Strategies that combine self-reliance with support from others facilitate choice.

(5) Observing, where possible and appropriate, the behaviour of other individuals helps to ascertain routes, terrain and procedures. This includes listening for auditory clues as to the location of specific buildings, escalators, and other significant landmarks.

(6) Proceeding with care and deliberation in unfamiliar situations, maintaining concentration at all times to avoid accidents.

(7) Provided due care is taken, shadowing other individuals who are proceeding in a particular direction towards a required destination can be helpful. It is important, however, to be aware of the potential dangers of following others, for example, when crossing roads.

(8) Requesting and/or obtaining physical positions of advantage in all circumstances. Individual requirements will vary, but a choice should be made with the objective of maximizing sensory input. For example, selecting appropriate positions on public transport, in restaurants, in meetings and lecture theatres.

(9) Identifying places by learning their particular characteristics in terms of layout, shape, architectural features, light sources, etc. facilitates general orientation.

(10) Deliberately taking time when entering environments – including new places – to assimilate information. The visual scanning undertaken by sighted individuals as part of the process of assimilating new visual information is a technique that is often unavailable to visually impaired people.

(11) Utilizing Gestalt principles facilitates recognition and information processing (see Chapter 2), for example, identification of a bus number at a distance far greater than that at which the number could be seen clearly.

(12) Memorizing information relating to the characteristics of people and the environment facilitates future identification. Footsteps, perfume and voice are often distinguishing features of individuals, and floor texture, ambient sounds, and spatial characteristics help to differentiate environments. It is useful to acquire as much information as possible from whatever source.

Sensory strategies

Utilizing input from all other senses compensates considerably for visual impairment. Such sense data are often ignored and it is helpful to learn to attend to them. All the remaining senses can be exploited effectively. The redirection and selection of attention comprises a skill that may require specific teaching. This should occur as part of a visually impaired child's educational process; in an adult, it is recommended that these skills are taught as soon as possible after deterioration in vision has been identified. Continual encouragement to practise, including feedback, should be given. It is equally important not to destroy concentration by permitting sensory 'overload' from one of the remaining senses. For example, the use of a personal stereo when travelling could act as a distracter.

(1) Sound

Sound may be divided into two categories: (a) ambient and (b) self-generated.

(a) Ambient sound

Existing sound can be utilized by identifying:

(i)   the direction of the sound source
(ii) the approximate distance between oneself and the sound source
(iii) the identity of the sound source

Dodds (1988) describes a further way in which the environment can be acoustically structured: 'sound shadowing'. When a large object is situated between the traveller and the sound source, its identity is revealed by virtue of the fact that it modifies the sounds of approaching sound sources. (The presence of a bus shelter is detected by shadowing the sounds of oncoming traffic.)

(b) Self-generated sound

Many visually impaired travellers deliberately utilize self-generated sound and learn which sounds provide the most useful acoustic information. In contrast to ambient sounds, those that are self-generated provide a relatively reliable source of sensory information. It is possible to develop a keen sense of obstacle awareness through 'echo-location', a technique that serves to increase the visually impaired traveller's preview of the immediate environment (Dodds, 1988). Dodds describes echo-location as a phenomenon whereby the brain picks up 'differences in the time a self-generated sound leaves the traveller and the time at which it arrives back at his ears'.

Sound signatures

Dodds (1988) further describes the nature of 'sound signatures' and states that many visually impaired people utilize these unique characteristics of sound to identify aspects of their environment. Sound emanating from, for example, the soles of the shoes, is structured in a similar manner to visual information and it is possible to develop this skill with practice. Sound waves are, however, less specific than light waves.

(i)   Developing active listening skills generally assists negotiating the environment. The capacity to pay attention to sound, from whatever source, and to interpret and understand its significance is crucial.

(ii) Identifying and locating extraneous sounds facilitates orientation in an unfamiliar environment. These sounds also act as sources of information relating to the occurrence of events too distant to be identified visually.

(iii) Some visually impaired people have found various sonic appliances to be helpful in certain contexts. Familiarization with the range of products available will facilitate choice. These devices are under constant development.

(iv) Regular use of a cassette tape-recorder, pocket memo or computerized note-taker with synthetic speech can be a helpful memory aid. Examples of use include: talking maps, personal notes, general information.

(2) Touch

(a)   The use of tactile input in identifying ground surfaces can usefully supplement sonic input. For example, identifying different ground textures using sensory input from the soles of the feet facilitates orientation. These differences can be valuable landmarks in both the internal and the external environments.

(b)   Reduction of sensory input by wearing thick rubber or platform-type soles or other thick-soled shoes or boots may cause problems because these impair sensory input and can disturb balance. Any uncomfortable footwear acts as a distracter to concentration because it offers too much tactile input.

(c)   Orientation can be increased by utilizing the known positions of the sun and air currents in buildings. Sensitivity to the movements of those who are acting as guides and increased sensitivity to the movements of others facilitates getting about in a large crowd.

(d) For some young, elderly and newly visually impaired people, manual contact with objects and items along routes, such as walls and bannisters, induces security. Although such strategies are often vigorously discouraged in many educational and vocational institutions for visually impaired people, the needs of the individual will always be the criterion by which the choice of strategy is made.

(e) Touch can be utilized for object identification. Additionally, learning any tactile communication method, such as the Moon or Braille system, enhances communication potential and may be invaluable if sight is reduced to the extent that communication by touch is the only alternative to sound. The increasing availability of raised maps and diagrams has proved invaluable. They represent useful learning tools in a wide range of academic and vocational subjects. They are helpful in facilitating orientation and mobility and in enhancing the visually impaired traveller's 'cognitive map' of a route (Dodds, 1988).

(f) Using an appropriate appliance, a long (white) cane for example, is often a crucial factor in gaining access to the environment (see Dodds, 1988). Interpretation of tactile information from the cane's tip is the underlying principle here.

(3) Smell

Utilizing the sense of smell can help to identify objects and places. Learning the significance of different smells facilitates orientation in both external and internal environments. 'British Rail travellers hoping to reach Euston at least know where they are when they grind to a halt alongside the McVitie's factory!' (Disabled Living Foundation, 1991).

(4) Taste

Developing the sense of taste helps to improve skill in ascertaining the quality of food and drink.

Psychological strategies

These are strategies designed to enhance a person's general psychological safety and security. They are valuable in reducing anxiety and stress levels thereby removing some of the emotional distractions that may arise during the course of everyday experiences. Some emotional energy may still be expended in worrying about the outcome of events, but this should be less disabling. The aim is to channel this energy into the positive management of the immediate situation so that a successful outcome of events is much more likely. As Dodds (1988) suggests, control over the environment can be exerted.

(1) Although debate continues, it is believed by many visually impaired people that 'being open about impairment is the only way to deal with the experience of disability' – but it is acknowledged that in the present climate this strategy is not easy (Barnes, 1996). Experience suggests that it is helpful to inform peers and educational staff of the existence of a visual impairment. The impairment may or may not be obvious but, with specific reference to partially sighted individuals, Morse, (1989) cites research conducted by Glass (1970) which led him to recommend 'that low vision persons develop skills in communicating experiences with significant others. In all cases, however, it seems sensible and helpful to attempt to describe, briefly, the particular impairment and its significance.'

(2) Anticipating the nature of situations facilitates the development of appropriate personal strategies in advance.

(3) Asking others to address everyone by name facilitates general communication. Use of eye language often obviates the necessity to identify participants in a one-to-one or group discussion by name, but, if such cues are missed, visually impaired people are placed in an embarrassing and disadvantageous position. Generally, everyone should be encouraged to use names; visually impaired people are usually concerned to learn and use the names of those with whom they come into contact.

(4) Avoiding potentially difficult situations in which visual impairment becomes the centre of other people's attention and interest reduces embarrassment. For example, some people might consider it to be more appropriate to choose a restaurant with 'at table' service rather than to battle with a self-service system. This has the added advantage that requests can be made for the menu to be read and, if necessary, for specific dishes to be described. Some visually impaired people prefer the food to be cut before it is served and this request can be made to the person waiting at table.

(5) Arranging meetings where possible, in specified, easily identifiable, or familiar, places reduces anxiety. To be in control of such organizational matters is preferable than to be at the mercy of someone else's choice. Arriving early for appointments, either with an individual or with a group of people, alleviates the fear of being unable to recognize them. Alternatively, it may be useful to remain in a predetermined place and ask others to meet there.

(6) Attempting to secure a position of physical advantage by arriving early for group meetings facilitates choice of a seat in an advantageous position – for example, if residual vision is to be maximized and put to effective use in optimum lighting conditions. Some visually impaired people prefer to sit by a door so that manoeuvring about the room is easier after the meeting. Arriving early also facilitates the identification of other participants: it is not helpful to be confronted by crowds of unknown – or even familiar – people.

(7) It helps to be polite but firm with members of the public from whom instructions or directions are being sought. The variety of responses to requests for assistance can vary, reactions including apparently aimless gesticulation, referring the visually impaired traveller to a distant information board or screen, or rushing to find the nearest wheelchair! It is recommended that offers of genuine help should always be accepted. If inappropriate assistance is offered, it behoves the visually impaired person to exercise diplomacy in specifying precisely the kind of help required. The public cannot be expected to understand the

nature and practical significance of a particular visual impairment unless they receive the opportunity to learn. This does not mean, however, that the rights of visually impaired people should be infringed and this point should be diplomatically made. For example, it is commendable that Gatwick Airport provides a Special Assistance desk for the benefit of all disabled travellers, but it is not acceptable when, for their own convenience, staff choose to take a route to the aircraft that by-passes the duty-free area (Disabled Living Foundation, 1991).

(8) Adopting an equally forthright approach when being asked to join a gathering, for example, in a pub, is also empowering. It can be extremely difficult to identify a specific group of people, especially in a crowded and/or dimly lit room, and matters are simplified by asking one of the group members to act as escort to avoid the potential embarrassment of joining the wrong group. Alternatively, some partially sighted people may find it possible to follow one of the group members visually towards the rest of the group. This identifies its precise location, which can then be remembered.

(9) When joining a community for the first time (for example, when entering college), it can be worthwhile to make an effort to enrol in particular interest groups. This guarantees meeting others with similar interests, which provides a good topic for conversation and a foundation for potential friendship.

(10) Habitually using amenities such as toilets when they are available before embarking on unfamiliar journeys is a rational way to avoid unnecessary anxiety and discomfort. There is nothing worse than being unable to locate such facilities when they are required.

(11) It is advisable to anticipate items that are likely to be needed before undertaking an unfamiliar journey. This avoids the possible difficulty of having to locate appropriate shops in an unfamiliar environment.

(12) Clearly identifying personal belongings such as luggage facilitates its retrieval, following air travel for example. Most cases look identical or disconcertingly similar as they revolve

relentlessly on the carousel and much time and anxiety can be saved by attaching a brightly coloured or distinctively shaped label or some strapping to personal luggage. This technique is useful even when assistance is sought in retrieving such items.

Cognitive strategies

(1) Being willing to learn new behaviours prepares a visually impaired person for the life-long requirement of flexibility and adaptability. The ability to develop these characteristics facilitates mobility and promotes independence. This is associated with being able, selectively, to switch attention from one stimulus to another at will so that only relevant stimuli are processed.

(2) There are many advantages to the cultivation of good problem-solving skills, especially given the sensory deficit that visually impaired people experience. Such skills are useful in the educational context as well as in many aspects of domestic, social and personal life.

(3) Learning is associated with the development of short-term and long-term memory, which is facilitated by the 'rehearsal' and 'chunking' of information (Dodds, 1988).

(4) The process of note taking is facilitated if skills are developed which capitalize on the memory's natural tendency to organize, store and retrieve information in categories (Buzan, 1982).

(5) With specific reference to education and employment, the development of efficient note taking skills is part of good time management.

(6) Gestalt principles may be utilized by developing pictorial or diagrammatic representations of information.

(7) Where appropriate, a portable computerized note-taker, pocket memo or small cassette tape-recorder can be used to store short items of information such as notes, messages, addresses, telephone numbers and shopping lists.

(8) If seminar presentations are to be given, advance preparation is recommended, especially in relation to memorizing the material to be presented. It is also helpful to anticipate additional issues

that might arise in relation to vision as well as others relating to the organization and delivery of the material.

(9) If interviews are to be attended, advance preparation is also recommended in relation to personal presentation, journey plans, and anticipation of interview content, especially where this might relate to disability issues. This is particularly important for appointments that may be stressful, for example, those dealing with health, education or employment.

General strategies

Many of the strategies described above come together under this heading in the following general ways.

(1) Be well informed of the range of goods and services available to visually impaired people and how these may be accessed. Knowledge of and ability to utilize the system will increase life choices and promote autonomy.

(2) Select equipment/appliances/adaptations that actually serve the purpose for which they were intended and whose controls are simple to operate without undue reliance on sight.

(3) Label all personal items with easily identifiable tags to facilitate identification and retrieval.

(4) Keep items of similar generic nature in different containers. For example, pills could be stored in containers of different sizes or shapes. The risk of unnecessary and potentially serious accidents should thus be reduced.

(5) Develop and memorize a safe storage plan for domestic and personal items and maintain a tidy and well-ordered environment in which items are easily located and retrievable.

(6) Developing the capacity of memory is generally useful. It may be helpful to keep to familiar routes. This does not imply, however, that exploration of new ones should not be undertaken; rather, such exploration should be postponed until times when there is no urgency to use a particular route or routine.

(7) Counting and memorizing steps, doorways and turnings on routes, as long as caution is exercised, will help to increase safety and assist mobility and independence.

(8) In all contexts, be conscious of the importance of regulations relating to health, safety and welfare. As a routine, familiarization with the locations of fire exits, escape routes and evacuation procedures is crucial, as is acquaintance with any modifications of standard procedures which may apply to disabled people.

(9) Develop the powers of concentration and memory. Tasks that originally appeared tedious and difficult will, eventually, become automatic.

(10) Adopting a logical, methodical approach to all tasks promotes efficiency. This will result in developing and memorizing a safe storage plan for personal, domestic and other items.

Experience suggests that techniques to improve levels of assertiveness are particularly helpful in developing effective personal strategies. Being assertive – and not passive or aggressive – is empowering because it enables people to get what they want from situations. Books and courses on assertiveness training are widely available; some counsellors also provide individual assertiveness training sessions. It is important to emphasize that the development of personal strategies requires commitment: practice is better than avoidance. Difficult tasks will always remain difficult unless they are practised.

References

Barnes, C. (1996) Visual impairment and disability, in *Beyond Disability: Towards an Enabling Society* (ed. G. Hales), Sage, Thousand Oaks, CA, 36–44.

Backman, O. and Inde, K. (1979) *Low Vision Training*, LiberHermods, Malmo.

Buzan, T. (1982) *Use Your Head*, British Broadcasting Corporation, London.

Chambers English Dictionary (1988) W. & R. Chambers, Cambridge and Edinburgh.

Disabled Living Foundation (1991) *Visual Handicap: A Distance Learning Pack for Physiotherapists, Occupational Therapists and Other Health Care Professionals*, DLF, London.

Dodds, A. (1988) *Mobility Training for Visually Handicapped People: A Person-Centred Approach*, Croom Helm, London and Sydney.

Dodds, A. (1993) *Rehabilitating Blind and Visually Impaired People: A Psychological Approach*, Chapman & Hall, London.

Filip, S.H., Aymanns, P. and Braukmann, W. (1986) Coping with life events: when the self comes into play, in *Self-Related Cognitions in Anxiety and Motivation* (ed. R. Schwarzer), Lawrence Eribaum Associates, Hillsdale, NJ.

French, S. (1992) Equal opportunities? The problem of time. *New Beacon*, **76** (896) 97–8.

Glass, E.J. (1970) A working paper on pyscho-social responses to low vision, in *Proceedings of the Low Vision Conference, San Francisco* (ed. L. Apple).

Hamlyn Encyclopaedic World Dictionary (1976) Hamlyn, Feltham, UK.

Ighe, S. (1993) *What You See and What You Do Not See: Information and Assessment Material for People with Low Vision*, Siv Ighe, Atherstone, Warwickshire.

Morse, J.L. (1989) Psychosocial aspects of low vision, in *Understanding Low Vision*, 2nd edn (ed. R.T. Jose), American Foundation for the Blind, New York, pp. 43–54.

Royal National Institute for the Blind (undated) *Low Vision Training Pack*, RNIB, London.

Throughout this book, emphasis has been placed on the fact that a registered 'blind' person may possess some residual vision. In the UK, less than 5% of 'blind' people have no perception of light. Of the remaining 95%, almost all can orientate themselves to some extent using residual vision. Two points emerge from this information (Cullinan, 1986):

- what the individual is able to 'see';
- what use s/he makes of this vision, that is, how functional it is.

These points were discussed in Chapter 2.

It follows that a large percentage of visually impaired students in further and higher education will have some level of functional vision. The intention here is to discuss general principles associated with improvement of vision which will hopefully be of value to a wide range of students affected by a variety of eye conditions. At the same time, however, it is important to remember the potential danger of making generalizations concerning the requirements of these students. Ultimately the emphasis is on the individual and it is essential to adopt an open minded and flexible approach. Consequently it is strongly recommended that the student be consulted in each instance.

Students will have varying levels of understanding of the nature of their visual impairment and so will require different degrees of guidance from relevant practitioners in order to be prepared to make informed choices with regard to low vision equipment.

Low vision assessment

Some students may already have undergone a low vision assessment before commencing an educational programme. If so, they will probably be in possession of any low vision equipment required for everyday use, and possibly for their chosen study methods. This may not be the case, however, and a student might consider that some input from an assessment of functional vision would be helpful in deciding on appropriate low vision equipment, particularly in relation to the course being undertaken. It is also important to note that this assessment may be required as part of the application process for the Disabled Student's Allowance in higher education. The following information is intended to give an overview of the steps required to obtain and access the assessment, as well as some indication of what might be involved in the actual procedure.

It is important to realize that the provision of low vision services varies from area to area. Undoubtedly there are centres of good practice, but these are not available everywhere. The following material should at least inform students and staff in further and higher education of the provision that it is possible to access and so encourage a questioning approach if local services appear to fall short of this standard.

It is unlikely that a visually impaired student has arrived at the stage of undertaking tertiary education without having visited an optometrist (optician). Within the National Health Service (NHS) system, however, it is necessary to be referred to a consultant ophthalmologist in order to organize a low vision assessment. This referral can be provided either by the optometrist or by a GP. If the student is currently a patient of an ophthalmologist, it may be possible to request an appointment directly via the secretary.

A visit to the optometrist for an eye examination could prove to be useful. It is possible for some degrees of reduced vision to be corrected adequately by the use of spectacles, contact lenses or, for those already in possession of such items, a straightforward change in prescription. This would preclude the need to take the matter further. If this were not the case, however, referral to an eye clinic or hospital should be the next step offered. (With regard to cost, registered blind or partially sighted clients are entitled to a free NHS sight test and full time students under 19 years of age qualify for vouchers towards the cost of any necessary spectacles.) Once the student has been seen by the ophthalmologist, a referral can be made for the assessment for low vision equipment, which can be carried out in the hospital low vision clinic, at private opticians or in specialist low vision clinics, depending on local availability.

Some low vision equipment is available on prescription through the Hospital Eye Service. This system is free and the equipment is provided on a loan basis. Closed circuit televisions (CCTVs) are not normally included in this system. CCTVs can be used to produce magnified images of pictures, text and solid objects on a television monitor. More information can be found in Chapter 8.) If equipment is not provided through this channel, it can be purchased from some high street opticians and specialist outlets.

If for any reason, a person seeking a low vision assessment experiences any difficulties in obtaining a referral, it may be helpful to contact a specialist worker for visually impaired clients (known as a Rehabilitation Worker or Rehabilitation Officer). The local Social Services department or voluntary associations for visually impaired people usually employ these workers. They have an understanding of low vision issues and can help in obtaining appropriate referrals. If the choice is made to seek a low vision assessment without going through the referral system (that is, by attending a private optician), it is important to realize that the student may then be liable for all costs incurred, including those for any equipment (Royal National Institute for the Blind, undated).

Assessment procedure

Initial interview

The person carrying out the assessment should introduce him/herself and explain the purpose and the content of the assessment. Legally, records need to be kept for this type of procedure, and so certain information will be asked for, as follows (adapted from Royal National Institute for the Blind, undated):

- general details such as name and address, etc;
- eye condition (right and left);
- details of doctors, opticians or rehabilitation workers seen, dates of appointments or previous assessments, dates of any previous eye surgery, etc. as relevant;
- medical and functional history of vision;
- spectacles and other low vision equipment already in use;
- visual ability (near, distance, fields);
- lighting – this should include questions relating to good/poor lighting conditions for that particular person, both indoors and outdoors, as well as lighting for specific tasks;
- mobility – questions here relate to any mobility equipment currently used, such as a cane or guide dog;
- main difficulties – this item should be explored carefully and led by the visually impaired person (rather than all the suggestions being made by the interviewer);
- any other important points or comments;
- *agreed* action plan.

The above information gives a general indication of the areas that may be covered, but this will vary according to local procedures.

Once the interview has been concluded, the assessment itself should take place and this will include a number of areas.

Visual acuity

This involves testing for sharpness and clarity of vision. It is important that measurements are taken for both distance and near vision purposes. Questions should be asked about any low vision equipment used at present and how they help in defining objects at a distance.

An example of a test that can be used for this is the Snellen test chart (see Figure 6.1). This should be familiar to everyone, as these charts can be seen in any optician's clinic. Each row of letters on the chart represents a calculated distance at which the letters should be recognized with unimpaired vision, for example, the top letter should

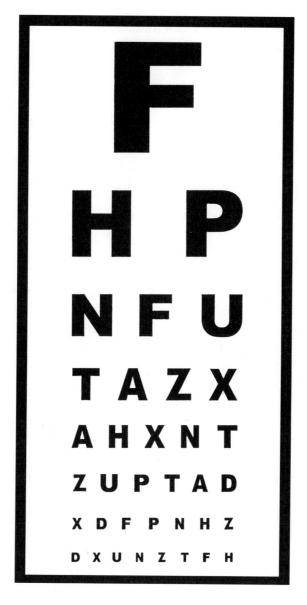

Figure 6.1 Scaled-down Snellen card for use at 10 feet (3 metres).

be seen clearly by someone with full vision standing at a distance of 60 metres (the subsequent rows should be seen at 36, 24, 18, 12, 6, 5 and 4 metres respectively).

The client is positioned at a calculated distance from the chart and is asked to read the letters, starting at the top and working down until it is impossible to read any further. Vision is recorded in the following way. The first number is 6 to represent 6 metres from the chart and, if the person tested could read only as far as the row of letters designed to be read at 18 metres, the vision would be recorded as 6/18 (average unimpaired vision is 6/6). This means that the person can see at 6 metres that which a person with average unimpaired vision can see at 18 metres.

If problems are encountered with glare or reflection, the lighting conditions may be altered or tinted spectacles may be offered.

Peripheral field testing

There are a number of factors that can indicate that a person has a field restriction, including: body posture, angle at which the head is held, changes in position of the head while in a viewing situation, mistakes in detecting words or letters, and difficulties in recognizing contours and shapes. Factors such as these relate to both peripheral and central restrictions.

These could have implications for a student on an educational programme ranging from aches and pains due to adoption of particular postures to difficulties in accessing print. The student may also have difficulty in seeing everything that is going on in the classroom or could have problems participating in activities such as sport.

The 'confrontation' method allows the assessor to obtain a rough peripheral field assessment without the use of expensive equipment. The assessor sits facing the client at a distance of 1 metre. The client is asked to cover one eye and to fix his/her gaze on the assessor's nose or eye. An object, such as a baton or pen light, is held approximately halfway between the client and the assessor to ensure that it can be seen. It is then moved from peripheral positions (12, 3, 6 and 9 o'clock) gradually towards the centre and the client is asked to indicate when it can be detected. Both eyes are tested in this way. A larger number of starting positions may be used if required (Carter, 1983; Royal National Institute for the Blind, undated).

Near reading vision

This is a test performed to ascertain how well someone can access information through print. Questions may be asked regarding how much reading the student undertakes currently in relation to how much has been undertaken in the past. It would also be useful to know how much the student may need or would like to undertake in the future. The student's preferred medium should also be noted. It is important that a record is made of any low vision equipment used at present and how much it facilitates reading, if at all. It is also relevant for enquiries to be made about any problems with glare or reflection and how these are usually resolved, if at all.

The test is then undertaken. Text in a range of type sizes on a standard card is shown to the client and s/he is asked to find the one that can be read with comfort. This should be recorded. The client is then asked to read a few words out loud. The procedure is repeated with gradually decreasing print sizes until the smallest working size is reached. The acuity of close vision is expressed as the smallest size of type that can be read in the normal reading posture of 30–45 cm from the eyes to the reading material (Disabled Living Foundation, 1991). The test may then be carried out again under different lighting conditions to ascertain the optimum lighting for that person for accessing text. If a client has difficulty in reading print, this may indicate a loss in the central field of vision.

The type used on the card in this test is described by printers as 'points' – for example 12 point, 14 point, 16 point – the system being based on the Times roman typeface, for which the abbreviation N is used (see Figure 6.2; Ford and Heshel, 1995). A description of N/point sizes can be seen in Table 6.1.

Lighting

Lighting is discussed in Chapters 7, 9 and 10 with regard to the environment, widening participation and accessing the curriculum, but it is also an area that needs to be considered in a low vision assessment. Even if low vision equipment is used, the lighting in a particular situation could cause difficulties. The assessment should

Table 6.1   Description of N/point sizes

N72 print or 72 point = 1 line only within one vertical inch of text
N48 print or 48 point = 1 1/2 lines of print within one vertical inch
N36 print or 36 point = 2 lines of print within one vertical inch
N24 print or 24 point = 3 lines of print within one vertical inch
N18 print or 18 point = 4 lines of print within one vertical inch
N12 print or 12 point = 6 lines of print within one vertical inch
N8 print or 8 point = 9 lines of print within one vertical inch

ascertain the level of natural light preferred by the client and what situations cause difficulties – such as bright sunlight, low light levels and night-time conditions.

Lighting is a key factor in the use of residual vision: too much or too little will restrict visual acuity and reduce function. This is particularly relevant when undertaking close work, which is very relevant to a student about to commence an educational programme.

The 'lux' is an international unit of illumination. Close work requires from 250 to 1000 lux, depending on the fineness of the work involved. In daylight this level of lighting should not be a problem; near a clean window, the light ranges from 1000 to 2000 lux. Activities taking place at a distance from the window, however, may need artificial lighting to augment the level of illumination.

In artificial light, fine work or continuous reading may require a reading lamp as well as the usual ceiling or wall lights. It is useful to keep the room lights on however, as this reduces the marked contrast between the bright light on the work and a dark background, which can be fatiguing for the eye muscles.

The lighting assessment is a fairly simple procedure. It is essential that the assessor ascertains what tasks the client needs to carry out; for example, for a student this would include reading text and producing written work. An area is prepared with appropriate materials and the client is seated comfortably with available lighting falling on the surface or task. The light should not cast the person's shadow across the task. Using a lamp, the client is asked to adjust the position and brightness to suit personal requirements. The task should then be performed for a short time and a light meter used to measure the light falling on it. This should be carried out while the client is in the position required to execute the activity. Changes can then be made in the position and intensity of the light to ascertain whether functional vision can be improved. Intensity can be changed by using a dimmer switch or by altering the distance of the lamp from the surface. The latter method makes use of the inverse square law: halving the distance of the light source from the surface increases the intensity fourfold (see Figure 6.3). Different lamps may also be tried with varying types and colours of bulbs. Visually impaired students often need to get very close to the light source while working, and so 'cool wall' lamps are often recommended to decrease the risk of burns. These lamps incorporate fluorescent tubes and are available from many shops and office suppliers. Constant feedback from the client is essential for the assessment procedure to be effective.

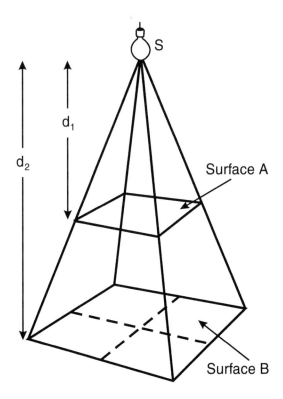

Figure 6.3 The inverse square law.

It is generally accepted that many people with a visual impairment require 50–100% more light than those with unimpaired vision (although in some cases more subdued lighting is preferred). With the increase in numbers of older learners it is also pertinent to note that, on average, twice as much light is required at 60 years of age as is needed at 40 years (Royal National Institute for the Blind, undated).

Selection and demonstration of low vision equipment

Following the assessment, the assessor and client should have the opportunity to decide on the most appropriate low vision equipment for the particular person and his or her circumstances. The most important factor on which to base any decisions are the specific uses to which the individual wants to be able to apply her or his available residual vision.

Equipment should then be selected and demonstrated. The client must be given the opportunity to try a range of equipment and to practise with it. The reading matter used should be representative of that which the client will be accessing using the equipment. It is important to note that some equipment used to improve access to print cannot comfortably be employed for great lengths of time, for example, portable CCTVs such as the EezeReader. With this in mind, a record should be made of how long the client is able to spend reading using this method, and whether it has, in fact, extended the pre-assessment comfortable reading time.

Low vision equipment

Spectacles

If spectacles are prescribed for a user with a visual impairment, it is important that s/he understand the reason for and purpose of the prescription, for example, whether it is for near distance or distance vision. Indeed many people will require separate pairs of spectacles for each of these purposes and contrasting frame design and/or colour helps to differentiate them.

Glass lenses are superior in terms of image clarity. Plastic lenses are, however, very robust and lighter. Whatever their composition, spectacles should always feel comfortable and fit well. Slight problems with fit can effectively alter the intended prescription of the lenses and can cause visual discomfort. Tilting of the frames or frames that are very loose and consequently slip down the nose can be very irritating.

Good spectacle care is essential. A case is usually supplied and it should be used for storage purposes to avoid scratching (especially of plastic lenses) and chipping. If not kept in the case, it is unwise to place the spectacles – lens down – on any surface, even temporarily, as they can be easily damaged. An efficient temporary measure is to keep the glasses around the neck; chains and cords designed specifically for this purpose are commonly available from high street opticians. This also helps people to avoid the problem of being unable to see where they have left their glasses.

Although probably rather obvious, it is worth mentioning that to gain maximum advantage from spectacles, the lenses should be kept clean at all times. Warm water with the addition of ordinary detergent is adequate for the purpose and a soft polishing cloth is provided with spectacle cases. It is also possible to purchase microfibre cloths from opticians that are very effective for polishing lenses between washes.

Contact lenses

One of the many disadvantages of high-powered spectacle lenses is the alteration of image size, although users' vision does adapt to this. If someone has a uniocular problem, contact lenses may provide an effective solution. In some conditions (keratoconus, aphakia – see Appendix B), correction of visual acuity by contact lenses is better than that by spectacle lenses. Contact lenses give the wearer an increase in the peripheral visual field, which may be obstructed by spectacle frames. This can be an advantage in general mobility as well as in sporting and recreational activities. Furthermore, many individuals choose contact lenses as they are perceived to be aesthetically more acceptable than spectacles.

Increasingly all lenses are being made out of plastics that are gas permeable. The older 'hard' lenses were impermeable to gases and so tended to cause a lack of oxygen to the cornea that resulted in blurred vision and the appearance of haloes around lights. The newer hydrophilic 'soft' lenses are much more comfortable to wear and cause less inflammation. Some people, however, are unable to tolerate even these.

Soft lenses, although preferable due to their gas and liquid permeability, have the disadvantage of absorbing and retaining bacteria, thus increasing the risk of infection, although prescription of antibiotic drops can help to combat this problem. These lenses also attract and retain protein particles, causing the surface to become cloudy. They are relatively fragile and may tear, dehydrate or quickly discolour for no apparent reason. Discomfort after 3–4 hours' wear, due to dehydration, can be relieved by regular use of drops. It is now possible to obtain disposable lenses that are discarded after a week or even a day, which may help to alleviate some of the above problems. It is possible, however, that these would not be suitable for use by people with some types of eye condition.

Whatever type of lens is chosen, scrupulous attention to hygiene is required at all times to avoid infection. Cleansing methods and routines vary, but adherence to the instructions should avoid problems. As with spectacles, contact lenses should be stored appropriately and care taken to ensure that right and left lenses are correctly inserted into their respective containers to avoid later confusion. Regular check-ups at a contact lens clinic are essential to ensure that the prescription remains correct.

Optical low vision equipment

These can be defined as 'optical appliances which augment reduced visual acuity *after* correction with conventional spectacles' (Disabled Living Foundation, 1991, emphasis added). Users include those whose vision is impaired and who are unable to obtain acceptable visual acuity with standard equipment (that is spectacles or contact lenses). Such people may or may not have a field loss. Optical appliances of this kind range from simple to sophisticated: the former are generally readily available; the latter require an appropriate practitioner's prescription.

After a low vision assessment, the following points should be considered when recommending optical low vision appliances (Disabled Living Foundation, 1991):

- No appliance replaces lost sight.
- The power of scanning print is lost: reading is word by word or letter by letter.
- They are job specific: different tasks require different appliances.
- As the magnification of the lens increases, the diameter decreases, hence a magnifier to cover the whole page in a book is likely to have very low magnification.
- The distance of the magnifier from the object varies with its power: the more powerful the magnifier the closer it must be held to the object to be viewed.
- Low-powered magnifiers can be moved a certain amount and will still retain maximum magnification, but with high powered ones this is not possible as focus is critical.
- The field of view of a magnifier can be increased by moving the eye closer to the lens without sacrificing maximum magnification.

Simple hand magnifiers (see Figure 6.4)

These are readily available from high street outlets. One of the disadvantages is that the user needs a steady hand. It may be impractical for a student to use one of these for protracted periods of study as holding the magnifier can be very tiring, so causing distraction. Cheaper versions also tend to cause distortion at the periphery of the image. More expensive versions are designed to reduce or eliminate this problem.

Stand magnifiers

Fixed focus. The magnifying lens is fitted into the stand at a specific height that places it within its focal length, so reducing possible distortion (see Figure 6.5). The stand is designed to remain in contact with the page and so is relatively stable. Some of these

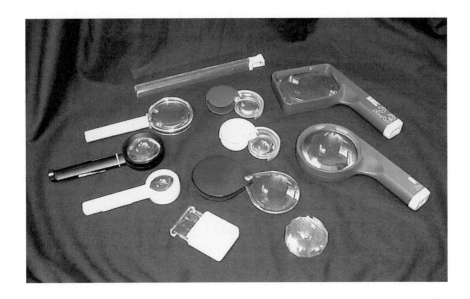

Figure 6.4 Hand magnifiers.

magnifiers incorporate illumination, whereas others require external lighting such as an angle poise lamp, the positioning of which needs to be carefully considered (see earlier under Lighting). Bringing the eye closer to the lens can increase the field of view.

Variable focus. Here the lens is fitted into an adjustable stand, so providing more flexibility for the user. This type of magnifier was originally designed for workers in industry who required augmented vision to undertake fine tasks. Some can be suspended around the neck for convenience. In general, the levels of magnification obtained from these appliances are fairly low, but their use is often facilitated by in-built illumination.

Spectacle magnifiers/microscopes and telescopes

This type of equipment is usually available only on prescription although some varieties can be purchased from specialist photographic dealers.

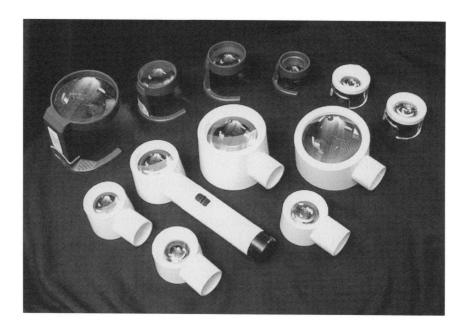

Figure 6.5 Stand magnifiers.

Spectacle magnifiers/microscopes. This simple form of microscope consists of thick, convex, high powered reading lenses. The magnifiers can be single focus or bifocal and their appearance resembles that of standard spectacles. Their advantage over standard spectacles and stand magnifiers is that they provide the user with a wider field of vision. They are most valuable if long periods of reading are required but the working distance is short (that is, the student would have to bring the text very close to the eyes), especially in the high powered models. Binocular vision is possible only with low magnification, which could be a disadvantage if a great deal of study is to be undertaken.

Telescopes. These are the only type of distance appliance available and can be monocular or binocular. It is possible to obtain models that are spectacle mounted or that clip on to spectacle frames. Other models are hand-held monoculars that can be attached to a ring to be slipped over a finger, and binocular telescopes with a neck cord. Telescopes for near vision (for reading), intermediate vision (for typing or reading music) and distance vision (for looking at black/white boards, overhead projections, etc.) are available. They may be prescribed as separate appliances or, in the case of some distance models, the lens can be focused to the required distance. Some have the option of adding auxiliary lenses on to the base unit. Binocular vision is obtainable at lower magnification.

The principle disadvantage of these pieces of equipment is that they are unsuitable for constant use when moving around. They disturb the user's perception by altering spatial relationships between objects as well as reducing the peripheral visual field so that a 'tunnel vision' effect is experienced. All telescopes are relatively heavy and may cause discomfort if used over long periods. They are also expensive. Many people consider appliances of this type to be aesthetically unacceptable and feel conspicuous when using them (Disabled Living Foundation, 1991).

Light-related equipment

Lighting has been explored in a number of sections of this book where problems with lighting levels and glare are discussed. Generally it is the light from above or the side that proves to be the most troublesome source of glare. Many visually impaired people find this extremely disabling but its effects may be reduced or eliminated by the use of an eyeshade, brimmed hat or sun visor. Alternatively, sunglasses or tinted prescription spectacles may help, although they have the disadvantage of reducing overall illumination and contrast. If sunglasses are used, it is recommended that those permitting 20–30% of light transmission be selected. Lenses that react to different light levels may be of particular help to people whose adaptation to such alterations is poor.

Reading stands

These are extremely valuable in that they enable the user to place the reading material in a comfortable and visually advantageous position (see Figure 6.6). The back and neck ache that visually impaired people often experience after long periods of study may be alleviated by regular use of a reading stand, which can also be used for writing.

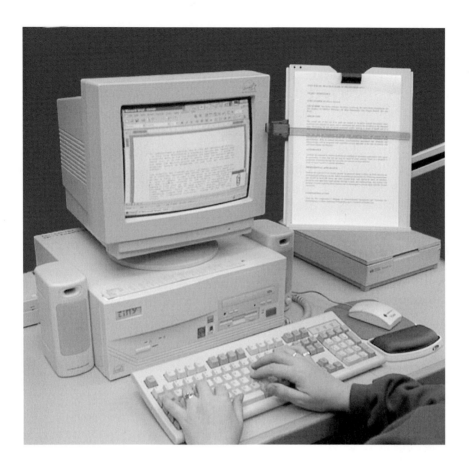

Figure 6.6 Reading stand.

There are many varieties of stand commercially available (usually from office suppliers), with a range of useful features such as in-built lighting, adjustable height and angle, clamps and line rulers. Some can be attached to desks, so facilitating simultaneous reading and typing/writing. Portable models are available that can be used while travelling.

Labels

Labelling items facilitates their identification and many visually impaired people devise labelling systems to suit their individual needs. There is an almost endless variety of materials that can be utilized for labelling purposes. Colour, shape, patterns and/or surface texture can be helpful depending on specific requirements. Students may find it useful to devise labelling systems to facilitate filing of course materials, notes and so on.

It may be advantageous for students if adapted labelling systems can be used in areas such as libraries and practical rooms. It is important to discuss requirements with individual students, as some may prefer notices with enlarged text whereas others may find plastic tape Braille labelling more helpful.

Tactile indicators

There are a number of products available that enable tactile indicators or labels to be added to items or equipment.

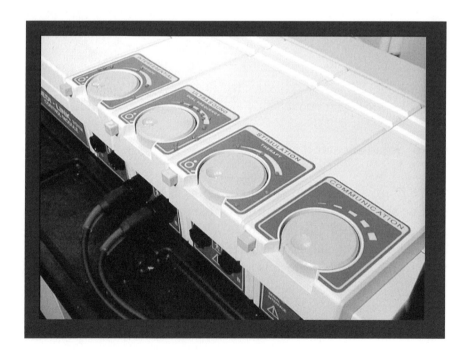

Figure 6.7 Hi Marks used to indicate dial settings.

Hi Marks

This is a bright, fluorescent paste sold in a tube with a thin nozzle. The paste can be squeezed out on to different surfaces in dots, lines or various shapes, taking approximately 3 hours to dry. This gives a bright visual, as well as tactile indicator, which can be felt as well as seen. Hi Marks has proved to be extremely popular as a means of marking items. The uses to which it can be put are numerous and are limited only by the imagination and dexterity of the individual. For example, it can be used to label items such as machine controls (see Figure 6.7) or specific keys on computer keyboards. It could also be helpful in constructing raised maps or diagrams.

Bump-ons and Locator-Dots

These items consist of premoulded shapes, available in a range of sizes and colours that can be stuck on to surfaces as tactile indicators

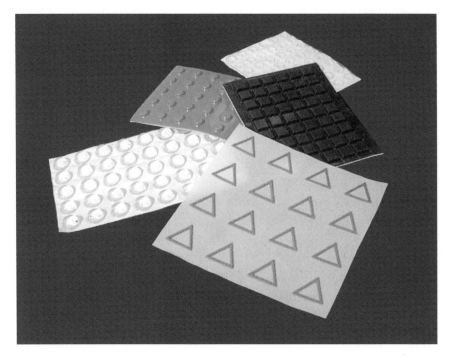

Figure 6.8 Bump-ons.

(see Figure 6.8). Bump-ons come in dayglo orange, black or transparent varieties. Again they can be used to mark a variety of everyday items such as keyboards or machine controls – for example, commonly used settings on a photocopier (see Figure 6.9). Locator dots are transparent with a much smaller bump (see Figure 6.10), which are useful for marking items such as keyboards, central heating or hi-fi controls.

These and other labelling items are available through organizations such as RNIB.

Assistance with mobility

White canes

These are designed specifically to assist mobility for visually impaired users, both partially sighted and blind. They are lightweight pieces of

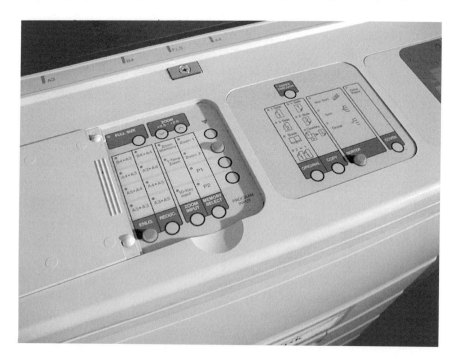

Figure 6.9 Fluorescent Bump-ons used to mark photocopier controls.

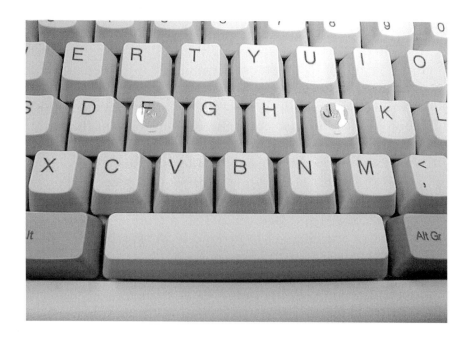

Figure 6.10 Locator dots on keyboards.

equipment, constructed of composite fibre, which can be folded down to fit into a pocket or bag for convenience (Cotton, 1997). There are three different types.

The symbol cane. This is available in a choice of lengths and is essentially intended as a signal to others that the user has a visual impairment. Some models have a reflective surface. (A red and white banded cane is used by people who are deafblind.) The symbol cane has a limited use in identifying obstacles ahead and can be used without special training (Cotton, 1997; Ford and Heshel, 1995).

The guide cane. This is longer and sturdier than the symbol cane. It can be used to locate obstacles and give some indication of the immediate surroundings. Generally, people whose residual vision necessitates that they use tactile methods of orientation would be likely to find this type of cane useful. Again, specialized training is not necessary.

The long cane. This is a longer cane than the previous one but the length is selected to suit the user's height and stride length (as a rough guide, a cane of this type usually reaches approximately mid chest height when held upright). Some training with a rehabilitation worker is required in order to perfect the technique of using this piece of equipment. The user holds the cane in front of the body at an angle of approximately 30 degrees to the ground. On walking forward the cane is moved from side to side in an arc extending a few inches beyond the width of the body in order to 'pre-view' the ground one or two paces ahead. The cane is swung to the left as the right foot steps forward and vice versa. This technique gives warning of obstacles and of any changes in ground level (Ford and Heshel, 1995).

If a student feels that she or he may need to learn long cane technique to aid mobility in the new college environment, it is recommended that training takes place before the commencement of the academic year. Once lectures start, there may not be the time or opportunity for this as it can take several weeks to perfect the technique, depending on individual requirements.

New developments. Recent research in robotics in the United States has resulted in the development of a prototype of the first robot cane for blind users. It is called the GuideCane and has been presented as the first step on the road to replacing guide dogs. The proposition is 'a computerized, sonar equipped navigation aid which detects obstacles in the user's path and automatically steers around them' (Parker, 1997). More work needs to be undertaken before this equipment is commercially available, as it is unable to detect overhead obstacles at present. Testing has shown that, after a relatively short time, users do become proficient with the GuideCane and are able to navigate at their normal walking speed. It is important to monitor the development of this type of equipment, as it could help to improve mobility levels significantly for some visually impaired users. It remains to be seen, however, whether current guide dog users would choose the GuideCane in preference to their dogs, even if the new equipment proves to be superior in mobility terms.

Guide dogs

There are currently over 4000 guide dog owners in the UK (Ford and Heshel, 1995), although, contrary to popular stereotypes, this makes up only a small proportion of the total visually impaired population. Any blind person over 16 years of age who is normally resident in the UK and able to use and care for a dog, can apply to Guide Dogs for the Blind Association (GDBA). Initial training in the care and effective use of a guide dog normally takes up to 4 weeks, and this is generally residential (there are a number of training centres around the country). In a few cases all or part of the training may be carried out at the applicant's home.

Once an application is made to GDBA and is accepted, there will usually be a waiting period of approximately 6 months before a dog becomes available. If the applicant has specific requirements, such as wanting a specific breed of dog, this period can be up to a year (Ford and Heshel, 1995) or possibly longer.

These factors need to be considered carefully by students if they choose to apply for a guide dog. It is unlikely that a student will have the time or opportunity to undertake the necessary training while involved in an educational programme. If a visually impaired person is considering applying for a guide dog as well as application to a course, it would probably be advisable to complete training with the dog before starting college, so allowing time for consolidation. If this is not possible, an alternative would be for the student to complete the first year of study and then to undertake the training in the summer break between years one and two of the course. In this situation, the student would already be familiar with the college environment and would not have to deal with too many new factors at the same time. GDBA do however, discuss the issues carefully with each applicant and any decisions regarding guide dog training are made in relation to the individual's situation and capabilities.

Factors that an institution needs to consider when interviewing and/or offering places to guide dog users are discussed in Chapter 9.

Electronic mobility equipment

Various types are available on the market. They normally use
reflected ultrasound to detect obstacles and nearby objects, and this is
translated into auditory or tactile (normally vibration) signals. The
design of individual equipment varies; for example, the Sonic
Pathfinder is mounted on a headband, the WalkMate has the
appearance of a walkman stereo and the Mowat Sensor resembles a
torch and can fit into a pocket or handbag.

Guidance systems

The React guidance system was officially launched at Queen Mary's
Hospital, Sidcup, in August 1997. This was designed in response to
RNIB research that highlighted the difficulties experienced by
visually impaired people in accessing buildings and services. It is a
radio frequency system that triggers speech from a beacon when the
user, wearing a React card, comes into range. It guides people to the
main hospital reception, so precluding the need to read signs when
in the new environment. From reception, volunteers guide visitors to
the appropriate area.

   This system has also been installed in other areas such as libraries
and civic offices; it is currently on trial for 6 months at Golders Green
tube station. An alternative system called Pathfinder is at present
being tested at Hammersmith bus/tube station; this system uses
infrared beams rather than sound (Lee, 1997).

Summary

This chapter has covered information about accessing and obtaining
a low vision assessment, as well as an overview of the general
procedure that occurs during the assessment. It has also given an
overview of the types of low vision equipment that are available for
visually impaired users. It was not considered appropriate in this
context to give details of manufacturers or prices, but this
information can be obtained from agencies such as RNIB and GDBA.

References

Carter, K. (1983) Comprehensive preliminary assessments of low vision, in *Understanding Low Vision* (ed. R.T. Jose), American Foundation for the Blind, New York, Ch. 6.

Cotton, C. (1997) Canes survey – an update. *New Beacon*, **81** (955), 10–12.

Cullinan, T. (1986) *Visual Disability in the Elderly*, Croom Helm, London.

Disabled Living Foundation (1991) *Visual Handicap: A Distance Learning Pack for Physiotherapists, Occupational Therapists and Other Health Care Professionals*, DLF, London.

Ford, M. and Heshel, T. (1995) *In Touch*, 12th edn, In Touch Publishing, London.

Lee, A. (1997) React – hospital leads the way with guidance system. *New Beacon*, **81** (956), 20.

Parker, C. (1997) Smart cane leads blind to safety. *The Times – Interface*, 10 September, 4.

Royal National Institute for the Blind (undated) *ESSN Low Vision Training Pack*, RNIB, London.

The environment

This chapter aims to give an indication of issues of access to the environment which need to be taken into account by institutions for students with visual impairments.

It is important that environmental issues should be considered for all disabled students. A user-friendly built environment frees the student from the unnecessary stress of attempting to negotiate inaccessible areas, so permitting greater concentration on academic matters. It is not possible, of course, to design any college, campus or building on that campus, to the exact specifications of every group of disabled users, each of which has its own access requirements. But if the commissioners of new buildings and the designers are sensitive and informed with regard to differing needs, it is possible to create environments that 'embrace and invite the widest possible range of users' (Barker, Barrick and Wilson, 1995). This type of inclusive design strategy moves a step further towards ensuring that disabling barriers are eliminated.

As discussed in other chapters, Further and Higher Education Funding Councils in England, Wales and Scotland have a duty placed upon them by the Disability Discrimination Act (DDA) to take account of the needs of disabled students. The DDA also builds on the Further and Higher Education Acts of 1992 which require further education providers to take account of these needs. Part of this responsibility requires institutions funded by these Councils to provide disability statements that give information about their facilities for disabled students. These statements may include descriptions of the general environment on the college campus. The information should be widely available, in a range of formats, in order that any potential applicant can obtain an indication of each institution's provision for visually impaired students. There should also be a note of the names and telephone numbers of staff who can be contacted about the stated provision. This allows discussion of particular issues that are of importance to individuals in relation to accessing both the built environment and the courses offered by the institution.

The campus

The majority of further and higher education institutions are not in the fortunate position of being made up of new buildings, or even of being purpose built for their current usage. It is unlikely, therefore, that many permanent environmental features can be changed. Some adaptations and modifications can, however, be introduced in an attempt to make the campus more user friendly for visually impaired students. These can often be simple and economic to put into practice. The principle underlying the following suggestions is to create an environment in which disabling barriers are reduced to the minimum. It is extremely important that design changes are practicable and useful, enabling and/or empowering to the user (Barker, Barrick and Wilson, 1995). It is, therefore, recommended that the opinions of a range of visually impaired users are obtained during the design and planning stage of new buildings, or before changes are made to existing premises. (NB, It is important to canvas the opinions of a range of users, as the design adaptations made for a person with one type of visual impairment may not be ideal for others.) In the interests of furthering understanding of the requirements of visually impaired students and staff, it would be useful to request feedback from them some time after the new building is occupied or the modifications are implemented. It is regrettable that the latter is not common practice at present, as this type of feedback would enhance planners' and designers' understanding of disability issues. Although it is important to be realistic about what can and what cannot be changed, it may be helpful to consider the issues from an idealistic perspective.

A good design is one which enables a disabled person to gain access to, and move around within, a building freely, independently, safely and with peace of mind. The care and attention to detail that is necessary when designing for the needs of disabled people will in fact enhance both the functional efficiency, and the aesthetic appeal of the premises for all users. (Barker, 1992)

It is strongly recommended from the outset, that the design approach should be to design for all, that is, inclusive. Consideration should preferably be given to the needs of disabled people at this stage, as making changes at a later date can be time consuming and more expensive than if the modifications had been incorporated from the beginning. If an institution is commissioning new premises, it is useful to plan ahead and design for possible future extension. This automatically builds in flexibility, so allowing review and modification to occur further into the life cycle of the building, rather than the design being finite once construction has begun.

Users and the environment

It is inevitable that, however carefully a campus is designed, it will not be ideal in terms of the requirements of each individual user. Everyone, whether visually impaired or fully sighted, will fall somewhere on a continuum in their ability to orientate themselves within an unfamiliar environment.

Most fully sighted individuals will be able to cite instances in which they have found orientation difficult. For example, using the Underground system in London, when exiting Chancery Lane station, it is very difficult to work out where you are until you become familiar with the area. There are four possible exits, no obvious street signs, the traffic is heavy and everyone is in a hurry. Which way to go? This is the experience of someone with full sight; the disorientation may well be increased significantly for someone with a visual impairment.

Another example of this problem with orientation in an unfamiliar environment may be experienced in buildings designed with recurrence of regular principles. This occurs in some hospitals where the wards are arranged around a square courtyard with one ward on each side of the square, or a number of wings leading away from a common central area. Each of the sides or wings is essentially identical and confusion about one's exact location occurs very easily. These problems can be compounded if the building has multiple floors. There may be visual clues such as signs or different patterns on the curtains around the beds – but these are often not significant enough to prompt the realization of being in the wrong place.

Again, difficulties of orientation for a visually impaired user are compounded by this type of design, however well developed his or her innate ability to find their way around unfamiliar environments. If the 'recurrent principle' type of design is planned or is already in place, it is helpful to build in or to add some means of clearly differentiating between areas.

Someone with full sight can often see at a glance how to get from A to B and can then progress towards the identified target without necessarily being conscious of the specific route. This method is often not available for a person with a visual impairment. This is not to say, however, that the use of significant landmarks is a totally impractical way of negotiating a new area. For example, sometimes a particular shape of building, a clear sign or a coloured door can indicate the initial position of the person, the route to be taken or attainment of the target.

Similarly, some visually impaired students and staff may find maps useful in negotiating a new environment. Even if a print map is not totally accessible, the concept of having a map-type image in mind may aid orientation enormously for some people. Many large complexes already have maps located around the grounds and buildings to facilitate route finding for visitors. These may not be accessible for all visually impaired users. It is therefore recommended that some other method is easily available. This could be an enlarged copy of the map in print, a relief version or directions on cassette tape. The method used to read directions on to cassette tape is important. Most people have had the experience of asking someone the way to a specific place and being no clearer as to how to get there by the time the instructions are complete. If directions are to be made available on cassette tape, therefore, it may be advisable to seek advice from an organization such as RNIB about the appropriate method of describing the relevant information. This could have staff training implications.

As a general rule, it is probably true to say that it is easier for someone with a visual impairment to negotiate buildings and open areas that are angular rather than curved. Curves can be disorientating. This is also true for other areas; for example, a blind swimmer may find it easier to navigate in an Olympic-type, oblong swimming pool than in the irregularly shaped pools of the type seen in many leisure centres.

It is important for visually impaired people to attend carefully to incoming stimuli and to continue to be observant, even when familiar with a specific area. Senses other than sight can be useful in negotiating new environments.

It may be possible to locate certain areas by smell. An obvious example might be the college refectory or café, but the location of other areas, such as the chemistry laboratory on campus, the hydrotherapy department in the hospital or the bakery in a row of local shops, can be pinpointed by the additional use of the sense of smell.

Many visually impaired people are sensitive to the amount of echo present in any area they are negotiating. This can be a help or a hindrance to successful route finding. In very large open areas outside or large rooms with high ceilings (such as gymnasia) there may be few objects from which the sound can bounce back. This can make orientation more difficult. Another situation in which problems may occur is in a busy area of the college, particularly if there are long corridors, high ceilings and no carpets. There will be too many echoes and this can be very confusing. Conversely, if there is wallpaper on the walls (or even carpet in some instances), all the floors are carpeted and the windows are curtained, there will be very little echo. It may be difficult for a visually impaired person to orientate him/herself in this type of environment, as it has a degree of soundproofing. Some rooms, such as lecture theatres, may in fact be partially soundproofed. But this can be helpful, as it minimizes incidental noise, so facilitating concentration on academic matters.

In general, it is useful to visually impaired students and staff if various areas of the college have a certain amount of echo, although too many extraneous stimuli can be as disabling as too few. Some echo will facilitate identification of features such as open doors and items of furniture. It may also facilitate route finding and can help with the location of people and objects in the area. Up to a certain threshold, increased echo can give a visually impaired person considerable information about a particular environment.

These factors could be considered at the design stage of new buildings or during refurbishment of college premises. It may not however, be possible for any practical measures to be taken to alter echo variation in existing buildings. But it is important for staff and students to be aware of the positive and negative aspects of this phenomenon and how they could affect a visually impaired user's ability to orientate him/herself within the environment.

General environmental points

Colour contrast

This issue is crucial in all instances in which a partially sighted person needs to negotiate a particular site or to access print information. If any colours used are too similar in tone, they will tend to blend into a single colour and so make it very difficult for a visually impaired person to differentiate between them. For example, pale blue and pale green are different colours but are very similar in tone, the same applies for dark red and dark green. Although different colours, they can appear very similar; it is the tonal contrast that is important, rather than just the colour contrast. This is an issue with regard to access to printed information, but it also has implications for exterior and interior design.

Recent research carried out at the University of Reading in collaboration with ICI Paints has investigated the most important sites within a building where colour contrast can be used for maximum benefit to visually impaired users. The authors also refer to a property known as 'luminance contrast' (Bright, Cook and Harris, 1997). Luminance is the intensity of light emitted from a surface per unit area in a given direction (*Concise Oxford Dictionary*, 1990). It follows, therefore, that if the luminance of one surface is of a different intensity to that of the adjacent surface, it will help visually impaired users to distinguish between the two. This property is due to a combination of factors such as the colours used on each surface, the finish (gloss, matt, eggshell and so on) and the lighting levels. Colour and luminance contrast together can therefore provide vital visual clues to a visually impaired person, particularly when entering a new environment.

These issues will be addressed in a little more detail later in the chapter.

Lighting

Lighting levels are an important consideration and, although they are not essentially related to college layout, accessibility is much easier if areas are appropriately lit. This needs to be considered carefully, as some partially sighted people experience night blindness when light levels are very low, that is, the eye cannot adapt to the reduction in light and so the amount of vision is reduced. Conversely, if some areas are very brightly lit or sunny, it can cause problems for those with photophobia. In fact, large amounts of light on any surface will cause colour contrast to reduce and glare to increase (Bright, Cook and Harris, 1997). This can be compounded further by glare from reflective surfaces such as shiny floors, glass or mirrors.

These issues may not be of great importance in a totally static environment with which the student is very familiar. Most areas of a college, however, tend to be very dynamic. The population moves around constantly and furniture and equipment never remain in one place for very long. Correct lighting levels in this type of setting, therefore, are essential in making the environment a generally safer place for all users.

Unfortunately, there is no documentation to which planners and designers can refer in order to find recommendations for appropriate lighting levels for visually impaired people. All of the codes of practice available relate to the needs of those with levels of vision in the 'normal' range. In fact, it would probably be almost impossible to define 'appropriate' lighting levels for all visually impaired people, as requirements vary enormously. There are, however, some general points that may aid designers in the task of ensuring that the environment is rendered as user friendly as possible, in lighting terms, for those with a visual impairment.

(1) The general level of lighting should be as uniform as possible and adequate for the needs of visually impaired people ('adequate' in this case refers to the quantity of light, which often needs to be greater, but care needs to be taken to avoid glare). Pools of light and dark should be avoided; for example, spotlights create intense pools of light surrounded by areas of comparative darkness; this can give rise to optical illusions and visual distractions (Bright, Cook and Harris, 1997) Shadows may appear to be solid structures, or shadow could mask a hazardous obstruction (see Chapter 2 for a more detailed exploration of optical illusions). A shadow produced by sunlight falling through a window can also be confusing, particularly as the edge of the shadow will move across a range of internal surfaces as the sun moves round during the day. Sudden changes in light level may also occur due to variable cloud cover. This can be a visual distracter (Bright, Cook and Harris, 1997). Curtains and blinds can help to negate these effects.

The area illuminated by a particular fitting should be evenly lit with no patterns of light to cause confusion. The fall-off at the edges of the area should be gradual and not sharply defined, as, again, optical illusions could occur. Consideration of the spacing between each light fitting and any lampshades used should help to avoid these problems (Barker, Barrick and Wilson, 1995).

(2) Glare should be reduced whenever possible, as it can cause visual confusion. Bright natural light falling through a window, glass entrance hall or glass-sided building can cause problems, as can light reflected from shiny surfaces such as tiled floors, glass, mirrors or walls painted with a gloss finish. In the first instance, blinds and

curtains are very useful for modifying lighting levels where natural light may cause glare. The use of this equipment introduces an element of flexibility into the environment, which can then be changed according to individual requirements.

In the second situation, a matt finish on walls and the avoidance, where possible, of shiny surfaces, plus diffused lighting, can decrease the amount of reflection.

On some courses, students are required to use visual display screens for protracted amounts of time. Care should be taken to supply correctly designed light fittings in any computer laboratories to avoid glare from the screens; this is important for all users but particularly so for those with a visual impairment. If it is impossible to fit appropriate lighting or to modify existing fittings, computer filters can be purchased. These are placed over the screen and manufacturers claim that they cut out over 90% of the glare but do not affect colour or contrast.

(3) The choice of colour for the lighting should be considered. If the interior decor has been carefully designed with respect to good colour contrast, this can be totally negated by the use of inappropriately coloured lighting. The principles of basic physics apply here. Objects are visible because they reflect light that has come from the sun or some other light source – in this case, light fittings inside a building. The objects appear coloured because they reflect some of the colours in the spectrum and absorb others. For example, in white light (that is, full spectrum) a white chair appears white because it reflects all the colours of the spectrum, a black chair appears black because it absorbs them, but a red chair appears red because it reflects the red light and absorbs the rest. White light, therefore, is the most appropriate variety to use to avoid colour confusion. If coloured lighting is used, however, objects may appear to be entirely different colours to those seen in white light. For example, a red chair will still appear red if illuminated with yellow light (since yellow light is a mixture of red and green light, the red of the chair can reflect back the red elements of the yellow light). But the same chair will look black if illuminated with green light (green light contains no red elements and so the chair absorbs it all) (Pople,

1982). These are fairly extreme examples and it is clear that interior designers rarely use such primary colours in their lighting. They serve to illustrate the principle, however, and it remains true that some colours used in lighting can mask or affect natural tones, and so reduce visibility. This should be avoided whenever possible.

(4) It is possible to fit dimmer switches, which can be useful for some visually impaired people, depending on the level of lighting they prefer or find most comfortable. This means that the same light fitting can suit a range of requirements for different students. This relates to the earlier point of introducing flexibility and adaptability into the environment whenever possible.

(5) Where the level of general lighting is unsuitable for a particular situation, it is useful to offer a variety of options such as a change of bulb, filters over the light source or a range of lamps and/or illuminated magnifiers appropriate for specific task lighting where necessary. If a lamp is used, the light source, the task and the student's head are in very close proximity. Because of this, it is advisable to use equipment that does not reach a high surface temperature, for example, a compact fluorescent lamp. Lamps of this type also have a hood that avoids glare. This is helpful when the student is working very close to the light source as mentioned in Chapter 6.

(6) Light levels can be improved by painting walls and ceilings a light colour and by ensuring that windows are cleaned on a regular basis. Lights that produce flicker can adversely affect vision; therefore, it is advisable to check that any fluorescent tubes used are not at the end of their useful life. Accommodation to different levels of lighting may be slower for some visually impaired students. It is therefore advisable to avoid turning lights on and off whenever possible. For example, some teaching staff turn the lights off when the overhead projector is being used. If the transparency is of good quality, there should be no need to do this. If the lights are kept on, this avoids problems with accommodation and reduces glare from the screen.

Location and layout of the college

If new premises are to be built, it is important to consider location
with regard to amenities, facilities and public transport links. Many
visually impaired students rely heavily on public transport in order to
travel to college and work placements. If possible, the approach to
the college from nearby bus stops or bus/railway stations should be
flat. Ideally the need for the student to negotiate cluttered areas or
very busy roads should be kept to a minimum. Once on campus, it is
helpful if the site itself is flat. If changes in level are unavoidable,
then clearly marked ramps and steps, both with handrails, will ensure
improved accessibility for all disabled students, staff and visitors. An
overall simple and logical layout will help visually impaired students
to memorize routes for negotiating the area.

Approach to the buildings

It is advantageous if the paths around and approaching the buildings
are level, have an even surface and are of a material that is non-slip
when wet. If paths have too great a camber, they can cause a blind
person to deviate inadvertently from the correct route. Any gaps
greater than 5 mm between the slabs of a paved path may cause
someone to trip. It is very helpful if the edges of paths are clearly
defined by a contrasting colour and/or a change in texture, such as
gravel or grass. Handrails can also be useful to indicate the edge of a
path or ramp. Again, clear colour contrast will make it easier for a
visually impaired person to locate the rail (Barker, Barrick and
Wilson, 1995).

Drainage grilles

If drainage grilles need to be present in the path, they should be offset
if possible, and the gap between the bars should be no greater than 13
mm. This will reduce the possibility of trapping the tip of a long cane,
or tripping over the grille, which could cause a fall. Problems such as
this will also be reduced if the bars of the grilles are at right angles to
the general direction of travel (Barker, Barrick and Wilson, 1995).

Tactile surfaces

Paving and other surfaces may have different tactile patterns that can indicate particular features. An example of this is the 'modified blister' pattern commonly used to indicate the edge of a pavement at pelican crossings, and to warn that there is no kerb (it is dropped to facilitate road crossing for people in wheelchairs or pushing prams). Most members of the public are familiar with this idea. Other examples of situations where this type of tactile finish can be of use are: to alert a visually impaired person to the top or bottom of a flight of stairs; to indicate a particular route; or to denote a 'crossover', which is where motor vehicles cross a pedestrian walkway.

Bollards

Bollards are features found in many pedestrian areas, including college environs, where they may be used to prevent motor vehicles entering a certain area, or as decoration. They can, however, be very hazardous to someone with a visual impairment if not clearly marked. In order to enhance their visibility, bollards should be colour contrasted with the paving. A band of contrasting colour around the neck of the bollards can also improve visibility. For obvious reasons, they should not be linked together with chain or rope.

Other outdoor features

Other outdoor features such as seating, signposts and rubbish bins need to be considered. They may constitute hazards if they are actually on the path itself, particularly if they blend into the background. To avoid these problems they should be positioned off the walkway (but adjacent to it) and should be of a contrasting tone or colour.

Consideration needs to be given to facilities for guide dogs. Ideally part of the grounds should be made available as a 'relief area' and a dog run. The location of this area needs to be communicated to any students, staff or visitors who are guide dog users. The route to it should be clear and easily negotiated.

Plants

The presence of plants and trees enhance the aesthetic appeal of any location. They help to soften the lines of the built environment, giving an attractive and welcoming appearance. Depending on the choice of plants, particularly with regard to colour and shape, they can sometimes help visually impaired people to orientate themselves in an area. The principles of colour contrast can be utilized here by choosing different tones of green for the planting. If the design of the site does include any vegetation, care should be taken with regard to both the positioning and the planning of maintenance of the plants. Overgrowth on to walkways and overhanging branches can make negotiation of routes difficult and may cause injury. Many plants also drop leaves, seedpods, cones and so on. This can make footing treacherous and uncomfortable. Because of this, plants should:

(1) be chosen carefully to avoid those which shed such items; or
(2) be planted far enough away from paths to negate the problem; or
(3) be pruned back from the edge of paths, and any material that is shed should be regularly cleared away.

Open spaces

Large open areas are usually considered to be desirable features in the design of buildings, as they can give a pleasant impression of space, light and airiness. This can, however, be a disadvantage for people with a visual impairment. Finding a route across a large space can be difficult, if not almost impossible, particularly if there are no clear landmarks. There is no suggestion that open areas within buildings and colleges should be abolished because of this. It is important, however, for planners and designers to be sensitive, and to provide distinct features with the use of contrasting colours and textures. These can be used to indicate specific routes across the space, and to denote locations for particular use, for example, seating areas. Any changes in level, involving steps or ramps, should also be clearly marked using both visual and tactile methods.

It is important to indicate clearly any objects that project into the open space or that are free standing within it. Examples of these are staircases, pillars supporting higher levels of the building, canopies over doorways which may have support struts, any decorative features such as statuary or fountains, and so on.

If any building work is being carried out on campus, it is important that the workmen do not leave equipment or rubble in areas where a visually impaired person may inadvertently walk into them. This should be carefully monitored, possibly by a member of staff from Estate Services or the equivalent. It is strongly recommended that this person has specific responsibility for ensuring that any building work carried out on site does not impede the mobility of or potentially endanger staff and students with disabilities. Another hazard to be avoided is that caused by ladders left protruding from the back of a van or lorry, usually at head height.

Features of buildings

The entrance is probably the most crucial feature on the exterior of a buildings which needs to be readily identifiable by visually impaired students. For all users, it should be easy to recognize, simple to negotiate and, ideally, should look welcoming. Elements mentioned earlier, such as colour contrast and a different tactile surface underfoot, can help to indicate the presence of the entrance.

An overhead canopy may be fitted to protect users from the rain and to decorate or highlight the door. If struts or columns support this structure, they should be of a contrasting tone or colour to the background and must not obstruct entry. Given that some visually impaired people experience difficulties at night, the area under the canopy should be well lit. This lighting will also help users to identify the position of the door from a distance.

Glass doors and glazed panels can be difficult to see. If the entrance is just one more sheet of glass in a large expanse of a glass-sided building, it may be almost impossible to distinguish. It is an important safety feature to highlight any glazed panels with a coloured strip or motif at approximately eye level. The doors should have further identification that may include previously mentioned features such as colour/tonal contrast, lighting, tactile changes underfoot, and so on. Any door furniture should be in a logical position and of a contrasting colour or tone.

Doormats can be useful in identification of door position, but may also be a hazard. They are often set into the floor and this avoids the problem of tripping.

If a building is still at the design stage, the doors can be planned to be a convenient width for any users with different requirements. The Building Regulations state that a minimum of 800 millimetres width is necessary for users in wheelchairs to pass through freely. For visually impaired individuals, however, there may be other considerations. The width necessary to allow free passage of a person plus guide dog is 1.1 metres and for a person using a sighted guide a width of 1.2 metres is needed (Barker, Barrick and Wilson, 1995).

The type of external door used also needs to be considered. If finances permit, automatic doors are certainly the most convenient. They allow easy access to the building for all users. Non-automatic doors with a hinge on one side are usually relatively easy to negotiate, although this does become more difficult for those with guide dogs or sighted guides. If they are fitted with door closers, the spring should not be so strong as to cause problems to users. Revolving doors are particularly difficult to negotiate and should not be used.

All institutions have to be very security conscious, as theft of expensive equipment and personal belongings is an all too familiar occurrence. To this end, many external doors are fitted with entry devices of various sorts, for example swipe cards or intercoms. If this is the case, the equipment chosen should be logically positioned and clearly indicated. If a student is required to punch in a code, the buttons need to be large and the numbers clear. Braille labels or raised characters may need to be added for any Braille users.

The threshold of any external doors should be flush with the floor. If this is not possible, any features standing proud of the floor surface should not exceed 15 mm (Barker, Barrick and Wilson, 1995).

Steps and stairs

Steps and stairs can be difficult to negotiate. If the goings and risers are the same colour, they may appear as a flat surface or a slope to some visually impaired people. Conversely, if the floor covering is highly patterned, it can cause visual confusion, particularly when trying to identify the edge of each step. This could have health and safety implications. If possible at the design stage, curved staircases should be avoided. It is very important that the goings and risers are uniform and any stairs and steps are well and evenly lit. It is advisable that the edge of each step (the nosing) is a clearly contrasting colour. The nosing strip should be a thinner line than the step itself, otherwise it is possible for a person with partial sight to confuse the two. As mentioned earlier, changes in the floor surface, such as tactile warning strips at the top and the bottom of flights of stairs, give another indication that the stairs are there.

Some designers, who are presumably aiming for a very light and airy atmosphere, use translucent materials to form staircases in some public areas. These are extremely difficult for anyone with partial sight to identify, as it is not clear where each step begins and ends. They therefore constitute a hazard. Due to the materials used these are often open-plan stairs, which are also problematic.

Continuous handrails of clearly contrasting colour or tone should be fitted, preferably on both sides and continuing on to the landing areas. The rail should have a ridge or other tactile feature to indicate the approach of the first or last step. Another helpful point is for the floor number to be clearly indicated by a sign at the top and bottom of the staircase. Raised characters of no less than 100 millimetres height (2 millimetres proud of the background) will assist a visually impaired person to identify which level s/he is on. Contrast in colour and tone between the background and foreground of the sign is essential (Barker, 1992).

Interior design

It is advantageous for doors, architraves, walkways and railings to be in contrasting colours and tones relative to the background to facilitate their identification.

As alluded to earlier, it is helpful if the walls and ceilings are decorated in pale colours to maximize available lighting and to even out its distribution. Matt, eggshell or silk finishes create less glare than gloss, although a matt finish would be the surface of choice. Patterned wallpaper can cause visual confusion and may act as a distracter. It may make identification of items adjacent to the walls difficult, for example, the location of items on a shelf, signs or noticeboards. A small pattern on the wallpaper is often acceptable and less distracting, as it may appear plain to someone with partial sight. Items such as switches, sockets and pull cords should contrast with the background for easier identification.

Doors and other features such as dado rails, door frames and skirting boards should contrast clearly with the colour of the walls to assist in identification and to help with navigation. A consistent choice of colours may help students to locate features that occur regularly, such as doors. It may also be possible to use some colour coding, for example, to differentiate toilet doors from classroom doors. Bright, Cook and Harris, (1997) found that, given a number of options, most visually impaired people expressed a strong preference for the whole door to be a contrasting colour or tone to the wall rather than for only the architrave to be different. This makes identification of the feature as 'a door' much easier.

Any door furniture should be clearly contrasting, and this includes any signs or numbers that the student may need in order to identify a specific location. The colour and shape of the handle help to indicate the presence of a door and the way it opens. Contrasting finger or push plates near the handle and kick plates at the bottom of a door are also useful indicators (Bright, Cook and Harris, 1997).

Contrasting colours and/or tones should be used for floor coverings to differentiate them from the walls and doors. Again, bold patterns should be avoided to reduce visual confusion, to make it easier to see any items on the floor and to help with relocation of objects. A highly patterned carpet could hide a small object inadvertently dropped on to the floor. This is an example of illusion and camouflage, as discussed in Chapter 2. Furniture should also be of a contrasting material to help with identification. Patterns may be quite useful here as long as they do not create the illusion of the chairs blending in with the floor covering.

Bright, Cook and Harris, (1997) have found that, when navigating around a building, many visually impaired people use residual vision to obtain information about their surroundings. To do this the scene is scanned, usually by looking downwards and not more than 2 metres in front. Consequently, to assist negotiation of an area, maximum benefit from using colour or tone contrast is gained by targeting its use up to 1.2 metres above floor level (approximately handrail or dado height), with special attention given to the junction of the floor with the walls.

As mentioned earlier, generally reflection should be minimized by avoiding shiny walls and floors whenever possible.

Interior designers, to give the impression of more space, often use mirrors. The use of too many mirrors, however, can be very confusing to people with a visual impairment, who may mistake the image for real space and walk into it. If mirrors are to be used, full-length ones should be avoided and a contrasting frame fitted to help in identification.

Good colour/tone contrast is of paramount importance in the identification of features in all areas, not least in relation to interior design. These contrasts, however, should not result in a garish decorative scheme. Remember that tone is the key and so, for example, light grey walls with a dark grey carpet will be eminently visible and clear to many students with a visual impairment. Some contrasting colour could be used for woodwork, light switches, and furnishings, to provide a well co-ordinated but visually clear impression.

Signs

Visibility

A sign should be highly visible and not surrounded by other items that would distract attention from it. It should be in a prominent position and the design should be bold. The positioning of signs can be included in the planning process of any new buildings.

Clarity

The layout and design of the sign must be clear, as should the message itself – simple, short and easy to understand.

Position

Signs at a height of 1.75–2 metres above ground level are usually satisfactory for adults, but for children or wheelchair users a height of 1–1.5 metres may be more useful. Depending on the size of the text (see below), a visually impaired person may have to get closer to the sign in order to read it, so this should be considered when deciding where to place it (Barker, 1992). Generally, in order to facilitate reading, the signs should be as near to eye level as possible.

Lighting

Signs must be adequately lit at times when natural light levels are low. Care should be taken to ensure that the light source is positioned away from the sign and shielded in order to avoid glare.

Style

Ideally the lettering on signs should be clear and simple, for example, Universal bold in lower case letters. Each letter should stand alone and italics are better avoided.

Colours

The optimal choice is a strong background colour such as black, dark blue, dark green, with light lettering such as white or yellow. This combination reduces glare.

Size

Approximately 70% of visually impaired people are able to read 50 millimetre letters at a distance of 1.5 metres, and 200 millimetre letters at a distance of 5 m and so on, provided there is good lighting, colour contrast and style. (See Barker, 1992.)

Signs as described above can be provided (and, if necessary, Braille signs can be added) for classroom and office doors and lifts. Speech output in lifts to announce the floor and important areas on that level can also be useful. The control panel is easier to use if it is illuminated and readily distinguishable from the rest of the decor. Raised characters or Braille can be used to indicate floor levels.

If Braille is to be added to signs as a general rule, there are a few useful points to remember:

- One-word signs can use Grade I Braille, but for longer messages Grade II should be used (see Chapter 8 for an explanation of Braille grades).
- The sign needs to be positioned so that the Braille user can approach it easily and get near enough to touch it.
- The Braille should be placed high enough on the sign that it can be read without the reader having to crouch.
- If the Braille is interspersed with the visual text, it is easier to locate if the sign has small notches at the side to indicate where each Braille line begins.

Some large, new complexes have lines painted on the floor or walls, or coded signs, to indicate the routes to specific areas. These features may be helpful to some people with visual impairments. The extent to which such features facilitate access may depend on levels of colour vision, but as emphasized before, the contrast between foreground and background colours and tones should always be high.

Classrooms

For many visually impaired people, familiarity with the environment reduces stress levels and facilitates concentration on academic matters. In the ideal situation it is recommended that a minimum number of classrooms should be used, to enable the visually impaired student to become familiar with their layout. It is also helpful, where possible, for the principle of consistency to be applied when allocating rooms for each week.

Issues of lighting and contrast again apply. The matter may need to be referred to Estate Services if there are particular problems in some rooms. Difficulties will be kept to a minimum if attention is given to making the environment as flexible as possible from the design stage onwards.

Lecture rooms

Because of their relatively permanent features, lecture theatres may pose a few problems of access. Older institutions often have dark wooden steps which students have to negotiate in order to reach their seats. It may be necessary to mark the nosing of these steps to facilitate access to the room for students with a visual impairment. If the student uses enlarged sheets of paper and/or equipment such as a laptop computer, tape recorder or task lighting, s/he may choose to discuss specific requirements with staff. This could involve sitting in a particular position in the room near to electrical sockets and having an extension lead supplied by the technical department. An additional desk may be provided to increase the work surface.

In non-tiered classrooms, many institutions seem to favour stackable chairs with quite small, swing-over desks. These can cause problems in two ways. Firstly the chairs will inevitably be in different places every time the students enter the room; secondly the size and position of the desk is often inadequate, particularly if the student is using a tape recorder or other equipment, and/or enlarged (A3) sheets of paper. Although little can be done about the furniture being moved, it is helpful if the student is informed of the situation. As already mentioned in the case of tiered lecture theatres, following discussion with the student, the choice may be to offer a separate table and chair in the room for the student's personal use. This would provide a larger surface area on which to work.

It may be necessary for some students to approach text very closely in order to read it. This can cause pain and tension in the neck and back due to poor posture. If this becomes a problem, the student might wish to consider the use of an adjustable height desk and/or an inclined surface on which to place written work. A reading stand can also be useful to hold books and papers in a convenient position, particularly if entering material on to computer.

Practical rooms

Some courses involve work in laboratories or practical rooms. The student should be given the opportunity to become familiar with the layout of the rooms and, if appropriate, storage areas for personal equipment should be offered. If any apparatus is set out for a specific class, it may be useful for the student to have access to the room before the beginning of the session in order to become familiar with the general layout.

It is important to ensure that any items of electrical equipment, such as overhead projectors, are safely positioned. Flexes should not trail on to the floor or be stretched across an area where students have to walk. This has general health and safety implications but could prove to be particularly hazardous for a visually impaired person. Liaison with technicians may be helpful, and contact can be made with Estate Services and health and safety officers as appropriate, to ensure good health and safety practice throughout the institution.

Summary

This chapter has considered issues relating to the environment in a college campus which should be taken into account when facilitating access for visually impaired users. As stated earlier, some of this has taken an idealistic perspective. It is suggested, however, that many of the ideas are not outrageous and would not necessarily be prohibitive in terms of financial and human resources, particularly if implemented from the outset or built into regular maintenance schedules. The design suggestions and modifications are inclusive, aiming to produce an environment where disabling barriers are reduced to a minimum. It should be safe, welcoming and, above all, practicable for use by the widest possible range of students and staff in a college setting.

References

Barker, P. (1992) *Key Features of Good Design*, RNIB Mobility Unit, London.

Barker, P., Barrick, J. and Wilson, R. (1995) *Building Sight: A Handbook of Building and Interior Design Solutions to Include the Needs of Visually Impaired People*. RNIB, London.

Bright, K., Cook, G.K. and Harris, J. (1997) Project Rainbow – colour and contrast design guidance. *Access by Design*, **72**, 11–14.

Concise Oxford Dictionary (1990) 8th edn, Clarendon Press, Oxford.

Pople, S. (1982) *Explaining Physics*, Oxford University Press, Oxford, pp. 182–5.

Access technology | 8

This chapter gives a brief overview of the access technology available for visually impaired users in post school educational settings. It is beyond the scope of this book to give detailed information about specific products and manufacturers, but this can be obtained from organizations such as RNIB, members of the National Federation of Access Centres (NFAC) or possibly from resource centres run by local societies.

The term 'access technology' is used here in its widest sense as meaning any technological equipment that can facilitate visually impaired students' access to the educational environment. The technology under discussion can be used to do this in a number of ways. First, teaching and support staff can make teaching and learning materials available via technology and can also produce materials in a range of accessible formats. Second, access technology can be used to provide an alternative means of reading and writing for the visually impaired student. Third, it enables the student to access independently the vast amounts of information available, particularly any that is stored electronically such as that on the Internet and on CD-ROM (compact disc – read only memory). It has also increased the accessibility of much text-based information with the advent and improvement of optical character recognition (OCR).

Although technology can be a key factor in facilitating access for visually impaired students to many courses, it must be remembered that it is not a panacea for all curricular barriers that may be encountered at college. It is also very important for teaching staff to realize that they still have a duty to provide material in appropriate formats. They must not expect the students to take on the responsibility for dealing with all the access issues related to teaching and learning materials, just because they may have some technological equipment.

Each institution should be responsible for deciding on the technology that needs to be made available in the library or learning resource centre in order to facilitate access for visually impaired students. There is the option of loading some types of access technology, such as screen enlargement systems and speech output, on to a computer network that will enable students to use electronic mail and Internet facilities if they wish. This will be of particular importance if parts of certain courses are presented to students and/or assessed electronically. These issues should ideally be considered in overall institutional policy, in consultation with the disabilities coordinator or learning support tutor. RNIB operates a 'Partners in Access' scheme that seeks to meet institutions' specific technology requirements by providing appropriate equipment. In return for this the institution is required to purchase a package of staff training to raise awareness of visual impairment issues. Further information can be obtained from RNIB ESSN (Employment and Student Support Network).

Once equipment and systems are in place, information about them can be included in the disability statement. It is also extremely important to ensure that all staff members know what equipment is available so that they can make effective use of it and direct students to it as necessary. When the financial implications of installing access technology are being considered, it is important to remember that some money will be needed to provide staff training and to allow for maintenance of equipment. There is no point having a plethora of high-tech equipment if no one can use it.

Assessment

Low vision assessment has already been covered in Chapter 6 and assessment of educational needs is discussed in Chapter 9. It seems appropriate, however, to include some brief mention of assessment here in view of its paramount importance. Depending on their previous experience and background, some students will arrive at the institution with an excellent knowledge of available technology, and may indeed already own the requisite equipment for accessing their chosen course. This seems, however, to be the exception to the rule. Many students arrive with little, if any, knowledge on these matters and very few have any equipment of their own.

Access technology tends to be expensive and so it is vital that the student should be offered an assessment, in order that any equipment purchased is relevant and appropriate for his or her requirements.

Fetton (1996) refers to a checklist of points which can be used during an assessment to ensure that the introduction of new technology is successful. Although his focus is on school children, some of the points that can be modified for further and higher education settings are identified below:

(1) What are the student's curriculum access requirements?
(2) What factors are likely to affect the student's ability to develop any new skills in relation to new communication methods and/or the operation of new equipment?
(3) In what particular ways could technology be used?
(4) Which input, storage and output features are the best match for the student's needs and abilities?
(5) Which equipment offers the right combination of input, storage and output features?
(6) What entry-level skills are required to manage the selected system?
(7) Are there any initial or ongoing training requirements for the student and/or staff if the technology is to be introduced successfully?
(8) What are the implications of the technology for the organization of the student's work and study strategies?
(9) Will the introduction of new technology change the level and/or nature of support that the student may require?
(10) What level of technical support (if any) will be necessary to introduce and maintain the technology?

There are two important issues to highlight here. One is the need for training, which may be necessary for the student and possibly for staff members. There is no point in carrying out an assessment and providing equipment if the student is subsequently unable to use it. Training is available from some suppliers but this may be very general and focused on technical points rather than educational requirements. There may be someone available on site who is able to provide help or it may be necessary to contact an organization such as RNIB to make use of its network of Technical Consultants within ESSN, who are available to provide training. There is usually some cost involved, which will vary depending on who carries it out. Any training provided should be specific and needs led, with careful referral to the results of the assessment to ensure it meets the requirements of the individual student. It should not include the whole range of technical features of the equipment in question, but should focus on the specific purpose for which the technology was recommended (Fetton, 1996). Depending on the particular student, there may be a need for some follow-up after the initial training.

The second issue that deserves brief attention is technical support. Equipment can sometimes go wrong, or, after some experience, the student may wish to change the set-up. Often the technology becomes vital for the student's continued full participation in the course, and so it is important to ensure that there is someone available to provide technical help as necessary.

This type of technical support may involve the following activities:

(1) General administration and maintenance of equipment.
(2) Building up a stock of equipment to be used as replacement items while personal or institutional equipment is under repair.
(3) Administration and upkeep of any loan stock.
    (a) If possible it is helpful to have some loan stock available in a designated area so that students can hire or borrow this in the short term in order to try it out in the academic setting before buying their own.
    (b) It may also be useful as a stop gap, as there is often a delay before students can access funding at the beginning of a course.

   (c) Finally, having some equipment available may make it possible to provide access technology for those students who do not receive any funding.

(4) A technician is able to keep up to date with suppliers and any new developments in the access technology field.

(5) Finally, students and staff may require ongoing technical support once the initial training has been carried out, as well as help while practising new skills.

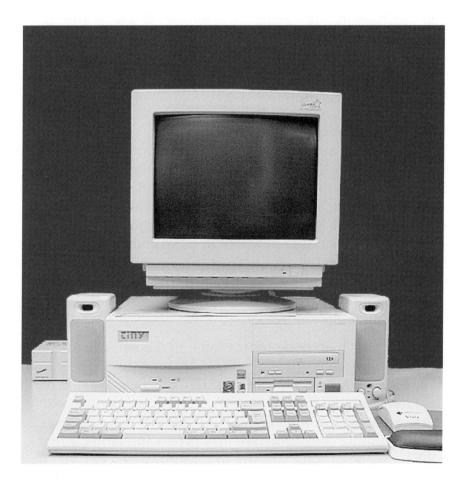

Figure 8.1   Desktop computer.

Computers

Inevitably, much of the access equipment discussed in the ensuing sections is computer related. The advent of the computer plus its commonly available accessories, and the apparently exponential rate of their development have made a great contribution to the accessibility of material for visually impaired users. This section gives a very brief overview of the types of computers and accessories that are often found useful by students in various college and work placement settings.

The type of computer with which most people are familiar is the desktop which, as its name suggests, is for use on a desk and so is non-portable (see Figure 8.1). It has the capability to accommodate a large number of accessories. This is probably one of the most common items purchased by students with access to funding such as the Disabled Student Allowance (DSA). The equipment is usually sited at the student's home or hall of residence and is used for producing written work and for accessing text.

The other type of computer that may be useful to visually impaired students is the laptop (see Figure 8.2). This is a portable piece of equipment and so can be used both at home and in lectures, either attached to the mains supply or using integral batteries that are usually rechargeable. Portable PCs vary in size and capability but some have equal processing power to desktop computers. Palmtops are the smallest computers available at present and many people use them as personal organizers. For visually impaired users, however, the screens of laptops can be more difficult to access than those of desktops, for the following reasons:

(1) Many screens have poor contrast due to the use of liquid crystal technology. This is not always the case, however, as some laptops now have colour screens with contrast almost as good as desktop monitors.
(2) The smaller size of screen and consequently reduced text size – although some companies are now producing larger screens which may be of sufficient size to cater for a percentage of visually impaired users, with or without the requisite access technology.

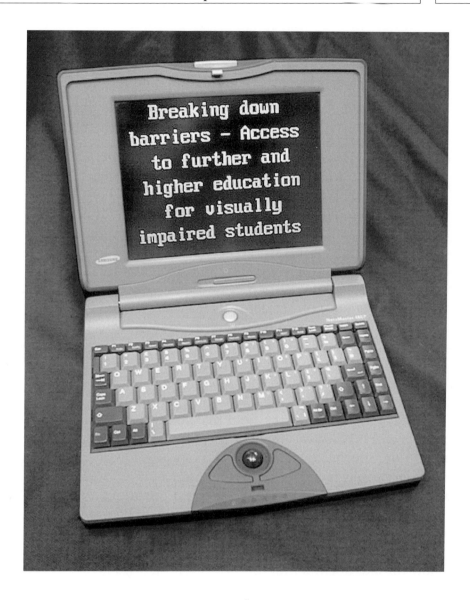

Figure 8.2 Laptop computer.

(3) Layout.
(4) Decreased backlight.

If students still consider laptops to be the most appropriate equipment for their requirements, access technology is available which can be used to overcome these difficulties to a certain extent. It is important, however, that commercially available equipment is considered, particularly by partially sighted people with a considerable degree of useful vision. The assumption should not be made that because someone is partially sighted he or she will not be able to use non-specialist equipment.

Earlier computers used DOS (Disc Operating System) and all of the associated software was based on this. More recently, DOS has been superseded by Windows, which is a graphical system that has allowed greater standardization in software operation. It is, however, designed as a very visual computer environment based on a screen made up of hundreds of tiny dots (pixels) as opposed to the text-based DOS applications, meaning that screen readers can no longer read exactly what is displayed on the screen (Morley, 1995). It also uses an on-screen pointer controlled by a mouse to highlight icons, which enables navigation around the system. This has proved to be a barrier to people with a visual impairment, many of whom still use DOS, which allows easier access. Until fairly recently, there seemed to be a general feeling that most visually impaired people would never be able to work with Windows, but there are now a number of developments in the field that should encourage prospective users. Windows 95 includes a limited text enlargement system and the specialized access technology is gradually improving, which will hopefully facilitate its use by more students with a visual impairment. Morley (1995) has produced an introductory guide in a variety of media, to help visually impaired users to access Windows. Manufacturers are also becoming more aware of disability issues and are working with developers of access systems as well as producing more appropriate documentation for non-sighted users.

Accessories

Monitors

Desktop computers have monitors of a standard size included in the price. These are usually high-quality, 14 or 15-inch, colour screens with good contrast. They are large enough for use by a percentage of visually impaired students. Personal experience, however, indicates that more partially sighted students are able to use computers satisfactorily without the need for additional access technology if standard monitors are replaced with larger ones, for example, 17, 20 or 21-inch screens. These do, however, tend to be more expensive (see Figure 8.3).

A 20-inch monitor offers approximately 1.5–2 times the magnification of standard size monitors. It is advisable for a student to view a monitor before purchase if possible. The points to check are brightness, clarity and amount of flicker – the latter should be minimal. Two other useful features are a tilt and swivel base and a non-glare screen (RNIB Employment Development and Technology Unit, 1997a).

It should be noted that if the student's preference is to access material on the computer via methods such as speech or refreshable Braille line, the size of the screen may be irrelevant.

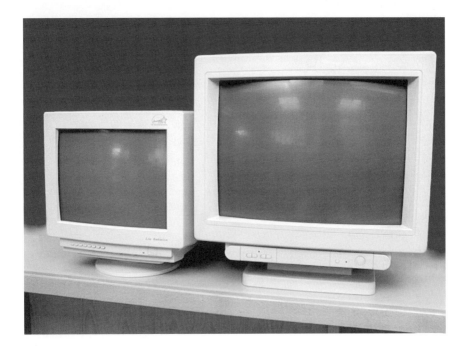

Figure 8.3 Comparison of monitor sizes.

Printers

If a student has a computer, it will be necessary to have access to a printer in order to produce any written work. The two main types are inkjet (or bubble-jet) and laser printers, which both produce good-quality, high-contrast print. Inkjet printers tend to be rather slow but produce letter-quality print at low cost (see Figure 8.4). The print produced by laser printers (see Figure 8.5) is the best quality. These are faster than the inkjet printers, but tend to be more expensive, although prices are becoming more reasonable. Inkjet printers are smaller and lighter, which may be an advantage to students who have to move around. There are also portable printers available, for example those designed for use with a laptop that can

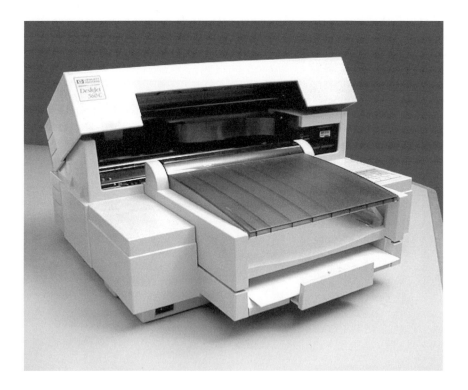

Figure 8.4 Inkjet printer.

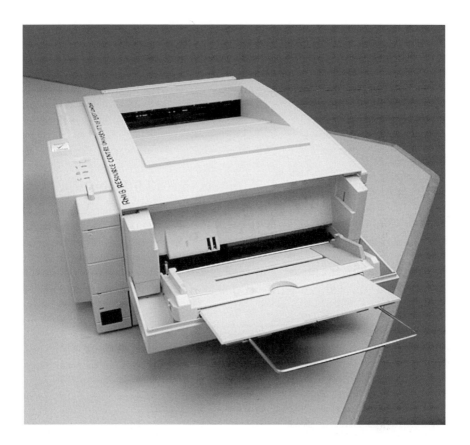

Figure 8.5 Laser printer.

be carried in the same case. This could be particularly useful to students on work placements.

Depending on the student's requirements, some important features to look for if purchasing a printer may be the range of fonts/print styles it can produce, the range of point sizes (size of character available) and whether it can print graphics (RNIB Employment Development and Technology Unit, 1997b). These features can be explored during an assessment or by asking manufacturers for demonstrations of printouts.

Colour printers are also available. Some partially sighted students should have the option to purchase this equipment if they have the available funding, particularly in the situation where access to text is facilitated by the use of specific colours. This would usually be an inkjet printer as laser colour printers are still expensive. If the students have no funding for this equipment, then they should have the opportunity to access a colour printer on the college site if one is available.

Scanners

These are devices that enable computers to read information from paper (printed text or graphics) and then to display it on screen (see Figure 8.6). The technology used to produce the image on screen is known as an optical character reader and comprises two components:

(1) A scanner, which can be flat-bed (that is, the image is placed face down on a glass sheet while the scanner scans it – rather like a

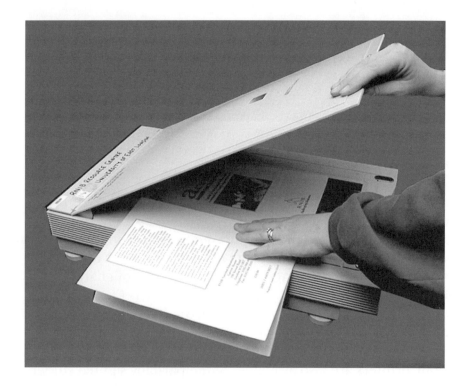

Figure 8.6 Flat-bed scanner.

photocopier) or hand held (here the device is placed on and moved over the text to be read). The latter kind is more difficult to use and practice is necessary.

(2) Recognition software which converts the scanned image into a computer-readable file (RNIB Employment Development and Technology Unit, 1997c).

The text stored in this way can then be manipulated using word-processing software or communicated to the student using a screen enlargement system, speech output or refreshable Braille line.

CD-ROM

Many computers now have integral CD-ROM drives as part of the purchasing package. If this is not the case, these can be bought as separate units. The CD-ROMs themselves are fairly robust plastic discs capable of storing large amounts of data. This data can take the form of text, graphics, animation, sound and video images – hence the term 'multimedia'.

There are large numbers of CD-ROMs available commercially, containing a huge diversity of information including games, encyclopaedias, design programmes (for example designing greetings cards or the layout and content of a new garden), educational programmes and so on. A large number of software programmes are also now loaded from CD-ROM rather than from diskette as in the past. As well as providing multimedia information, many of the discs also permit interactive use and provide a means to manipulate the computer environment.

In order to make full use of CD-ROM, a computer needs facilities for sound and video output. If a student or institution already has equipment without these accessories, upgrading is possible. This may be necessary if a course is utilizing this type of technology as a teaching method on a regular basis.

There are some access issues here for visually impaired students. As mentioned earlier, graphical user interfaces such as Windows are not as easy to access as DOS at present.

Enlargement systems

There are a variety of ways in which text and diagrams can be presented in an enlarged format. This is useful to some partially sighted students in facilitating access to general information as well as teaching and learning materials.

Paper based

Probably the least technical way to provide enlargement of standard print or diagrams is by the use of a photocopier. Material presented on sheets of A4 size paper can be enlarged to A3. The pros and cons of this method are discussed in Chapter 10. Some partially sighted students may find the provision of material in this medium satisfactory but it should be discussed with the individual.

A second way to provide enlarged text is by using a larger font size when printing a document from a computer file. This is more satisfactory for many students, as it dispenses with the need to manage very large sheets of paper. This method of producing enlarged text usually proves quite easy provided the computer and printer used have the requisite functions. (See Chapter 10 for information on alternative page layout. For further detail on printing large characters using a personal computer and a printer see RNIB Employment Development and Technology Unit, 1997d).

Closed Circuit Television (CCTV)

A CCTV is a piece of equipment made specifically for readers with a visual impairment, and many partially sighted people find them valuable. They can be used to support reading, writing and in some cases keyboard input when linked to a PC. Pictures, text and solid objects can be placed under the camera and a magnified image appears on the monitor or television screen. Magnification up to ×75 is possible but it does take practice to master the technique of reading with a CCTV.

Many CCTVs are available on the market, offering a wide range of features. There are a number of different varieties:

(1) Non-portable designs are meant for use on a desktop or work surface (see Figure 8.7). These usually have a built in camera and a moveable X–Y reading table that allows the position of the book or

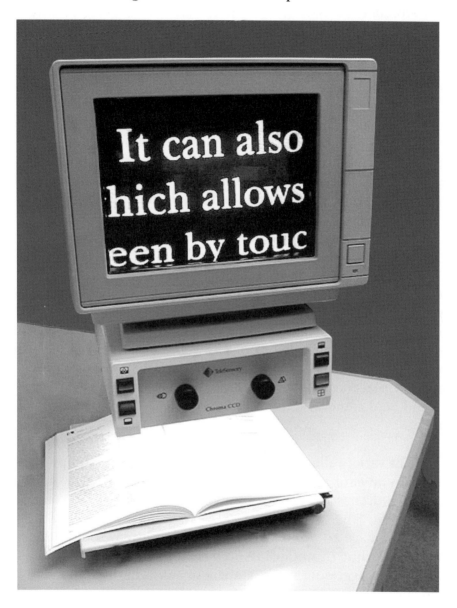

Figure 8.7 Desktop CCTV.

object to be changed easily. They normally offer a range of between ×5 and ×35 magnification, although this will depend on the distance between camera and the object or text as well as the size of the display screen.

The image on the display screen may be colour or monochrome. The black and white systems have the option of reversing the polarity, that is, switching foreground and background colours to give light text on a dark background or vice versa depending on user preference. They may also have a feature that allows shades of grey to be switched out, so giving a more sharply defined picture.

Colour displays often have an option that allows switching of foreground and background colours. They may also feature colour pairing, in which one colour is automatically changed to another, so for example a red diagram under the camera can be changed to blue. The latter feature may be useful for those visually impaired people who see some colours better than others.

(2) Portable CCTVs may have an integral screen or be designed to plug into a standard television. They are normally black and white (or black and some other light colour such as amber, green or cyan) with the same facility for change of polarity as the desktop versions. The cameras vary; some are hand-held (see Figure 8.8) and others are clamped or placed over the text in a similar way to a magnifying glass. The hand-held cameras tend to be more difficult to use than the static ones.

(3) The last variety allows the user to share a personal computer display with an external CCTV camera. In some cases this would involve the purchase of extra software or hardware for the computer.

Some CCTVs have an option of changing the display so that there is a horizontal overline or underline on screen to assist reading along lines of text or accessing mathematical or other figure-based data such as spreadsheets. A number of the systems also allow blacking out or shading of the screen beyond the boundaries of these lines. This helps the user to concentrate on the relevant area of the text (RNIB

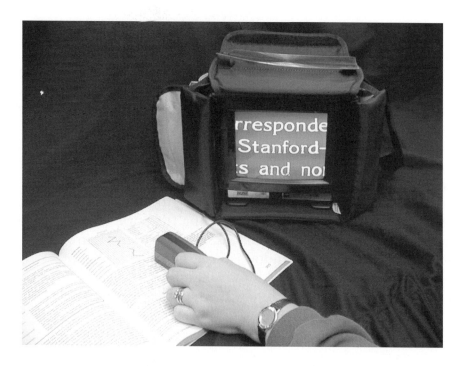

Figure 8.8 Portable CCTV with hand-held camera.

Employment Development and Technology Unit, 1997e). The CCTVs on the market vary considerably in price depending on whether they are monochrome or colour. The price also increases in relation to the number of extra facilities required in order to access text satisfactorily (Lodge and Arthurs, 1996).

It is important that the student has the option to see and test out a variety of the available CCTVs in order to ensure the most appropriate choice of equipment is made for individual visual needs and particular course requirements.

Screen magnification systems

As mentioned earlier, some visually impaired people may find the magnification provided by a large monitor on a computer to be satisfactory without the need for specific access technology. The advantage of this is that the whole screen can be viewed at one time.

If this does not provide sufficient magnification however, a screen magnification, system can be used.

Screen magnification systems are not stand-alone products. They are usually software programmes that increase the image of other applications running on a computer displayed on the screen. Some require the fitting of a PC card that needs to be installed into an expansion slot in the computer itself.

A disadvantage of these enlargement systems is that only a portion of the original screen image is shown at one time (see Figure 8.9). Most programmes offer the option of enlarging the whole screen or variable amounts such as a line for reading text, or a box that could be used with a spreadsheet or database package (see Figure 8.10). In these cases the magnified window is superimposed on the non-magnified display. This window will, under normal circumstances, automatically follow the focus of attention on the

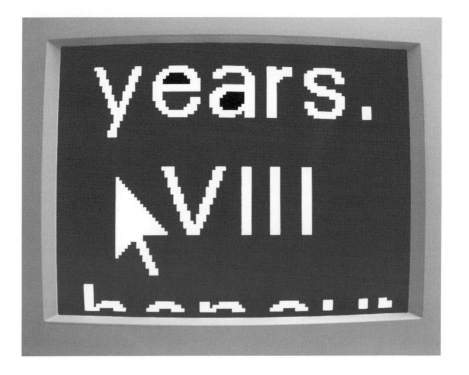

Figure 8.9 Enlarged text on screen.

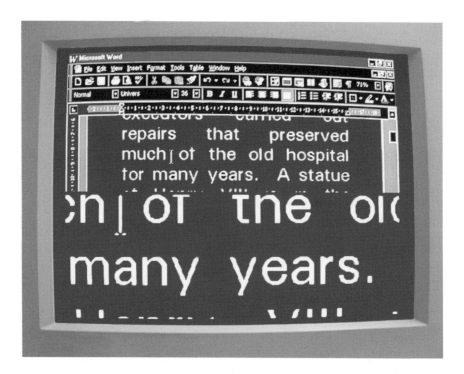

Figure 8.10 Split-screen enlargement.

screen, that is the cursor, mouse pointer or highlighted item. It is, however, possible to view other parts of the screen as required using the mouse or keystrokes. Most systems also have an adjustable-speed automatic scroll feature.

Some magnification systems, such as ZoomText and Lunar, also offer the facility to change the colour of text and background, giving a range of contrasts to suit individual requirements.

The choice of magnification system will depend upon a number of factors. First the visual ability of the individual student must be considered in relation to the available features of the chosen system. This again emphasizes the importance of a technology assessment. Second, the types of computer application with which the system will be required to work need to be ascertained. This is due to some instances of incompatibility; for example, some magnification systems are unable to enlarge graphics. It is important that this is checked before any purchase is made. If the system chosen is software only, it is usually possible to obtain a demonstration disk that will enable the student to try it with the appropriate packages. Finally, the student will need to learn some new skills in order to use the magnification system. The choice of system, therefore, may depend to a certain extent upon whether the user prefers keyboard or mouse controls, although some packages offer both facilities.

If the student's choice of equipment is a laptop computer, most software-only magnification systems will run on current portables (RNIB Employment Development and Technology Unit, 1997f). If funding is available, it is essential for the individual student, before purchase, to check the screen quality and size.

There are some magnification systems available for use with Windows. These work similarly to the DOS-based systems and most programmes will again follow the focus of attention on screen. This can usually be customized to suit individual preference. With some of these systems the on screen characters can look jagged on very high magnification, which could be a problem for some users. Those with a font-smoothing feature reduce this problem, making the characters easier to identify (see Figure 8.11).

As mentioned earlier, Windows 95 has a limited number of integral magnification features allowing most screen elements to be enlarged and appropriate fonts and font sizes to be chosen. This is not, however, equivalent to the specific magnification systems described earlier and does not give the same level of access or

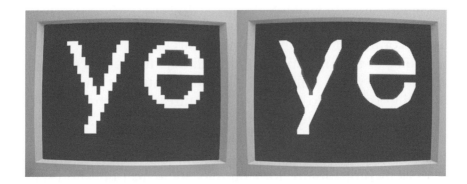

Figure 8.11 Font smoothing.

flexibility. Windows 95 also provides a means of changing the size, shape and colour of the mouse pointer on screen, as some users have difficulty locating its position. If this latter facility is not inbuilt, there are some programmes available that are written specifically for this purpose (for example the shareware package Meta-Mouse). Finally, Windows 95 provides a number of high-contrast colour schemes which some visually impaired users may find helpful (RNIB Employment Development and Technology Unit, 1997g; Lodge and Arthurs, 1996).

When purchasing screen magnification systems, institutions should look for those such as Lunar that can be loaded on to any existing network. This will enable some visually impaired students to use electronic mail and other services provided by the college in this way. If wider access of this type is intended by the institution, it is important to enquire about site licences, as these are required before the package can be made available to multiple users.

Speech systems

For some visually impaired students, the use of speech in various forms may comprise a major part of their study method. As discussed in Chapter 10, many students make use of cassette tapes for recording lectures and for accessing text when available. This is a relatively low-tech method and the most widely used, but it can be a useful adjunct to study. It does, however, have some drawbacks, as it can be slower than reading text, scanning is not possible and the method requires practice and concentration.

Some models of cassette recorder have special features added and are particularly useful for people with a visual impairment. These features may include tactile markings on buttons, large high contrast controls, pitch/speed control (to allow the tape to be played up to twice the speed at which it was recorded), pulsing or cue/review facilities for marking and quickly finding sections on a tape, two or four tracks for recording, and inbuilt microphones.

Other miscellaneous low-tech speech system equipment that may be useful to students on some courses includes devices such as talking calculators, a colour tester (reads out the colour of the surface on which it is placed), a talking compass and various Teletext readers (Lodge, 1996).

There are now more high-tech options for students to use in both college and work placement settings. Depending upon circumstances, they may also be suitable for use after qualification in some work situations. The options consist of electronic equipment that has speech output either as an integral part of the system or as an add-on feature. Voice recognition systems for computers are also gradually becoming more reliable and their development continues at a fast pace.

Some portable devices have inbuilt speech systems. They include both custom-designed note takers of various sorts and standard portable computers. It is also possible to add speech systems to desktop and laptop computers.

Speech systems for use with personal computers

These usually consist of two components; a speech synthesizer and a screen reading programme.

Speech synthesizers usually have an inbuilt speaker and headphone socket, which gives some flexibility as to where the system can be used (that is, the speaker could be used when the student is working alone, but the headphones are useful in examination situations or libraries). The speaker or headphones produce speech output from text sent to them from the computer. The synthesizer may be an external piece of equipment plugged into a computer port (see Figure 8.12), or a card that needs to be installed into an expansion slot inside the computer. The voice of the synthesizer can sound rather robotic and may, initially, be difficult to understand. Over time and with practice however, this becomes less of a problem. RNIB has produced a comparison cassette tape that gives examples of the voices of a number of the synthesizers. This may be useful to potential purchasers.

Screen-reading programmes send instructions from the user to the synthesizer. The software can be used in two modes; 'live' or 'review'. The live mode is interactive and so, for example, the words are

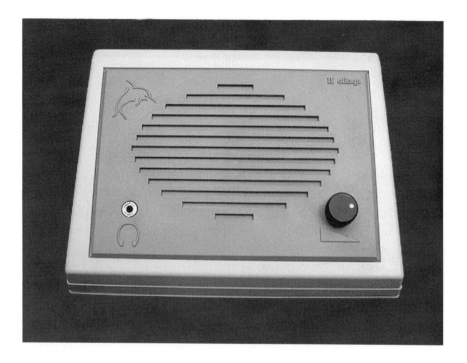

Figure 8.12 External speech synthesizer.

spoken by the synthesizer as a student enters text on to the screen. In 'review' mode, no changes can be made to the text, as direct communication with the speech system is frozen, but text already entered can be read.

(Many screen-reading systems are now designed to be used with both speech and Braille output.)

Typical features include the following possibilities:

- The whole screen is read out.
- Just one line is read out.
- One word is read out at a time.
- Individual letters can be read out or their phonetic equivalents.
- Capital letters, punctuation and symbols can be indicated.
- Speed, pitch, volume and tone can be altered for individual preference.

The text read by the system can come from a number of sources:

- entered by the student;
- from a file on a floppy disk (for example, lecture notes provided by a member of academic staff);
- from a CD-ROM;
- information downloaded from the Internet;
- text that has been scanned on to the computer and interpreted by an OCR programme.

Screen readers and speech synthesizers can be purchased separately, but many suppliers now provide complete speech systems that incorporate both as a package (for example the Dolphin Apollo system consists of an Apollo II synthesizer and Hal screen-reading software).

As with magnification systems, it is important to check that there are no incompatibilities between the speech system purchased for the computer and any other applications the student needs to use. Windows is a more complex system than DOS and is generally more difficult to use with speech, but the access technology is improving. As there are substantial differences between the ways in which Windows 95 and previous versions of Windows operate, it is essential to check with the supplier whether the speech system will work correctly. For example, at present a product such as Window Eyes works only with Windows 3.1; Jaws and Window Bridge work with both Windows 3.1 and Windows 95; ProTalk 32 is a screen reader for Windows 95 and Windows NT; and WinVision 2 works for both DOS and Windows 3.x. (RNIB Employment Development and Technology Unit, 1997h).

Some screen enlargement systems (such as ZoomText Xtra!) now feature fully synchronized magnification and screen reading systems. These have inbuilt Text-to-Speech software that supports all Windows soundcards, that is, they make use of the computer's existing sound card, so dispensing with the need to purchase a separate synthesizer.

Many new computers now have inbuilt capacity for multimedia use which includes a soundcard. If both the soundcard and the speech access software chosen are SSIL (Speech Synthesiser Interface Library) compatible, this would obviate the need to purchase a separate speech synthesizer, so saving around £400. The soundcard would, in this case, need to be dedicated to speech only and so would not be available to produce other sounds such as those normally heard in the Windows environment, or music. These details should be checked with the relevant manufacturers before purchase.

As with all of the equipment discussed in this chapter, the student will need some training. The amount of training and after-sale support offered by suppliers could be a factor in deciding which system to purchase. Training is also available from a number of independent trainers as well as organizations such as RNIB. As mentioned earlier, it is likely that any training will involve some cost and this needs to be remembered when considering financial implications.

Some of the speech systems can be used with laptop computers. An important point for institutions to consider is whether the software being purchased can be loaded on to the network; for example, this is possible with Hal. If students intend to use speech as a study method, when they attend for informal visits or interviews it may be useful to discuss the institution's facilities and to enquire about which systems, if any, are available on existing networks. Again, site licences need to be purchased for multiple users.

Speech output for portable computers and note takers

Most of the portable speech systems for laptop computers consist of battery powered speech synthesizers and screen-reading software. Some of the batteries are rechargeable. The available synthesizers can work with a variety of screen-reading programmes, although one type known as Arctic Transport has its own inbuilt screen-reading software. One make of synthesizer called Keynote Gold is different in that it is available on a credit-card size card that is inserted into the appropriate port on the laptop. It takes its power (a very small amount) from the computer itself.

There are a number of portable Braille displays for use with laptops, some of which incorporate an inbuilt speech synthesizer, for example, the CombiBraille 45 and the Alva Delphi Terminals.

There are also a number of note takers that have the facility of speech output. These pieces of equipment may be very useful for some students in that they can be used to take notes in lectures and practical classes. The various types of note taker offer a variety of functions, some acting as a personal organizer (including diary, word processor, telephone directory, calculator, clock, and file manager – for example the Aria), whereas others are more basic, simply being able to store information entered from the keyboard plus having the facilities of a talking clock, calculator and calendar (for example the Braille 'n Speak 2000).

There are other variations. Some note takers have speech only output (Aria, Type 'n Speak) whereas others have both speech and Braille output which can be used together or separately (Braille Lite). Other differences are found in the keyboards: some have a Braille keyboard (Braille Lite, Braille 'n Speak 2000) and others a qwerty keyboard (Type 'n Speak, TransType, Keynote Companion). Most of these note takers can be connected to a personal computer and/or printer (RNIB Employment Development and Technology Unit, 1997f).

Voice recognition (VR)

Voice recognition allows control of a computer by the use of voice; information can also be entered on to the computer by the same method. This has obvious advantages for visually impaired users. The systems are constantly being developed and refined and only recently have they become commercially available. The main reason for this apparent delay in availability has been the need for a fast PC, such as a Pentium or better. At the moment no VR system is 100% accurate and for the first time user the best that can be expected is approximately 80–90% accuracy. This sounds promising but it equates with having to repeat one or two words in every ten spoken into the computer, which may become extremely tedious. The average typing speed is 35 words per minute and so the VR system would need to match or outdo this rate in order to be commercially viable and practical to use. Once systems reach this rate there may well be more investment available from companies for further development.

All VR systems need training and become more reliable and accurate as this ensues. This training involves that of the user with the system and training of the system to the user's voice. The latter is the most important and the most time consuming. To obtain good results, 40–100 hours of training may be necessary. With the majority of systems, the user has to pause after each word and this may be difficult to judge in the first instance. This is rather an unnatural way to talk and may take practice. Consistency of the voice is also essential if good results are to be obtained. Volume and pitch are important and there may be problems if a user's voice temporarily changes, for example if someone has a cold or laryngitis. Anyone considering the purchase of a VR system needs to take into account the environment in which the equipment is to be placed. The systems are not intelligent and will try to recognize any noise picked up by the microphone; a noisy environment is therefore unsuitable.

VR systems have dictionaries that vary in size; for example among the main systems available at present, Dragon Dictate Solo has a 120,000 word dictionary, Kurtzweil Voicepad Pro has 200,000 words and IBM Voicetype has 30,000 words. With a smaller dictionary the likelihood of encountering unknown words increases, although new words can be added during use.

Although VR systems have definite advantages for visually impaired users, more development will be necessary before they can reach their full potential. At present, only Dragon Dictate Solo allows direct control of Windows and its applications (that is, commands such as Open File, Print, Close and so on). It also offers voice input into many Windows applications. Even so, the levels of accuracy are not yet good enough to allow full access for totally blind users. There may be problems of conflict with other access systems such as speech output, as PCs are not yet fast enough to cope with simultaneous running of a number of complex systems. There is also the issue of whether the VR system listens to the voice of the user or that of the speech output system. So more work will be necessary to iron out these problems. Voice recognition will, however, be an important development in improving access to PCs for visually impaired users (Guyver, 1997).

Scanners

Scanners are often an important part of the overall process of accessing text for eventual speech output (and also Braille output). They are devices that allow computers to read information from paper and then to display this on screen relatively quickly. This avoids the need to enter text by hand (Lodge, 1996). Scanners are used widely in desktop publishing, particularly for incorporating graphics into documents. The material to be scanned is placed face down on a glass sheet and the scanner 'scans' it in a similar way to a photocopier – in effect it takes a snapshot of the page. The information is then converted into a pattern of dots that can be interpreted by the computer (Arthurs, 1996). The OCR software is instrumental in this conversion, which then enables the computer to produce the text on screen. Once the process has reached this stage, the information can be enlarged as text on screen, read by a speech synthesizer, displayed using a refreshable Braille line, or produced on a Braille embosser or in a large font and different layout by a printer.

This technology is very useful in providing independent access to text-based information. Most scanners are relatively straightforward to use and have high success rates, but they do have limitations; for example, they are unable to access hand-written documents, some coloured text and dot matrix text. The success of the scan depends on a number of factors: the quality and capabilities of the equipment, the complexity and arrangement of the page layout, the font used, the quality of the original and the number of illustrations. The process is not always straightforward, as the conversion of the text may not be 100% accurate. If the original is of high quality with a clear font, no diagrams, no columns and no anomalies (for example, any extraneous marks on the page), then the OCR may be perfect. From experience, however, when accessing textbooks or journals, this is very rarely the case, and if the original is a photocopy with any grey shading or small black marks or lines, the scan can be seriously affected. A scan of a good photocopy of a journal article however, commonly reaches 75–80% accuracy. A speech synthesizer can read the text produced on screen but the student needs to be prepared to check for any inaccurate translation.

It is important to note how much longer it takes a visually impaired student to access text using this method than it takes a student with full sight to read it in the conventional manner.

There may be advantages for teaching staff in that if a bank of electronically stored information is gradually built up by scanning material used on a course on to computer, it could then be easily accessed and/or produced in a variety of formats (print, Braille, speech) as necessary.

Types of scanning system

Scanning systems are classified into two types: (a) those that can be added on to PCs, and (b) stand-alone systems.

The PC-based OCR systems vary in their capabilities and the equipment included in the price. Some provide software only and others include a scanner or choice of scanners, with the price varying accordingly. For example, OsCaR is a software-based DOS OCR package supplied (in the UK) with a flat-bed scanner. It works automatically with some speech systems (such as Vert) but may need changes in configuration in order to work with others. The Reading AdvantEdge is also a software based OCR system, but this can be supplied as software only or with a flat bed or Bookedge scanner (see Figure 8.13) as required.

The stand-alone scanner systems work without the aid of a computer but tend to be more expensive, as the microprocessors and speech systems are inbuilt. These also vary in capability and price. Many are able to store text for future use (for example, the Reading Edge can store about 150 pages, whereas the Reading ACE can store up to 15,000 A4 pages), but some do not have this capability and text needs to be downloaded to a PC for storage (for example, the Robotron Rainbow).

Some products, such as the Omni 1000, are sold either as stand-alone systems or as a software only package for installation on to a PC.

Standard OCR packages sold commercially for people with full sight are often accurate enough as text readers for visually impaired users. Many of the more recent ones operate only with Windows. The

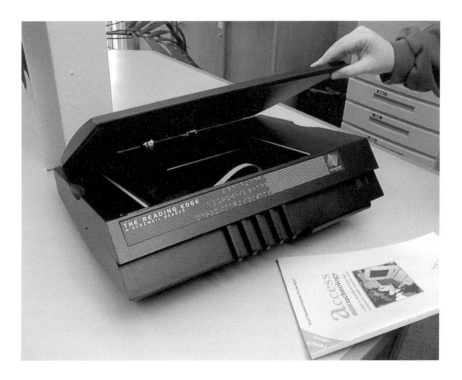

Figure 8.13   Bookedge scanner.

main advantage of these is the lower cost but, as they are designed for sighted users, they may be more difficult to operate for visually impaired people with little experience of this type of technology. (See RNIB Employment Development and Technology Unit, 1997c; Lodge, 1996.)

Braille systems

Braille is a tactile code used instead of print as a medium for reading and writing text. A relatively small percentage of visually impaired people use this method, most of whom have learnt the skill while at school, although some people who lose their sight later in life are able to attend Braille courses if they wish.

The letters in Braille comprise combinations of up to six raised dots arranged in 'cells' in a pattern similar to that on a domino. Devices used for writing Braille therefore have six keys each representing one dot in the Braille cell. The basic code is known as Grade I Braille, in which each letter of the alphabet is represented by a particular pattern of dots. Most experienced braillists, however, use Grade II Braille, which is a type of shorthand where many common words are represented by particular 'contractions' or smaller combinations of dots and cells. Use of this method can increase the speed of note taking considerably. Using a Braille keyboard (see later) can be faster than using a qwerty keyboard.

There are other Braille codes, including one that uses eight dots, the extra two dots being used to show characteristics of the text that the six dots cannot represent. There is a computer Braille code (sometimes called Grade O) as well as codes for languages other than English. This latter point has implications for Braille users undertaking foreign language study as a new Braille code may need to be learnt before it is possible for the student to begin the course. Conversely, it may be possible to learn the new Braille code alongside the new language, but this would depend very much on the capabilities of the individual student.

It can take a number of months to learn Braille and for many people it takes even longer to become proficient, particularly to reach a standard sufficient to be able to take an academic course. This is one of the reasons why it would be inadvisable for a student suddenly to decide to use tactile methods of study at the beginning of or during the course. If a student is aware that tactile methods may become necessary due to deterioration in vision or the nature of the course, it would be advisable for the learning of Braille to be undertaken before commencing an educational programme. There is likely to be little or no opportunity to do this once the course begins, although this will depend on the capabilities of the individual.

Braille can be used for a number of purposes. Students can access text directly from Braille books if available or from print by utilizing technology to be described shortly. Some students may choose to produce their work in Braille, in which case transcription will usually be necessary before marking can take place. Alternatively students can input material on to a computer using a modified Braille keyboard and the work can then be printed out as standard text. Finally, students may request that course material is presented to them in a Braille format, in which case academic staff would need to be aware of methods and sources of Braille production.

Braille production

The most basic method in common use for producing Braille is a portable mechanical brailler such as the Perkins (see Figure 8.14). This is a low-tech piece of equipment which, although relatively simple to use, is bulky, noisy and quite slow. Some visually impaired people, however, still use this type of equipment on a regular basis to produce small amounts of Braille. It is unlikely that this would be an efficient method for academic staff to use in the production of course material for students. If a student chooses to use a Perkins Brailler to

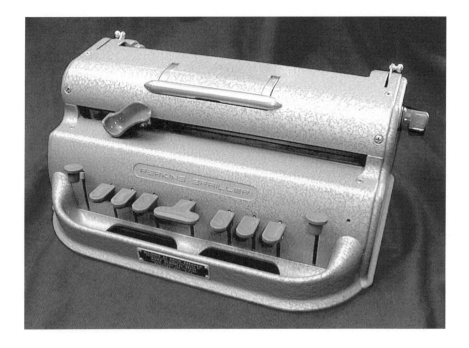

Figure 8.14 Perkins Brailler.

produce coursework or to answer examination papers in Braille, it is possible to produce a print version simultaneously by using a piece of equipment called the Braille 'n Print (see Figure 8.15). This is a mains driven device that forms a base for the Perkins and this is in turn connected to a printer (dot matrix or daisy wheel).

Braille is more conveniently produced on an embosser (see Figure 8.16) that prints Braille output from text entered on to a computer. This connects to a computer or note taker in the same way as a conventional printer but produces the Braille by punching dots on to paper. Before the text can be embossed however, it has to be converted into Braille format by translation software.

Embossers

When choosing an embosser, the most important factor to consider is the purpose for which it will be used, that is, whether the intention is to produce small amounts of Braille occasionally for one or two

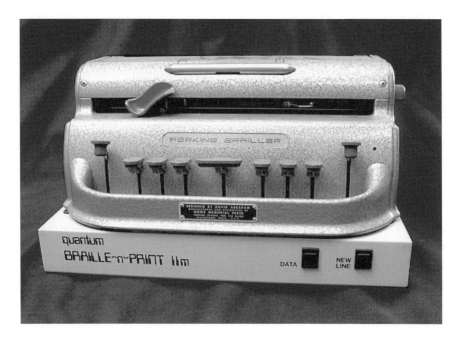

Figure 8.15 Braille 'n' Print.

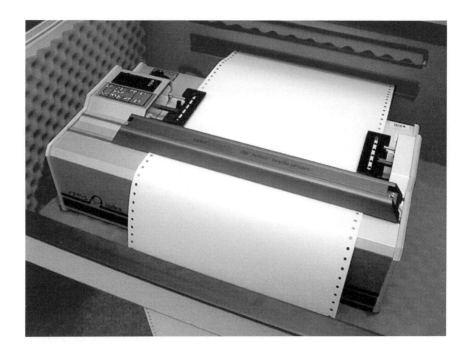

Figure 8.16 Braille embosser.

people, or large-scale Braille production for a larger number of recipients. Embossers range from cheaper, slower models more suitable for individual use to the fast, heavy-duty machines required for regular high-output brailling. The latter are inevitably more expensive. Most machines can be configured to print six or eight dot Braille (RNIB Employment Development and Technology Unit, 1997i).

Embossers differ from one another in the following ways:

- Speed – measured in characters per second (cps), which can vary from 10 cps to 200 cps in the heavy-duty models.
- Graphics capability (that is, the ability of the embosser to use the Braille dots to produce tactile graphics or ink graphics together with the Braille – specific software is necessary for these functions).
- Weight.
- Size.

- Sideways embossing capability (for wide lines such as program listing or spreadsheets).
- Price.
- Interface (parallel or serial).
- Noise levels.
- Quality of Braille – the type of paper used will also affect this.
- Ease of operation – this is particularly important for totally blind users with regard to loading and aligning paper and control of the machine. Some models have audio messages to alert the user to faults.
- Variable impact for different paper weights.
- Single or double sided embossing.

Some embossers are portable (such as the Blazie Braille Blazer) or transportable (the Romeo) wheras others (such as the Index embossers and the Juliet) are larger and need permanent sites. As mentioned earlier, prices vary depending on capability; the heavy duty embossers, which may be more suitable for institutional use, are, inevitably, more expensive (Hampson, 1996; RNIB Employment Development and Technology Unit, 1997i).

Acoustic hoods

Embossing Braille is a very noisy process, which could be disturbing if the machine is housed in the same room as people working or studying. It is therefore advisable to obtain an acoustic hood to keep the noise to a minimum.

Translation software

As noted earlier, in order to be able to produce Braille on an embosser from a computer, translation software is necessary. The software chosen will depend upon whether the individual can read Braille or not and on the nature of the material to be embossed. Most printed material can be accurately translated by the software. If a particular layout or specialist characters are needed however (for example, mathematical or scientific notation), it may not be suitable.

More sophisticated software will be necessary for translating this type of material, for example Braille Maker Professional, which allows translation of information such as mathematical formulae and different languages. Again, the more sophisticated the software, the higher the price.

Braille labels

It may be useful in some instances to provide tactile labels and these can be produced in Braille on clear or coloured tape.

Braille note takers

Students who are Braille users may find it helpful to purchase a Braille note taker. This can be taken into class or work placements so that notes may be stored to be accessed later for personal study. It is worth pointing out the usefulness of Braille note takers for taking down information 'in the dark', for example, in a classroom that has been blacked out for showing slides. Some partially sighted people may be braillists and it is not wise to assume that, because someone has reasonable vision and generally uses 'sighted' study methods, she or he does not write and/or read Braille. The note takers can be classified according to the type of keyboard and these are briefly described below:

Mechanical Braille keyboards

These are becoming rather outdated but probably the best known of these is the Perkins Brailler, which was mentioned earlier.

Electronic Braille keyboards

Note takers with electronic keyboards support the typical layout for keying in Braille, that is, six keys and a space bar (see Figure 8.17). Some also have features such as cursor keys, function keys or a Braille display. The note takers are very light and portable due to the presence of the Braille keyboard and the absence of a screen,

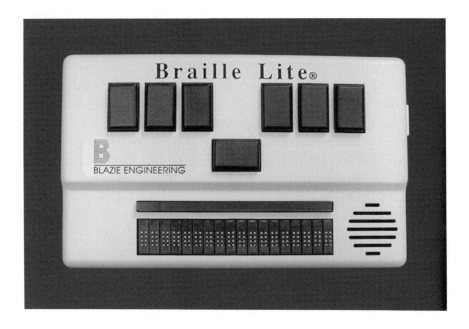

Figure 8.17 Braille keyboard on Braille Lite note taker.

meaning a lighter and smaller battery can be used. This feature makes these pieces of equipment very useful in class or on work placements.

There are a small number of Braille keyboards available that can be connected directly to a PC, for example the Braille In. This has a ten-key Braille keyboard (eight Braille keys, one for each of the eight Braille dots in computer Braille plus a space bar for each thumb). It can emulate all the key combinations on the qwerty keyboard.

Electronic qwerty keyboards

Braille can also be entered using a qwerty keyboard but this requires a software programme. Six keys of the qwerty keyboard are designated as Braille keys. Although it is possible to do this, it is unlikely this feature would be found on the small portable note takers.

All of the electronic note takers have a variety of functions, some of which were mentioned in the section on speech output. As a reminder, some of these functions and features are mentioned below (along with some additions relating more specifically to Braille):

- Word processing.
- Spell checker.
- Diary, telephone directory, calculator, clock, and file manager.
- Some allow the user the choice to key in Grade I Braille, Grade II Braille or computer Braille, whereas others are more limited.
- Serial/parallel ports allowing communication with a PC, printer, modem or Braille embosser
- ROM for reading long documents. Some note takers have the capacity for transferring parts of a document loaded into the ROM into RAM (random access memory) for editing.
- Speech output.
- Refreshable Braille display (plus speech).
- Rechargeable battery.
- External disk drive.
- Memory card.

It is important to remember that not all note takers have all of the above features. If a student chooses to use any available funding to purchase one for study purposes it is important to check carefully with manufacturers about specific features. These are relatively expensive pieces of equipment with prices varying according to individual requirements; for example, if an external disk drive is necessary the overall package will cost more.

A more sophisticated machine is the David. This cannot really be classified as a note taker but more appropriately as a Braille computer and, due to this, the price is even greater. It has a 44-cell refreshable Braille line and is compatible with PCs. It has the facility for speech as well as Braille output and has an inbuilt Grade II Braille translation program. It is possible to connect the David to a standard monitor and keyboard. Text can be produced in print or on a Braille embosser. Finally it can act as a Braille display for standard PCs. (Hampson, 1996; RNIB Employment Development and Technology Unit, 1997f).

Since this equipment is so expensive, the need to offer students assessments becomes even more imperative if they are likely to need anything of this sort. If a substantial number of students attending the college are likely to need this type of access equipment, it may be necessary to consider an institutional purchase rather than each student trying to access funding to buy individual machines. There may be funding issues here, given the present financial climate, but this should be considered in overall institutional strategy for improving access for students and staff with disabilities.

Electronic Braille displays

In general terms, an electronic Braille display is a tactile device placed under a conventional qwerty keyboard which enables the user to read the computer screen display in Braille (see Figure 8.18). Referred to as refreshable Braille lines earlier in the chapter, they are also known as paperless or soft Braille displays. There is a variable number of Braille cells – 20, 40 or 80 – and, given that each line on a

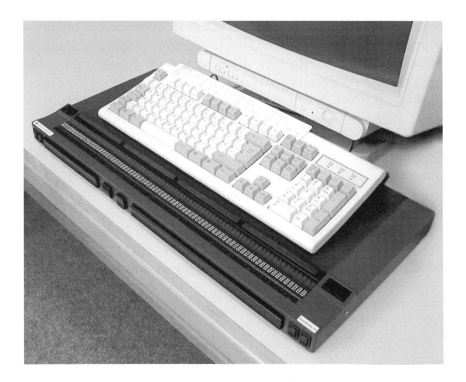

Figure 8.18 Electronic Braille display.

standard computer screen consists of 80 characters, they can show, respectively, a quarter, a half or a whole line at a time. The 20 and 40 cell Braille lines can be used with laptop computers.

Each cell on the Braille line comprises six or eight pins, which may be metal or nylon. These are controlled electronically and move up and down to change the Braille version of characters shown on the monitor as the user moves around the screen. These Braille displays are usually used to read text although in some cases they can provide access to graphical screens such as those used in Windows programmes.

There are a number of electronic Braille displays available. These are similar, but have slightly different functions and capabilities. Some of them are mentioned below:

- Additional cells to display information about screen attributes (for example, colour) and display status.
- Buttons to move the Braille display to different areas of the computer screen.
- Touch-activated cursor buttons next to each Braille cell to route the cursor to different areas of the screen.
- Eighty cell displays which can be divided (40/40 or 20/60). This can display information presented in columns or it can be used to monitor a separate part of the screen such as the status line.
- Separate function keys used to control and programme the operation of the display.
- Integrated qwerty keyboard and Braille display.
- Inbuilt speech synthesizer and screen reader.
- Internal rechargeable battery when used with laptop computers.
- Access to Windows via software such as WinDOTS, JAWS for Windows, Window Bridge, ProTalk and so on.

As for the note takers, not all Braille displays have all of these features. It is important for potential purchasers to check carefully all of the relevant details with the manufacturer before choosing their equipment. If the details are too confusing for those with little experience, an organization such as RNIB can offer advice.

The prices for these Braille displays are high, with 20 and 40 cells being somewhat cheaper than 80 cells. They may cost more than available funding allows for; for example, a student who is able to access the DSA would find the equipment allowance insufficient to purchase a Braille display (Hampson, 1996; RNIB Employment Development and Technology Unit, 1997j).

Accessing the Internet

For a large percentage of the population, using the Internet is becoming a common way of accessing vast quantities of material on all subjects as well as allowing almost instant communication with users anywhere in the world. It can be used in many ways, for example:

- sending and receiving messages via electronic mail;
- browsing, disseminating and retrieving information;
- keeping up to date with the news;
- discussion forums;
- communication with special interest groups – for example, there is a news group dedicated to blind computer users;
- accessing the World Wide Web – a huge collection of multimedia pages on almost every subject.

A large percentage of the information on the Internet is contained in electronic text files, meaning that it is very accessible compared with other media, such as books. It is also delivered direct to the user via the computer and so is a much faster and efficient method than physically going to the library.

Many institutions already have the facility for staff and students to access the Internet via the local network. Depending on circumstances, some students may find it advantageous to have this access from home also. If so, certain equipment will be necessary, comprising a computer and a modem – either internal or external. The modem enables the computer to send and receive data via a telephone line.

Once the equipment is in place, the user needs to connect to an Internet Service Provider (ISP). An ISP is a company providing a computer that the user connects to over the telephone line which acts as a gateway to the Internet. These companies differ in the services they provide and the way that they charge. There may be an initial set-up charge, but for some this is free. They provide software for accessing the Internet and instructions on how to install and set it up. There is then a monthly charge and this can vary depending on the services the user wishes to access. It is also important to remember the telephone bill, as the user will be charged for the time spent connected to the Internet via the telephone line.

The installation of software necessary to set up the Internet account as well as that of the preferred access system may require the assistance of a sighted user. But once this is in place, blind and partially sighted students should be able to proceed independently (Murnion, 1996). As with any technology, new users will need to practise, explore and experiment in order to become proficient in surfing the Net.

Apart from the points mentioned above regarding the amount of information available and the speed and convenience with which it can be accessed, for visually impaired users there can be tremendous advantages in using the Internet. As the information is electronic, the visually impaired user can be much more independent, not needing to rely on others to put material on tape or to scan it and produce it in Braille. The time delay involved in these processes is also avoided, as is the problem of identifying where specific information is held on a tape. Information can be easily retrieved on to the screen and accessed via the methods discussed in this chapter, such as screen magnification and speech. The relevant items can then be selected and saved on to the computer, to be produced in print of an appropriate font size or Braille as preferred (Murnion, 1996; Bosher, 1996).

Some courses may have part of their material available on the Internet, which could improve access for visually impaired students either in college or from home. Teaching staff sometimes make their lecture notes available in this way and indeed some assessment may be carried out electronically.

There is concern that access to the World Wide Web will be difficult for blind and some partially sighted users due to the large amount of graphics, visual displays and animation contained in Web pages. Most of the information is, however, plain ASCII text. By switching off the graphical part of the Web browser, the user can download Web pages much more quickly (Murnion, 1996). A free guide to the Internet and how to access it has been published for blind and partially sighted people by RNIB. Contact RNIB Customer Services for further information.

For the design of Web pages, there are a number of guidelines available that will help to make these pages as useful to the visually impaired user as to the person with full sight. A version of these can be found in Murnion (1996) or can be obtained from the RNIB Website (http://www.RNIB.org.uk). Advice for Website designers on good practice for visually impaired users can be obtained direct from the Website Editor at RNIB. There is a large amount of work being carried out internationally addressing accessibility for people with disabilities on many levels. There is a Web Accessibility Initiative (WAI) at the World Wide Web Consortium (W3C) and work is being done in partnership with many organizations around the world. Information can be found at the Website http://www.w3.org/WAI/References/.

Tactile diagrams

Some students may find tactile diagrams helpful as an adjunct to other study methods. They may help to provide a spatial element which can be useful to some visually impaired people. Their production, however, can be difficult and time consuming. This needs to be taken into account by staff, that is, sufficient time must be allowed for the production of diagrams (whether produced in house or by an external agency) and they should be prioritized in order that the student receives those that are most relevant.

For some partially sighted users it may be helpful to have relief versions of the diagrams that the rest of the students in the group receive. For those with less vision, however, it may be necessary to modify the diagrams before they can be effective. This could be a matter of straightforward simplification and the addition of Braille labels or it could entail redrawing and the addition of specific points of reference and textures. Complex shapes are difficult to recognize unless this type of modification is made (Hinton, 1988). In fact, some visually impaired people – including the totally blind – may not find diagrams helpful at all because they have had no experience of using them. It is always important for discussion to take place with all visually impaired students to ascertain what they would find useful.

The most common methods of producing tactile diagrams are 'swell paper systems' and 'vacuum forming'.

Swell paper systems

These systems require special paper (commonly referred to as 'swell paper') on to which diagrams can be photocopied. These should normally have undergone some modification before this stage is reached. The paper is then passed through a fuser (see Figure 8.19) which resembles a sophisticated grill. The heat causes the part of the

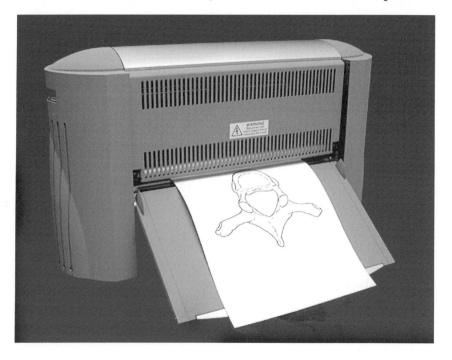

Figure 8.19 Fuser.

paper covered in the black lines to swell, so raising the diagram. An advantage here is that the production of the finished product is relatively fast. The lines are black on a light coloured paper, so giving good contrast. The relief, however, is all on one level, which could cause confusion. Some differentiation between areas of the diagram can be achieved by using patterns such as dots or cross-hatching. This needs to be used carefully, though, otherwise it could be disorientating for the user.

Vacuum forming

The second method of producing tactile diagrams is by making an original diagram, and then an image (or many images) of this can be created by warming sheets of plastic and using a vacuum to suck this on to the original (see Figure 8.20). Once the plastic has cooled, the raised image remains in place (see Figure 8.21). The advantages here are that diagrams can have multi-level relief and that differently textured materials can be used to make the original. Many copies can be made and the originals can be used for many years. From personal experience, however, construction of the original diagrams can be extremely difficult and can take a very long time. The time and effort involved, therefore, have to be weighed against the perceived benefit to the students.

Machines such as the Thermoform (seen in Fig. 8.22) and the Braille reproduction 350 may, however, be extremely useful in producing multiple copies of Braille text from an original card copy. The plastic sheets used have the advantage of being light and relatively easy to store. There are disadvantages, however, which include the following:

- The sheets are very slippery.
- The size is inconvenient, as they are square, not A4.
- If holes are punched in the sheets for the purpose of storage in a file the plastic tends to tear easily.
- For those partially sighted people who read Braille visually as opposed to manually the contrast between the raised dots and the plastic sheet is minimal, making them more difficult to see than raised dots on card.

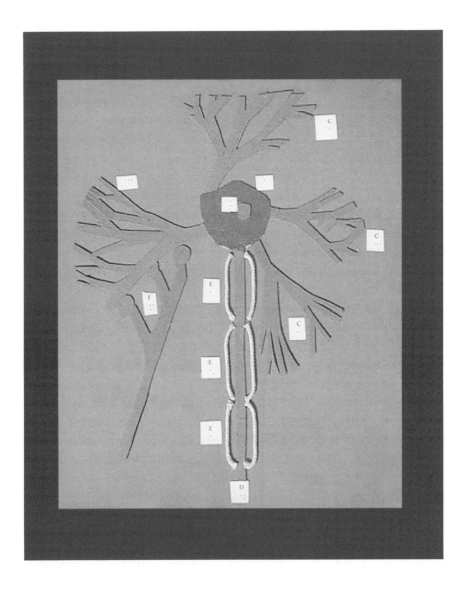

Figure 8.20 Vacuum forming: original diagram.

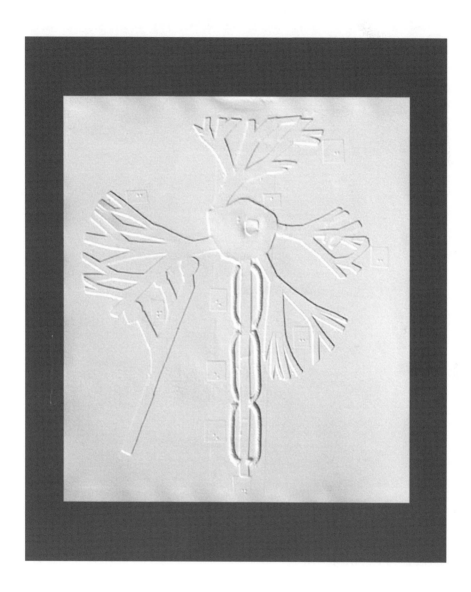

Figure 8.21 Vacuum forming: plastic copy.

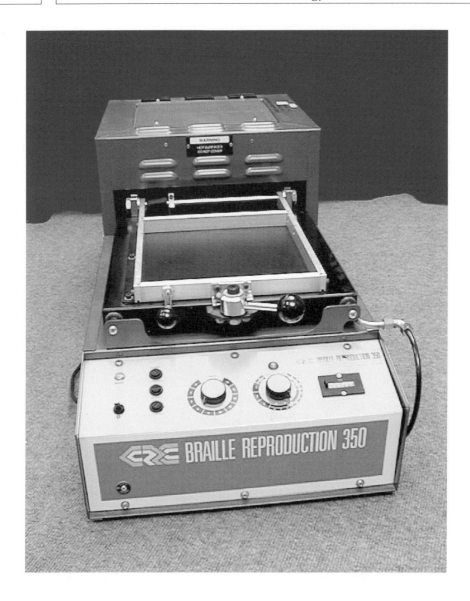

Figure 8.22 Thermoform.

Summary

This chapter has presented an overview of the range of access technology currently available. It is not possible or appropriate in this context to give detailed information about products or manufacturers. This information is freely available on request from agencies such as RNIB.

References

Arthurs, J. (1996) Computers and accessories, in *Access Technology: A Guide to Educational Technology Resources for Visually Impaired Users*, RNIB, London, Ch. 2.

Bosher, P. (1996) Opening electronic highways, in *Access Technology: A Guide to Educational Technology Resources for Visually Impaired Users*, RNIB, London, Part 2.

Fetton, E. (1996) The role of technology, in *Access Technology: A Guide to Educational Technology Resources for Visually Impaired Users*, RNIB, London, Ch. 1.

Guyver, P. (1997) Voice recognition – just hot air? Unpublished paper, RNIB Physiotherapy Support Service, London.

Hampson, M. (1996) Braille systems, in *Access Technology: A Guide to Educational Technology Resources for Visually Impaired Users*, RNIB, London, Ch. 4.

Hinton, R. (1988) *New Ways with Diagrams. Thermoformed Tactile Diagrams: A Manual for Teachers and Technicians*, RNIB, London.

Lodge, J. (1996) Speech systems, in *Access Technology: A Guide to Educational Technology Resources for Visually Impaired Users*, RNIB, London, Ch. 5.

Lodge, J. and Arthurs, J. (1996) Large display systems, in *Access Technology: A Guide to Educational Technology Resources for Visually Impaired Users*, RNIB, London, Ch. 3.

Morley, S. (1995) *Window Concepts: An Introductory Guide for Visually Disabled Users*, RNIB (for the GUIB Consortium), London.

Murnion, S. (1996) *A Guide to Internet Access for Visually Impaired People*, Research Centre for the Education of the Visually Handicapped, University of Birmingham, Birmingham.

RNIB Employment Development and Technology Unit (1997a) Factsheet – Large monitors. RNIB, London.

RNIB Employment Development and Technology Unit (1997b) Factsheet – Printers. RNIB, London.

RNIB Employment Development and Technology Unit (1997c) Factsheet – Electronic reading aids. RNIB, London.

RNIB Employment Development and Technology Unit (1997d) Factsheet – Large print methods. RNIB, London.

RNIB Employment Development and Technology Unit (1997e) Factsheet – Closed-circuit televisions (CCTVs). RNIB, London.

RNIB Employment Development and Technology Unit (1997f) Factsheet – Portable computers and note takers. RNIB, London.

RNIB Employment Development and Technology Unit (1997g) Factsheet – Screen magnification systems. RNIB, London.

RNIB Employment Development and Technology Unit (1997h) Factsheet – Speech systems. RNIB, London.

RNIB Employment Development and Technology Unit (1997i) Factsheet – Braille embossers and translation software. RNIB, London.

RNIB Employment Development and Technology Unit (1997j) Factsheet – Electronic Braille displays and Braille keyboards. RNIB, London.

<table>
<tr><td>

Widening participation: a general perspective

</td><td>

9

</td></tr>
</table>

When any student begins a course of study, the experience can be overwhelming. There may literally be thousands of new students starting on the same day. There is a great deal of information to be absorbed, in a very short time; the environment is likely to be new and very different, as are the people. The student's questions may include: Where will classes be held? Where is the accommodation? How will I get there and back? What equipment do I need? What will the other students on the course be like? The experience is exciting but can also be bewildering and, for some people, rather frightening.

Many of the general issues that emerge in this new setting will be dealt with in Chapter 11. This is an extremely important area to consider because many students may need some additional support, such as discussion with personal tutors or guidance in dealing with finances, in order to be able to deal with academic issues against the backdrop of possible major changes in life events. This chapter will consider some contextual issues relating to the changes within further and higher education and will look at specific areas that are relevant to widening participation for visually impaired and other disabled students.

Curriculum issues

The ease with which curricula, in their widest sense, can be accessed has implications for all students at every level and from all backgrounds (see Further Education Funding Council, 1997). It may be true to say, however, that this is more of an issue for students with different requirements, for example, students with impairments. Areas such as the range of possible entry routes, the amount of flexibility available in the system, and sensitivity in design and delivery of the curriculum will all impact upon the accessibility of particular courses for particular students. If the ethos of a college is student centred and inclusive, 'then many of the potential barriers for students with . . . disabilities may not exist' (Booth, 1994). It is important that educational provision 'respects the present position and knowledge of the learners' (Clare, 1990). This is the ideal towards which colleges should be working. There is, in reality, a great deal of variability from institution to institution and even between courses in the same institution.

Over the past two decades there has been a definite shift in post-16 education – 'away from course-based and syllabus-led provision' (Clare, 1990). This seems to have been particularly marked in further education but is also filtering through to the higher education sector. There is now a greater emphasis on individualized programmes of learning and this requires attention to be given to different styles of organization, design and delivery of the curriculum. Above all, flexibility seems to be the most frequently cited core factor in meeting diverse learner needs (Clare, 1990; Faraday, 1996).

Entry routes

In both further and higher education, entry routes have become more flexible. Overall this enables students from a much wider range of backgrounds to access educational programmes at all levels.

In the further education sector, the FEDA (Further Education Development Agency) report *Developing FE* (Faraday, 1996) describes 'discrete' and 'mainstream' provision. In many colleges of further education, discrete provision was 'perceived as separate and described as coming under the auspices of a distinct Learning Support or Special Needs section' (Faraday, 1996). There is a general trend away from this approach to a more inclusive system where in most cases discrete programmes are used as launch pads from which students can gain access to the whole curriculum.

Ideally there should be a wide range of entry and progression points available to meet the requirements of learners and the variety of curricula on offer. This could involve pre-foundation work, foundation studies and/or extended entry routes focusing on student achievement. These strategies will smooth the transition process and aid in curriculum development. Implicit within this is the need for good staff awareness of disability issues, which may involve the provision of advice and support (Booth, 1994) and/or some training (see Chapter 12).

In the higher education sector, many universities in recent years have shifted their emphasis for entry requirements for undergraduate programmes away from A-levels, to other types of course and applicants' previous experience. The extent to which these changes in emphasis have occurred depends very much on the institution and on the requirements of the course in question. The types of entry requirement that may be considered include:

- National Vocational Qualifications (NVQs);
- BTech;
- access to Higher Education programmes;
- Prior Experiential Learning (usually assessed by the institution under the Assessment of Prior Experiential Learning (APEL) scheme);
- previous awards at certificate, diploma or degree level.

Most universities provide information and advice on these issues in a number of ways, which may include: various leaflets and guides (which should of course be available in a variety of media), a home page on the Internet, open days, drop-in sessions, direct contact with staff on particular courses or staff with special responsibilities in this area. For example, the University of East London has a Centre for Access, Advice and Continuing Education which is able to deal with enquiries of this sort.

Programme design

Some issues relating to programme design inevitably span both further and higher education, although, as discussed earlier, further

education seems to be ahead of higher education in working towards
widening participation and increasing inclusivity. A number of
strategies are already in use in some areas and these could be
considered by institutions working on increasing access to the
curriculum. Some possibilities are suggested below (adapted from
Clare, 1990; Booth, 1994; Faraday, 1996):

- student-centred ethos;
- negotiated curricula where the goals of learning and the means
  to achieve these goals are agreed in partnership with the student;
- sensitivity and inbuilt flexibility within the curriculum to meet
  diverse learner needs; ability to recognize the constraints and
  difficulties in people's lives and to adapt accordingly;
- individualized programmes of learning with specific action plans
  and mapping of progression routes allowing progression at
  different rates;
- modular programmes;
- open and distance learning options;
- accumulation of credits at the student's own pace and according
  to their needs;
- increased staff awareness;
- focus on transition and progression.

With specific reference to students returning to education while in
employment, a handful of universities in the UK have pioneered a
venture that leads to a master's degree or a diploma by Work Based
Learning. This aims to equip employees with the skills to sustain their
employability by learning new competencies.

> All students enter into a 'learning agreement'; the student,
> the employer and the university establish the purpose of
> the programme of study, the activities therein, support
> offered by the employer and the university, work that must
> be completed, resources available, learning outcomes and
> how these outcomes will be demonstrated. . . . The basis of
> this approach is to be flexible enough to be studied by any
> employee of any rank in any business, regardless of size or
> turnover. (University of East London Students Union, 1998.)

When the above issues are addressed, it also facilitates increased flexibility in attendance patterns, for example, part-time study. If some or all of these strategies are adopted, access to curricula at every level will be improved for all students and the barriers that particularly affect disabled students associated with more conventional programme design will be considerably reduced (see Further Education Funding Council (1997) for further discussion on widening participation).

Application

The first step in pursuing an academic course is often thought to be the application. It is important, however, for the potential applicant to undertake some preliminary investigation before this stage is reached. It is also essential that the institution presents a positive image. Skill (1997a) state:

> Disabled people are part of your institution's market and they need to be recruited like any other group. They need information about courses and facilities, a chance to visit, and the assurance that their application will be dealt with efficiently and effectively. Above all, they need to have the confidence that they and their disability will find a welcome at your institution.

For a visually impaired applicant, accessibility to any course begins with the prospectus. The information included here should be available to applicants in different media, for example, large print, Braille and audiotape. Some institutions additionally provide the content of the prospectus and other information on the Internet. This makes it available to a wider range of potential applicants and, as long as the Website is designed correctly, the content will be accessible to those with visual impairments (see Chapter 8 for information on where to find guidance on Website design for disabled users). The prospectus should contain comprehensive, unambiguous information, including details about the institution, its disability policy and general facilities. It should be welcoming and should include the institution's disability statement as well as the name of the member of staff with responsibility for disabled students. If a mechanism such as this is already in place when the applicant initially contacts the institution, it gives an indication of the overall philosophy and approach to disabled students. If this is not the case, the publicity department should take a careful look at the institution's promotional activities in liaison with staff responsible for students with disabilities and/or learning support tutors. Redesign may be necessary in order to inspire greater confidence in potential applicants with different requirements. A checklist for presentation of prospectuses and other recruitment material can be found in *The Co-ordinator's Handbook* (Skill, 1997a).

The Disability Discrimination Act places a duty on Higher Education Funding Councils in England, Wales and Scotland 'to take account of the needs of disabled students and to require institutions funded by them to provide disability statements' (Disability on the Agenda, undated). Further Education Funding Councils in England and Wales have a new duty placed upon them to 'require that further education colleges publish disability statements' and to 'report to the Government on their progress, and their future plans for providing education to students with disabilities' (Disability on the Agenda, undated). The disability statement should give information about facilities for disabled students at the particular institution. It may include information on the institution's policy towards disabled students and the names of those responsible for it, any special admissions arrangements and the complaints and appeals procedures (Disability on the Agenda, undated). A checklist for disability statements and other guides can be found in *The Co-ordinator's Handbook* (Skill, 1997a).

The Further Education Unit (FEU) (1992) advocates that each LEA and its colleges

> . . . will seek to ensure . . . working systems of advice and guidance for school pupils approaching the end of compulsory attendance (and) for adults in all parts of the LEA's area . . . incorporating full information about

education, training and employment opportunities available, together with support facilities for individuals with special needs.

These systems, plus the disability statements, should help to provide a better picture of available support in each area for prospective disabled applicants. Even so, within each institution, it may be that staff members in individual departments have a varying awareness of disability issues and different experience in supporting students with visual impairments. More information on ways to make courses and institutions accessible for individuals with disabilities can be obtained from Corlett and Cooper (1992). It is, however, essential that all 'front-line' staff – for example those in admissions, school liaison officers, those who meet students at open days or at events such as higher education fairs and careers fairs – know what facilities are available for disabled students. Ideally these staff should also have undertaken disability equality training (Skill, 1997a).

Pre-application information gathering

It might be useful for prospective applicants, at least to contact the admissions tutor of the course for which they intend to apply and/or the disability coordinator or learning support tutor (or equivalent). If there is no one with a specific remit for dealing with disability issues then Student Services or a welfare officer may be able to provide relevant information. A thumbnail sketch of the facilities available for students with disabilities at the majority of universities can be obtained from the following publication if the information is not already available in the prospectus of the institution: *Higher Education and Disability: The Guide to Higher Education for People with a Disability*. This is produced by Skill (National Bureau for Students with Disabilities) and CRAC (Careers Research Advisory Centre) (1997) and is updated every year. At the time of writing there does not appear to be a similar resource manual in the area of further education.

A preliminary information gathering visit to the college is recommended. This allows the student to explore the environment, to assess the accessibility of the site, to meet staff and students and to ask questions. The latter is particularly pertinent if there are visually impaired students already on any of the courses who could provide valuable information about college life. The applicant may wish to give the following information either before or during the visit to ensure that the appropriate support mechanisms are put in place (adapted from Skill and CRAC, 1997):

(1) the nature of the applicant's visual impairment;
(2) what the applicant's needs are likely to be to access the curriculum;
(3) possible modifications to the college environment;
(4) which buildings the applicant would like to visit;
(5) any specialist equipment needs.

More information on ways in which staff can prepare for an information visit is available in *The Co-ordinator's Handbook* (Skill, 1997a). This is important, as the student may be using the visit to decide whether to make an application to the institution and it will inevitably influence the final decision. With specific reference to visually impaired visitors, it would be appropriate to ask the applicant if any special assistance, such as access to space for exercising a guide dog, enlarged maps of the route to the campus, or verbal description of the route on tape, is required.

Some applicants may prefer to attend an open day. A prepared list of specific questions is valuable, particularly regarding flexibility of study, methods of teaching used and any support that may be on offer. If the applicant chooses to attend an open day, however, the most relevant staff may not be available and there will probably not be as much time for discussion, so a specific information-gathering visit is the most useful option. Guidelines on making open days accessible to all are available for institution staff in *The Co-ordinator's Handbook* (Skill, 1997a). Some applicants choose both to attend an open day and to make a visit individually, but this may depend on time and geographical location, particularly if they wish to visit a number of institutions.

Finding out about these issues is important, to see which college or university can best cater for particular visual needs, but these may not take precedence over all other considerations. For example, there is no point going to a college that has excellent support systems in place if it does not offer the course in which the student is interested, or if it is a considerable distance from the applicant's home if s/he wishes to study locally. Provision will vary markedly from place to place and even from course to course within the same institution. It is essential that all parties are realistic. Inevitably the fact that the person has a visual impairment will have implications that need to be considered at the time of application and during the course.

If students with visual impairments have been previously accepted on to particular courses, then it is possible that the staff will be more aware of the support needs of disabled students. It is unwise, however, to assume that this is the case. Experience indicates that some students have successfully completed courses despite the fact that they have received no extra help; conversely, there are students who have failed to complete due to the stress caused by trying to work without any support. It must be said, however, that there is a continuum of success and failure among students even when adequate support is provided, depending on individual abilities.

If prospective applicants carry out this pre-application data gathering – which can be done up to 2 years before the time they wish to start the course – informed choices about which institution to select can be made.

Clearing

In the higher education setting, it is true to say that a percentage of visually impaired students will enter courses via the Clearing system. In these cases, it is important to realize that the above processes will not have taken place with regard to the courses and/or institutions that the students eventually attend. This may have implications for the amount of support available and the general preparedness of staff in both academic and non-academic areas. This will be less marked if the college in question has an ethos of inclusivity reflected in the establishment of cross-institutional policies on services for disabled people (see Chapter 12).

Skill (1997a) suggest that a separate procedure needs to be established to cover the Clearing period. This might include the following considerations (adapted from Skill, 1997a):

- Clearing room staff need to be briefed about the facilities available for disabled students.
- Questions about any needs arising from a disability should be asked and responses entered on to the form completed by staff.
- A disability coordinator could be on hand to offer advice and information to students about how their needs might be met.
- Information packs could be prepared to be sent out during the Clearing period.

The application form

It is important for applicants to be sure of the entry requirements for the course in which they are interested, and that they are taking a pertinent course or are able potentially to fulfil the entry criteria.

There is usually space on the form for a personal statement that supports the application – it is recommended that this be used to full effect. The statement should give some general information to allow admissions tutors to gain an idea of the applicant as a well-rounded person, and, if appropriate, part of it can also be used more specifically. If a BSc (Hons) Physiotherapy degree is taken as an example, it is essential that the applicant shows some knowledge of the wide remit of the profession. Ideally each applicant should have carried out – or be intending to carry out – some sort of work experience in a range of physiotherapy situations, although it must be said that this type of experience is becoming less easily available. If this has not been possible they should at least have visited a number of areas in which physiotherapists work. If a student enters the course expecting it to be concentrating, for example, solely on the treatment of sports injuries, disappointment is inevitable. This could in turn lead to poor performance, or in the worst instance the student may leave the course altogether. Although physiotherapy has been used as an example, it is essential to find out as much as possible about any course before applying.

There is also space on the form for a confidential reference from a tutor if applicable. This gives information on the applicant's academic and personal suitability for the course and, if relevant, the predicted grades of exams to be taken.

Disclosure

It is not always easy for applicants to decide whether to disclose that they have a visual impairment. Application forms from UCAS (Universities and Colleges Application Service) do ask for a statement of disability and any support needs, but it is of course the applicant's choice as to whether to use this opportunity. The admissions tutor may be alerted to an applicant's disability by the confidential reference. In this case an option would be to contact the referee to ask that they discuss the desirability of disclosure with the applicant (Skill, 1997a). There are issues here. It could result in discrimination towards those who opt for disclosure, but this is becoming less common as more colleges realize that 'disability and inability are not the same thing' (Skill and CRAC, 1997). If a poor response is obtained from the institution it can alert applicants that this may not be an appropriate place to study.

For institutions without a centralized admissions process, establishing a procedure for identifying applicants with disabilities can be extremely difficult. A system needs to be set up to deal with this issue. It is useful to encourage the inclusion of appropriate questions on all application forms. The details of the system are, however, secondary to its being 'agreed, well understood and easy to apply in order that appropriate action can be taken as necessary' (Skill, 1997a).

It is recommended that disabled applicants declare their impairment (Skill and CRAC, 1997) although, of course, the choice remains with the candidate. Such declaration does mean that the applicant can discuss support issues with the college, such as volunteer readers and funding. It is better if the information comes from the applicant personally and not from a referee. Experience also suggests that it is helpful to submit an accompanying statement that gives specific information about the functional significance of the visual impairment. This provides written confirmation of the person's specific access requirements, which should have been identified during an initial visit. Such information acts as a tangible reminder to the institution of its duties and obligations and is useful, for example, when making preparations for the provision of an accessible interview. The document can be kept by both parties for future reference and is important if, for example, the student subsequently considers that certain access needs have not been met.

In the higher education setting, an applicant who is rejected on the grounds of disability is allowed to make another choice through the UCAS system. If a place is not offered because it is felt the appropriate facilities are not in place, this should be made clear to both the applicant and to Clearing (Skill, 1997a).

The interview

It is becoming much more common for students to be selected solely via their applications, but some institutions or some specific courses still carry out selection interviews, for example, this is compulsory when applying for teacher training. Interviews can, however, be limited to mature students and any applicants with disabilities, as it is perceived that there are particular issues that need to be addressed.

It is important to ensure that the basic practicalities of the interview are taken care of in advance, such as getting to the campus, finding the appropriate room and being able to participate fully in the process. This may involve telephone contact to pass on instructions or sending out extra information or information in various media. For example, if the journey to the college site involves changes of public transport and/or a short walk, a visually impaired candidate may require enlarged or raised diagrams of maps and possibly a taped or written description of the route. A Braille user may appreciate the information in a Braille format. The same media options should also be available for any documentation that is generally sent out to applicants. As mentioned earlier, some institutions may make this information available via a Website on the Internet.

Some interviewees may choose to be accompanied by a personal assistant or support worker, as this helps to reduce the stress of the situation. If this is the case it may be helpful to discuss how the institution can support the student's mobility needs around the college site. This is particularly important if it is remote from the student's residence or if the course involves travel to different areas. For example, some colleges are split into a number of sites or the course could require students to undertake placements in different locations, and it would therefore be appropriate to encourage the student to consider these issues. It is useful to know if the applicant is a guide dog user. If so, water and a place to exercise and toilet the dog will be necessary.

Lighting may also need to be taken into account. For example, if photophobia (pain caused by exposure to bright light) were a symptom of the applicant's visual impairment, a brightly lit or very sunny room could be disadvantageous. Changes in the lighting or the use of blinds or curtains can be considered. It is important that the interviewers do not sit with their backs to a brightly lit window, otherwise their faces will be in shadow and their expressions more difficult to see (for more information on lighting, see Chapter 7).

The main purpose of the academic interview is to allow a dialogue to occur between the applicant and the institution which enables each party to assess the other. On conclusion of this part of the interview, it is helpful to talk to the applicant about institutional policies regarding students with disabilities. This can facilitate discussion about features of significance to that particular person. The interview represents a continuation, in a more formal context, of the discussions held during any previous informal visit and provides a further opportunity for information gathering by the candidate and the institution. The disabilities coordinator or learning support tutor should be invited to this second part of the interview.

It may be necessary to allocate slightly more time for the interview process, as more issues need to be discussed. With regard to equal opportunities, it should be noted that no questions should be asked of the visually impaired applicant during the actual academic interview which are not asked of other candidates. Any discussion about visual impairment issues is for information-gathering purposes.

For clarity, it may be preferable to conclude the academic interview before moving on to these areas.

It is helpful if both the applicant and the interviewers are ready to talk about the visual impairment and its implications. From the staff point of view, the ease with which disability issues are explored will depend on previous experience. If no visually impaired student has studied on the course before, staff may have anxieties about difficulties that could arise, or about adaptation of teaching methods and materials. Conversely, if visually impaired students have attended the course, there may be questions relating to how the particular applicant's needs are similar or different. It is worth noting that the access requirements of a new visually impaired student may be very different from those of a student already on the course. It is important to avoid stereotyping of needs and, so rather than make assumptions from previous experience, the interviewer should ask the applicant about his or her needs.

It is recommended that the applicant should speak clearly about possible concerns and potential solutions (Skill and CRAC, 1997). If prior study has been undertaken elsewhere, it is helpful to discuss any successful strategies already used. It is also helpful for staff if the applicant clarifies what support would be expected from the institution so that successful completion of the course is more likely. Again, some of this information exchange may have been dealt with on a previous visit.

Some courses require interviewees to undertake other tasks or tests as part of the selection procedure:

- Applicants may be asked to complete a piece of written work, for example, a timed essay in response to reading a journal article on a specific issue. If this is the case it is important to ascertain the applicant's requirements in advance. This may involve: providing the question paper in a different medium, for example, large print or Braille; extra time for reading material and writing the essay; provision of a reader or amanuensis; altering the environment such as levels of lighting; and/or providing special equipment, for example, a closed-circuit television (CCTV) or a word processor with access technology such as enlarged text or speech output.

- Participation in group discussion. This usually involves a group of interviewees plus one or more members of staff. If the facilitator mainly uses eye contact with members of the group to guide the discussion, this would lead to the exclusion of any visually impaired applicants and so preclude their full participation in the selection process. A way of avoiding this is to ensure that the discussion is led by using the applicants' names.
- Other methods of selection may involve watching a videotape, finding the way around the college site using a map or interpreting diagrams. If these methods are impossible for the applicant to access they should not be used, as this would be discriminatory.

Ideally the design of any selection procedure should meet the needs of every applicant and should reflect the college's commitment to inclusivity. In practice, however, an interim solution would be to modify the current selection procedures in discussion with the applicant. This process will ensure that the visually impaired applicant is not disadvantaged in relation to those with unimpaired vision.

Although it is important for all disabled applicants to be aware of the specific entry requirements of their chosen course, it is equally important for the admissions process to be flexible and adaptable. As indicated in Chapter 4, some visually impaired people under-achieve at school, and institutions are encouraged to:

> . . . recognize learning from whatever its source without predicating the outcome. This celebrates the diversity of qualifications and experience which increased numbers of non-traditional students bring without relegating those experiences to deficit models of learning. (Wailey, 1996)

Preparation for taking a visually impaired student

This section is very brief and does not relate to teaching as this will be dealt with in Chapter 10. If the staff servicing a particular course have had little or no contact with people with visual impairments, it is useful for them to undertake some background preparation before the student arrives.

Assuming that members of staff are aware that a visually impaired student will be entering the course at the beginning of the next academic period, what can be done in preparation? (These academic periods will vary depending on the student's pattern of study; for example, it could mean the beginning of a year, a term, a module or a semester).

Communication is essential. The student should be the first source of information but there are a number of other contacts that can be made. It is useful to find out if there is a disabilities coordinator, learning support tutor or equivalent in post, or, if not, someone in Student Services or another department who has an overview and previous experience of supporting visually impaired students. It may also be helpful for staff to conduct a trawl of other courses to see if there is anyone else with experience. These contacts may be able to give advice about setting up support, or about support already in place, in that specific institution. Other possible contacts are Skill and RNIB Employment and Student Support Network (ESSN), which can give advice and may be able to provide some training for staff.

When one or more visually impaired students are registered on the course, it is essential for members of staff to take account of this fact. Again, this is where communication becomes particularly important among teaching staff and those who service a course from outside the department, such as external lecturers. Communication is also necessary with other personnel the student may come across, such as technicians and staff responsible for areas such as accommodation, the canteen, security/caretaking and the library or learning resource centre. Supervisors of any work experience placements the student may attend during the course should be contacted at the appropriate time. It is useful if one member of staff can take on the responsibility of acting as contact person who can disseminate information if and when necessary. This helps to avoid duplication of effort. In order for the entire process to be effective, staff training and awareness-raising sessions may be required.

It is worth checking with libraries and any learning resource centres to see if there is already any specialist technology available on site that could be utilized by the student. If not, a certain amount of equipment commonly found to be helpful could be purchased or hired. It is possible to obtain information on a wide variety of access technology from a number of sources such as RNIB (see Royal National Institute for the Blind, 1996a). Experience suggests that staff often find it very useful to visit a demonstration centre to see the equipment in operation. Students can also choose to do this either before or during the course if they are not already familiar with what is available.

Depending on the particular student, course material may need to be provided in an alternative medium. If this is the case it is advisable to prepare such material in advance. Some books and journals are already available in Braille or on audiotape from RNIB but the number of titles is limited. Recordings can be produced in advance for individuals on request, but this may take a number of months. Any book lists should be sent to the student as far in advance of the commencement of the course as possible. This allows time for texts to be produced in a suitable medium, or for the student to read the material in print. Methods such as reading enlarged text or using a closed-circuit television (CCTV) or a personal reader can be slow and take more effort and concentration than that needed by a sighted person reading from standard print (see Chapter 10). The above issues will be more problematic if visually impaired students enter college programmes unexpectedly, leaving very little time for preparation in advance. An example of this is when students enter higher education from the Clearing system. These problems will be compounded if a support network is not already in existence. Students with different needs may experience a sense of alienation and can feel disempowered if they perceive that support has been 'put in place for them'. It should be possible for the student to approach any member of staff (academic or other) to discuss specific solutions to access issues. If this type of dialogue is established then support is likely to be much more effective.

This emphasizes the importance of implementing a strategic approach to the provision of services for students with disabilities (see

Chapter 12). As implied in the above discussion, there will be time and financial considerations involved if visually impaired students undertake a particular course. This can include training, production of course material in accessible formats, and/or purchase of equipment.

Assessment of individual needs

One way of teasing out some of the issues within the educational context is to offer the student the opportunity to participate in a detailed assessment of his or her learning and study needs. Students have accumulated varying levels of knowledge and/or experience about these needs by the time they enter the academic programme. Some have already successfully used a variety of different study methods and equipment; others are less aware of the pressures involved in undertaking a course, the wide variety of study methods and the range of access equipment that could aid in their learning experience. Whatever level the student has reached, however, it is helpful if an assessment is offered to ensure that any strategies, support and/or equipment used or recommended are specifically tailored for the course to be undertaken. It is important, therefore, that the assessment is flexible enough to take the student's current situation and experience into account. If the student is moving into a different setting, for example from further into higher education, then some consideration may need to be given in order to modify previous support strategies.

The assessment

In the UK there are a number of agencies that can offer advice about, and/or conduct assessments. The learning support tutor or disabilities coordinator should be able to give local contacts, and Skill's Information Service can refer students to appropriate agencies who deal with assessment of visual needs. RNIB's Employment and Student Support Network can organize and undertake assessments for a student's learning support needs.

Throughout the UK there is a network of Access Centres which all belong to the National Federation of Access Centres (NFAC). Disabled customers may attend an Access Centre 'to evaluate (under guidance) a range of enabling technologies relevant to their learning or training needs' (National Federation of Access Centres, 1996). The staff in the Access Centres are able to carry out assessments and provide training for customers with any impairment, including visual impairment.

There are usually a number of stages involved in each assessment.

- Information gathering on arrival – about the person's level of knowledge and/or experience with different study methods and access technology.
- Identifying the person's specific needs in relation to the demands of the course being undertaken. This may involve the assessor contacting a member of staff from the course to gain an insight into any particular issues felt to be relevant. This stage can also include obtaining information about the student's expectations of staff in class, for example, the provision of photocopies of overhead transparencies.
- A range of appropriate equipment should be demonstrated and the student given the opportunity to try it out. This will facilitate the selection of the equipment considered by the student and the assessor to be the most useful.
- Following discussion with the student, a list of recommendations can be drawn up. These are included in a report of the assessment, which can be used by the student to support requests for finance and assistance, for example, a personal assistant.

The procedure for the assessment of educational needs for students entering further education is usually conducted under the auspices of the Local Education Authority (LEA). The amount of information available before the assessment will depend upon whether the student has already been issued with a statement of educational need. When supplementary information is required, the services of external professionals and agencies may be purchased. Where the recommendation is that the students enter specialist colleges, these institutions then become responsible for providing any assessments required (Further Education Funding Council, 1998).

Within higher education, the student may require an assessment of educational needs in order to apply for the Disabled Students' Allowance (DSA). This is a supplementary allowance intended to cover any extra costs or expenses that arise on the course because of disability (see Chapter 11). For further advice and information contact should be made with the institution's disability coordinator and staff at RNIB. There is usually a fee for the assessment, which the student may be able to charge to the DSA or other funding sources.

Transition matters

What is transition? Transition describes a phase in a person's life that marks the change from one social role to another. Examples include:

- from school to tertiary education
- from tertiary education to employment
- from employment to retirement.

'It is both a phase in time and a process of personal growth and development.' (McGinty and Fish, 1992.) Referring to the first two examples, McGinty and Fish emphasize that this is a particularly crucial period for people with disabilities:

> Effective transition should result in the development of the skills and knowledge appropriate for open employment, for an independent life, for a self-chosen range of leisure and educational pursuits and, above all, for social interaction, constructive self-advocacy and community participation. The achievement of these objectives may take longer for some individuals and some may require long-term support to sustain their achievement. (McGinty and Fish, 1992)

As McGinty and Fish imply, open employment may not represent a realistic option for some young disabled people, the quality of whose adult life will depend very much upon the availability of appropriate support services within the community. Sections 5 and 6 of the

Disabled Persons (Services, Consultation and Representation) Act (1986) were designed to enhance the effectiveness and coordination of services for all disabled people by emphasizing the need to respect their rights and to improve cross-agency communication. Although concerned with the transition from full-time education to adult life, the Act does not focus on employment or careers but addresses in particular the issues faced by those who transfer from school or college into the community (Skill, 1997b).

Since they came into force on 1 February 1988, Sections 5 and 6 of the Disabled Persons Act have been modified and changed by other legislation, guidance and regulations which are equally concerned to ensure that the rights of disabled people are respected. (See, for example, the Children Act (1989); the Further and Higher Education Acts (1992); FEFC Circular 96/01, cited in Skill, 1997b.) All these documents acknowledge the significance of the transition phase in the lives of disabled people, recognizing that such change can render them especially vulnerable to manipulation and control by well-intentioned parents, friends and professionals who act out of concern for their welfare. As McGinty and Fish (1992) emphasize:

> It is particularly important that limitations should not be placed on the choices and opportunities available to young people with disabilities when they leave school and before they have had experience of work and independent living. Professional and parental preconceptions about the effects of disabilities on adult life may limit expectations. Young people should receive education, training, real experiences and support for a sustained period before, if ever, options are closed. Not to do so may be creating additional handicaps to the quality of adult life.

College staff will encounter many older visually impaired learners who are either re-entering full-time or part-time education after having been out of the system for periods of varying lengths. These students may well need assistance with returning to study and with the transition from one life-style to another.

Some duties and responsibilities of which tertiary education providers should be aware

Sections 5 and 6 of the Disabled Persons Act, together with subsequent legislation guidance and regulations, aim to facilitate the transition phase between full-time education and adult life. In an attempt to reduce some of the disabling effects of impairment and to enable individuals to make informed life choices, specific duties and responsibilities are placed upon a number of agencies during various stages of a disabled person's school and college life. These are legally binding. Further information can be found in *Making Connections* (Disability on the Agenda, undated) and a detailed account is provided by Skill (1997b). Only a brief summary of those duties that are considered to be of particular relevance to providers of post-school education will be given here.

Section 5 of the Disabled Persons Act requires Local Education Authorities (LEAs) to fulfil three duties. The first two are associated with the identification of pupils as disabled who are described as having special educational needs and who have been issued with statements, including those who have become disabled after the age of 14.

> A transition plan should be produced at the first annual review after the person's fourteenth birthday. LEAs are responsible for drawing up the transition plan, ensuring that it works successfully and co-ordinating the work of other agencies concerned. It is helpful if, as a matter of good practice, the principles which apply to those young people who have a transition plan by virtue of their statement are also applied to those disabled people without statements. (Disability on the Agenda, undated)

The objectives of the transition plan, the issues that should be taken into account when devising, it and the processes involved are detailed in *Making Connections* (Disability on the Agenda, undated). The document lists the individuals who should be contacted (including lay and professional personnel) and gives guidance on how the plans can be used to meet the specific needs of a young disabled person. It also contains helpful practical advice, citing several individual case histories.

Under the third duty imposed by Section 5 of the Disabled Persons Act, the LEA must inform Social Services or social work departments of the date on which disabled pupils under the age of 19 are due to leave full-time education, including those pupils attending LEA and grant-maintained institutions. This must be done at least six months before the leaving date. Emphasis is placed on the need for effective communication between all agencies, which becomes particularly important if a pupil moves from one area to another. The Further and Higher Education Acts (1992) reinforce this obligation and emphasize the need for regular review of the anticipated leaving date. This in turn reiterates the requirement stipulated under Section 6 of the Act. Information about all students with special educational needs, together with details relating to their plans for continuing their education, must be passed to Social Services and social work departments by LEAs. If pupils transfer to further education, LEAs are not required to maintain the statement but have a legal obligation to ensure that, in advance of the transfer, the further education institution can meet the individual's needs. Local Education Authorities should give full details of all relevant statutory and voluntary organizations to the disabled person, offer advice and help people who have lived away from home.

> Successful transition planning will mean that young people have a clear understanding of how to continue their education after leaving school. Arrangements will be made by LEAs where they have a statement. Young people without statements will have the process managed by their school and the Careers Service. (Disability on the Agenda, undated)

The (1992) Acts additionally require further education colleges to inform LEAs about the numbers of disabled students in the further education sector and the dates on which they are expected to leave. This information must also be passed to Social Services or social work departments by the governing body of the further education college or, in the case of independent colleges, the Further Education Funding Council (FEFC) or the Scottish Office Education and Industry Department. (For further information and details about the ways in which guidance and regulations have modified the Disabled Persons Act, see Skill, 1997b. See also *Making Connections* (Disability on the Agenda, undated).)

Transition in practice

It is worth reiterating that the quality of transitional process dictates the way in which subsequent life experiences are managed. For example, a negative experience before entering tertiary education is likely to increase on-programme stress; a positive experience before entering employment will ensure that the disabled person is adequately prepared to take on the challenges of the workplace.

In view of the parameters of this book, two transitional phases of particular relevance are:

- pre-entry to tertiary education
- on exit from college.

Pre-entry issues have been discussed in the preceding sections. Consultation of the Reference Section of *Making Connections* (Disability on the Agenda, undated) is recommended for an outline of the statutory framework for the provision of services.

Difficulties associated with transition

There are a number factors that may hinder a smooth transition process. Some of these have been discussed above. The following is a summary of the major areas of difficulty that may be encountered (adapted from FEU, 1992):

- Different initial starting points for individuals.
- Continuity across the phases of transition.
- Inconsistent approaches to the person from agencies involved.
- The timescale of the transition process is often too short for the development of appropriate personal strategies.

- Lack of coordination between further education and other agencies.
- With particular reference to young people, failure to establish a successful tripartite relationship between the young person, parents and professionals.
- Underdeveloped self-presentation and self-advocacy skills.
- Categorical or individual thinking, that is, the person receives a prescribed package of services according to their 'disability' rather than according to their individual requirements.

On exit from college: some general guidelines

The effective implementation of the Disabled Persons Act (1986) and the subsequent legislation guidance and regulations that have reinforced its tenets is contingent upon the establishment and maintenance of excellent communication channels between designated personnel within all agencies (Skill, 1997b). It is important, therefore, that staff from schools, colleges, LEAs and Social Services departments are familiar with the various processes that should be followed in order to fulfil their duties to disabled service users. Staff should ensure that all relevant information is passed to the appropriate department and that it reaches the correct (named) member of staff on a predetermined date.

For full details of the processes applicable to school and college staff, see Skill (1997b). The following is a generalized summary of the information contained in that document:

- Familiarization with the legislation and guidance and the duties this imposes.
- Identification of one's personal role and the roles of other relevant personnel, both within and outside the institution.
- Identification of personnel who have specific responsibility for the implementation of all relevant legislation, including undertaking assessments, and informing such people, well in advance, of the students requiring assessment.
- Identification of all disabled students and their service requirements.

- Monitoring the progress of disabled students through the system, reviewing expected leaving dates and communicating this information to the Social Services department.
- Undertaking regular reviews of the needs of all students with disabilities.
- Creation of and/or familiarization with transition plans and their relationship to all relevant legislation.
- Communication and discussion with disabled students, their parents, friends, advocates and all others involved to ensure familiarity with, and understanding of, the transition process and all appropriate legislation, explaining how this can be of benefit to the student.
- Obtaining the consent of the disabled student and all other interested parties before transferring information between agencies.
- Informing Social Services departments of the dates of annual reviews, and passing on all information deemed to facilitate the assessment process.
- Informing Social Services departments of the anticipated leaving dates of disabled students under the age of 19 in full-time education.
- Informing Social Services departments of disabled students and details of their plans for continuing in education.
- If a student elects to attend a non-sector (specialist) further education college, informing the FEFC and supplying a copy of the transition plan.
- In the event of a student moving from one institution to another, transferring all relevant details to that institution.

Transition from college to employment: some procedural guidelines relating to visually impaired students

As indicated earlier in this chapter, it is fully acknowledged that some visually impaired students will leave further education to return to Social Services provision. Others may leave further and/or higher education without any prospect of employment in the area for which they have obtained qualifications. For many, however, paid employment is a realistic objective and it is hoped that the following summary of some of the important issues will be useful.

Unlike non-disabled students, those with a visual impairment may require additional periods of information gathering before taking up employment following tertiary education. As well as being encouraged to participate in any general careers guidance services and courses on preparation for work offered by the institution, blind and partially sighted people will need to consider issues such as appropriateness of career, likely attitudes of employers and colleagues, access, support mechanisms and the availability of human, physical and financial resources to enable them to carry out their first job. It has been demonstrated that visually impaired people face many barriers to securing and retaining paid employment (Royal National Institute for the Blind, 1996b) and concern about encountering discriminatory practices, both at the employment interviews and during their working life, is therefore likely to be high. Research also suggests that a greater percentage of disabled people in work elect to be self-employed than do workers in the non-disabled population (Royal National Institute for the Blind, 1996c) and a significant number of visually impaired students may prefer this option. Clearly, consideration will need to be given to a variety of issues, and liaison with personnel from a range of external statutory and voluntary organizations is recommended.

RNIB has set up a new vocational information service called GROW (Gateway to Reaching Opportunities for Work) on the Internet for visually impaired people and those working with them. This provides a number of information areas in relation to employment and can be reached on http://www.rnib.org.uk/grow/welcome.htm.

The Careers Service (see also Chapter 11) may be a useful agency with which to make contact because it assists disabled people 'until they are settled in their careers without age or time restriction' (Disability on the Agenda, undated). This service is required by contract to work in partnership with a variety of organizations and agencies, including colleges, LEAs, employers and Training and Enterprise Councils (TECs), and advisers should be able to offer practical help to individual students. Organizations such as RNIB, Action for Blind People and staff from the Employment Service will also be crucial for obtaining information and advice. RNIB's post-16 information service can supply telephone and written information on a wide range of employment-related topics including careers. An interview with an employment consultant from the ESSN or the Self Employment Development Unit (SEDU) can be arranged. It may be appropriate for the student to receive further specialized training and employment-related preparation before entering the job market. In this case, a course at one of RNIB's specialist colleges or rehabilitation centres may be considered.

Regardless of the student's choice of employment, it is important that contact is established with the Disability Employment Adviser (DEA) at the job centre closest to the proposed place of work. Disability Employment Advisers can offer advice and practical assistance on employment-related issues, including making arrangements for preliminary training and/or rehabilitation. Where additional specialist involvement is required, staff from the local Placing Assessment and Counselling Team (PACT) can be contacted and an assessment for the various components of the Access To Work (ATW) scheme can be conducted. The objective of the ATW assessment is to ascertain the visually impaired person's equipment and service requirements with specific reference to the proposed job. It is recommended that each ATW applicant should be fully conversant with the scheme's tenets to facilitate meaningful participation in any discussions and decision-making processes relating to equipment and service provision.

As has been noted elsewhere in this book, technological advances are continually being made and solutions to the access problems faced by visually impaired people are becoming increasingly available. It is not necessarily the case, however, that each blind or partially sighted person will be familiar with these developments, or with the variety of equipment currently on offer. The importance of making an informed choice of equipment before commencing employment cannot be over-emphasized and it is crucial that specialized information and advice is obtained to facilitate selection. A comprehensive list of factsheets are available from RNIB's Employment Development and Technology Unit (EDTU) and technical consultants can provide demonstrations and equipment assessments if required. Visits to specialized resource centres are also recommended. As important as making an informed choice of equipment is obtaining appropriate training to use it. The course should be tailored to meet the training needs of each individual, and excellent negotiating skills may be required to secure a course of adequate length. Training programmes are currently available from a variety of sources including RNIB and Action for Blind People.

If the prospective job requires the visually impaired person to move to a new environment, some preparation in terms of orientation and mobility is likely to be necessary. Guide dog users will need to familiarize the dog with the new surroundings, both at the place of work and in the local environment. Liaison with Social Services and/or Guide Dogs for the Blind Association (GDBA) may be useful in obtaining specific mobility and orientation training. It may also be helpful for the visually impaired person to make contact with the local blind society, the details of which can be obtained from RNIB's Voluntary Agencies Link Unit. Additionally, other voluntary agencies, clubs and organizations offering services and recreational facilities for blind and partially sighted people can provide an important introduction to the new community. RNIB's Holiday and Leisure service can provide further information. Local branches of support groups for people with specific visual impairments are equally important in providing information, general advice and counselling. Many blind and partially sighted people find membership of these groups to be extremely valuable.

References

Booth, C. (1994) Current developments for students with disabilities and learning difficulties in FE, in *Innovations in FE – Beyond Ramps and Rhetoric: New Challenges and Issues in Learning Difficulties*, Issue 1, Autumn, Staff College Publications Department, Bristol.

Clare, M. (1990) *Developing Self-Advocacy Skills with People with Disabilities and Learning Difficulties*, Further Education Unit, London.

Corlett, S. and Cooper, D. (1992) *Students with Disabilities in Higher Education: A Guide for All Staff*, Skill, London.

Disability Discrimination Act (1996) DL 60: Definition of disability. HMSO, London.

Disability on the Agenda (undated) *Making Connections: A Guide for Agencies Helping Young People with Disabilities Make the Transition from School to Adulthood,*

Faraday, S. (1996) *Developing FE – Assessing the Impact: Provision for Learners with Learning Difficulties and Disabilities,* Vol. 1, No. 3, Further Education Development Agency, London.

Further Education Funding Council (1997) *Learning Works: Widening Participation in Further Education,* FEFC, Coventry.

Further Education Funding Council (1998) Arrangements for students with learning difficulties and/or disabilities requiring provision in 1998–99. FEFC circular 98/03, FEFC, Coventry.

Further Education Unit (1992) *Supporting Transition to Adulthood: A Staff Training Package for Practitioners Working with Students with Severe Physical Disabilities,* FEU, London.

McGinty, J. and Fish, J. (1992) *Learning Support for Young People in Transition: Leaving School for Further Education and Work,* Open University Press, Buckingham.

National Federation of Access Centres (1996) Document two – constitution. NFAC,

Royal National Institute for the Blind (1996a) *Access Technology: A Guide to Educational Technology Resources for Visually Impaired Users,* RNIB, London.

RNIB (1996b) Blind in Britain: the employment challenge. Campaign Report No. 1, RNIB, London.

RNIB (1996c) Factsheet 4: Self Employment.

Skill (1997a) *The Co-ordinator's Handbook,* Skill, London.

Skill (1997b) *Successful Transitions: Implementing Sections 5 and 6 of the Disabled Persons (Services, Consultation and Representation) Act, 1986, Skill, London.*

Skill and CRAC (1997) *Higher Education and Disability: The Guide to Higher Education for People with Disabilities,* Hobsons, Cambridge.

University of East London Students Union (1998) MA/MSc or postgraduate diploma by Work-Based Learning – 'Lifelong learning for the millennium'. *Fuel* (UEL student magazine), (13), February, 7.

Wailey, T. (1996) Developing the reflective learner: learning development entitlement and APEL, in *Opening Doors: Learning Support in Higher Education* (eds. S. Wolfendale, J. Corbett), Cassell, London and New York. Ch. 3.

Suggested reading

Action for Blind People, Royal London Society for the Blind and Royal National Institute for the Blind (1977) *Quality and Equality: Good Practice in Vocational Training for Visually Impaired*, RNIB, London.

Garner, K., Dale, M. and Garner, S. (1997) *Education, Employment and Rehabilitation for Visually Impaired Adults: A Survey of Recent Research*, RNIB, London.

Royal National Institute for the Blind and Royal Association for Disability and Rehabilitation (1995) *Access to Equality: An Analysis of the Effectiveness of the Access to Work Scheme*, RNIB, London.

Simkiss, P., Garner, S. and Dryden, G. (1998) *What Next? The Experience of Transition: Visually Impaired Students, Their Education and Preparation for Employment*, RNIB, London.

Yates, L. (1998) *Supported Employment: Towards a National View*, RNIB, London.

<table>
<tr><td>10</td><td># Accessing the curriculum: specific issues</td></tr>
</table>

In contrast to the previous chapter the focus here will be on ideas and practical suggestions concerning the access needs of visually impaired people undertaking study in further and higher education institutions. It is hoped that these ideas will be useful both to visually impaired students and to staff involved in the provision of teaching and support services.

The student's access to the course itself will mainly be considered here, although some other aspects will be mentioned to put the course into context.

Audit: some introductory comments

It is important that institutions undertake audits of the facilities and services available to support students with disabilities within the college. An audit involves systematic evaluation of service provision in relation to measurable standards and can be used to initiate change. It should result in efficient and effective delivery of a quality support service for disabled students, but in order for this to take place there needs to be commitment on the part of both management and staff. If no work has been carried out in this area before, it will be necessary to undertake a pre-audit survey. This will examine existing facilities and services and allows a baseline to be established on which to set standards that can be used in a subsequent audit (Barnard and

Hartigan, 1998). Organizations such as RNIB may be able to help with these surveys and more information is given in Chapter 12.

The learning environment

The environment in which a student's learning occurs will differ enormously from place to place. On the whole, colleges and universities are very varied and there is a wide range of accessibility, due to age of buildings, layout and design. It still seems to be the case that architects rarely consider and/or act upon the access issues of the disabled customer when designing new buildings.

It is not always easy to ensure the accessibility of teaching areas for students with visual impairments at all times, as classrooms are used for a wide variety of different courses. There may, however, be some strategies that can be employed to attempt to overcome even the worst scenario. These are explored in Chapter 7.

Tour of the campus

Either before or at the beginning of the course (perhaps in the induction week or just before it), it is useful to provide a guided tour around the college site, whatever its design. This should concentrate specifically on the areas with which the student will need to be familiar and to which full access will be crucial. Examples might include: the canteen and other common areas, library, usual classrooms and lecture theatres, Students Union building, the route to and from the bus stop or tube station, and so on. A staff member, a student already on the course, a Students Union representative or the disability coordinator or learning support tutor could guide the tour. Some students may choose to recruit the services of a mobility officer. Directions may be available to supplement the tour, which might be in the form of a route map (standard size, enlarged or raised, depending on choice), written instructions (in print or Braille), audiotape instructions or a combination of these. If the college is split into different sites and the student is expected to travel between them, this information should be included on the tour with some description of possible travel options. The student may choose to be accompanied for the first couple of trips, but this might be unnecessary given that other students on the course are likely to be travelling at the same time. It is possible that a visually impaired student will not choose to participate in a guided tour, preferring to explore the campus independently. But the initial offer of assistance should be available.

Equipment

This issue will be dealt with briefly here – for more detail see Chapter 8. On some courses that involve the use of particular equipment, it is important that the visually impaired student has full access to each machine used. Accessibility will depend on the type of equipment and its intended use. Some equipment may be visually challenging or inaccessible, for example, machines with very small readouts or complex control panels with little or no labelling. This can be dealt with in various ways.

In some situations, it is recommended that the student should consider the adoption of a specific operational routine when using the equipment. This involves learning the position of controls on the machine and their function by using touch and/or residual vision. It may be useful to learn the specific sequence in which these controls are operated depending on their purpose.

Machines can be modified by adding extra labels (in large print or Braille) and by using such products as Hi-marks and bump-ons (see Chapter 6) to give a tactile indication of the position of settings.

Contrast and colour (as discussed in Chapter 7 and later in this chapter) are issues for the labelling on machines and readouts. Good contrast is helpful and it may be possible to modify equipment accordingly. Digital readouts vary in accessibility. Liquid crystal screens may prove to be difficult or inaccessible due to inadequate contrast and the student may seek assistance to read them. Machines with light-emitting diode displays in red or green can be more accessible depending upon the user's colour vision. It is possible to link some equipment to a large PC monitor with speech output that would enable the student to work independently.

There may be situations where it is impossible for the student to gain access to a piece of equipment even with modification. What happens in these cases depends on the outcome of discussions between the student and the course team:

- It may be decided that it is not an essential part of the course and that the practical element could be omitted as long as the theoretical basis is understood.
- It may be a piece of equipment that is used in a group. In this case the visually impaired student would still be able to participate, but one of the others in the group would assume responsibility for operating the equipment and recording any readouts.
- If the student is required to use the equipment and to lead the activity, this can be done with the assistance of another student, a member of staff or possibly a support worker. Here the student is expected to be familiar with and able to interpret the readouts, for example, the upper and lower safe limits on a monitor. An assistant may be asked to provide a commentary on what is occurring to these levels as the procedure is carried out, to enable modifications to be made as necessary.

Study space

Ideally, facilities should be available for students to undertake private study if there are gaps in the timetable. Space may be available in a library, learning resource centre or some other dedicated area. For a student with a visual impairment this might involve extra equipment, such as a CCTV, which tends to be quite bulky. Because some access equipment requires considerable space, extra room may be necessary. It is useful if the room can be locked or if there are staff available to police it, as the equipment also tends to be very expensive.

Staff

The overall tone of the learning environment is usually set by the staff. Many of the teaching strategies to be discussed shortly are essentially a matter of good teaching practice, which will benefit all the students in the group and thus improve the overall learning environment. There are, however, a number of strategies that involve some extra thought. If a lecturer considers these before coming into contact with the students, it is then possible to discuss them with each individual to ascertain which might be most helpful. If a flexible and non-confrontational approach is adopted, most access issues can be overcome or at least circumvented. It may be useful to offer the student the option of regular review sessions with the opportunity for discussion of these points.

It is essential that staff in the institution should participate in disability awareness training. This can be provided by such organizations as RNIB, the Centre for Accessible Environments or local disability organizations. It is possible that the Educational Development department (or equivalent) that is responsible for monitoring staff training may have a budget for provision of this type of awareness raising input.

Adapting learning materials

Accessibility to visually impaired users is the main objective for adapting learning materials. Some materials are readily made accessible; others can be partially adapted and others perhaps have to be used in different ways – or alternatives considered. The amount of work necessary for adaptation will depend very much on the type of course and the content, for example, is it mainly paper based or is there a large practical element? Some of the information given below will overlap with the section on teaching strategies.

Learning materials fall into a number of categories:

- Paper based – books, journals, diagrams, written course material and study guides.
- Audio visual – overhead transparencies, slides, videotapes, cassette tape.
- Information technology – computer based learning materials.
- Practical equipment – this will vary depending on the course.

Contrast and colour have been mentioned earlier, but these issues are also relevant to learning materials. Good contrast is very helpful. Some users prefer black on white; others find white too glaring. The use of coloured paper can make it very difficult to see text, although sometimes lighter colours such as yellow can reduce the background glare, making items on the page easier to decipher. Some colours may be more easily visible than others. These issues need to be investigated with the individual student to ascertain specific preferences.

Paper based

Written material is perhaps the easiest to make accessible although, depending on the subject matter, this will vary from course to course. Straight text can be adapted in a number of ways already mentioned.

Enlargement

Some visually impaired students can access most written material if it is enlarged. Using a photocopier is one method (although there can be some negative features here; see 'Alterations to layout' below). Success will depend on the original size of the text, the shape of the font used, the quality of the original text and the contrast.

Some journals and books are produced in small type (e.g. 10 point) and this may need to be enlarged further to make it clear. If the original is of poor quality, then the enlargement will also be poor and thus may not be readable.

An option here is to scan the material on to computer diskette, where it can be stored as a text file. The font style can be altered and increased in size and then reprinted. This may not, however, be a practical method to use for large amounts of text, as it takes some time and the file needs to be checked for mistakes because OCR systems are not perfect (see Chapter 8).

If teaching staff are producing their material on diskette it should be relatively easy to produce a version with an enlarged or modified font. The original document can then be kept and used from year to year. As a general guide, a 16-point sanserif font is usually accessible to many partially sighted readers, but this needs to be discussed with individual students. The font should be clear (for example, Univers or Arial) with no italics and should be presented in a mixture of upper and lower case. Fonts using just upper-case letters are difficult to read.

It may not be acceptable to enlarge hand-written material, as some visually impaired people find this difficult to decipher. Type is generally preferable.

Institutions usually have specific copyright licensing agreements (via the Copyright Licensing Agency) which allow the enlargement of greater amounts of material for private study use by students and staff with partial sight. For example, entire textbooks or journals can be copied as necessary.

Some students prefer to receive all material in standard size print (usually 12 point), which can then be enlarged as necessary using a CCTV. This may not, however, be appropriate if the text has to be read in class. But it should be noted that it is not always the case that bigger is better; this is why discussion with individuals is so important.

Alterations to layout

Some students may find that enlargement does not necessarily facilitate accessibility. If an A4 size document is enlarged to A3, there can be problems such as the difficulty of dealing with large sheets of paper in class and the storage of at least twice the bulk that other students receive. With the increase in size the lines of text become very long and this can cause scanning difficulties. Such problems can, however, be overcome.

As a general principle all work should be produced on A4 size paper but with larger font, so cutting down the overall amount of content on each sheet. Large amounts of information on one sheet can be daunting and the presentation may appear dense and cluttered, so inhibiting learning.

Another strategy that can facilitate access is to organize text into columns on a page; the shorter lines facilitate an increase in reading speed.

If text is fully justified (that is, has even left and right edges), this can be a problem to the visually impaired reader in two ways. First, the spacing between individual letters and words may be altered automatically to fit the text into the space, and second the even right edge makes it more difficult to navigate around the page. A helpful strategy, which avoids these problems, is to justify all text to the left only. This gives an even spacing between characters and words and an uneven right edge.

Headings and sections of the text can be emphasized by using bold or larger print. This enables identification of a new section, as headings are more easily differentiated. Some students find the use of colour extremely helpful, for example, headings or paragraphs in different-coloured print or coloured underlining. Paper with a matt surface should be used whenever possible, as a shiny finish produces glare that can reduce the accessibility of text.

Cassette tape

The process of transcribing printed text on to tape can be time consuming and therefore requires advance planning and preparation. If the text contains technical terms it may be necessary to use a reader who is familiar with the subject.

In order to produce high-quality recordings, there are certain guidelines to be observed when reading on to tape; these can be obtained from RNIB, who recommend that all staff should undergo training. If a book or journal is to be transcribed on to tape, permission should be obtained from the publisher.

Depending on the support network available at the institution, it may be possible for material to be read on to tape on site. Alternatively, an outside network of volunteer readers may have been organized. RNIB offers a professional transcription service, which will incur a cost. Individual students may request books to be read on to tape by one of RNIB's regional transcription centres. If the student is registered blind or partially sighted, there is no fee for this service.

Braille

The translation of written material to Braille text is relatively straightforward. The original should be either a clear copy in print or a file on floppy disk. Braille translation is done via a computer programme, so the text has to be entered into the computer in some manner, either from existing files on disk or via a scanner. The text may have to be formatted and then produced via a Braille embosser. The process can be time consuming. Unless an institution has its own equipment for producing Braille, the work will probably need to be sent away. Again, this requires advance planning and preparation to enable the student to access the material at the appropriate time during the course.

Just because someone is a Braille user does not mean that the most efficient way to make material accessible is to provide everything in Braille on paper. This is bulky and difficult to carry around. Storage is also an issue. Current technology permits the material to be provided on a disk which can then be downloaded and accessed via computers with speech output (for example, a desktop PC with a refreshable Braille line) and/or Braille/speech output note takers (for example, the Braille Lite). This means that the student could be given the material on the appropriate occasion – or preferably in advance to allow fuller participation in the session (see Chapter 8).

Diagrams and graphs may be included in the text to be adapted. Straightforward enlargement may be appropriate, although graphics may need to be enlarged more than the text in order to be decipherable. It is possible to produce diagrams with raised lines and this is helpful to some partially sighted individuals (see Chapter 8). Sometimes the diagrams need modification or simplification before they can be raised and given Braille labels for Braille users. Some people may not, however, be able to interpret diagrams at all and so it may be necessary to replace or supplement them with extra verbal or textual description. This is particularly pertinent if material is produced on tape or in Braille. In this situation, it is useful if the reader or Braille transcriber has some knowledge of the subject or access to someone who can interpret any graphics included in the material.

It is not possible to produce everything in accessible media, as new books and articles are being written all the time. It is also necessary for students to utilize a large number of textbooks and journals when producing course work or research projects for assessment. It is therefore advisable to implement some form of rolling programme, either in-house or by using services such as those provided by RNIB, to keep as up to date as possible with the tape and Braille production of regularly used learning materials.

Audio-visual

Many learning materials are now available in audio-visual formats, some of which are more accessible than others. Most lecturers use overhead transparencies (OHTs), and most visually impaired students cannot see them, even if they sit right at the front of the class. It is, therefore, useful to adopt the practice of producing copies for the students to have either before or at the beginning of each class (see below for more information).

Slides and video are often used in class. These again cannot be seen easily, if at all, by visually impaired students. Little can be done to adapt them, but there are strategies that can be used to facilitate access. The easiest one is to make the slides and videos available before and/or after the class. Working with video and slides in this way enables the user to gain undisturbed access to the information. In the case of slides, it is useful if an appropriate projector is available (that is, the type used for tape/slide presentations where the image is projected on to the inside of a small screen). If the institution has access to the requisite equipment, it is possible to scan slides into a PC using a film scanner and to store them as digital images. The images can then be displayed on screen and viewed by students in this way, or the material can be printed out on a colour photocopier in a variety of sizes as necessary.

This approach is not ideal, however, as it denies full class participation. For video, an alternative method is to set up a second screen in the classroom specifically for use by visually impaired participants. This has been found to be a successful method. Slides require more preparation. If slide images have been stored as described above, it should be possible to issue copies of the originals to each visually impaired student for use during the session. Depending on resources, the students may be allowed to keep these for personal study, or, if this is not possible, the images could be laminated and used each year. Alternatively a video camera can be trained on to the screen so that the image is available on a television monitor that can be positioned as required by the student. These strategies would probably involve liaison with the technical or audio-visual department as appropriate.

If the student has no residual vision, video and slide presentations could be totally inaccessible. This may not always be the case, however, particularly if there is a comprehensive commentary that accompanies the visual material. In situations where the visual material is not augmented in this way and the information is considered to be a crucial part of the course, some method must be found to make it accessible. The information could be presented in different ways; advice on this type of modification can be obtained from RNIB.

No adaptation of spoken information on cassette tape is necessary.

Information technology

A great deal of information is now available on computer especially with the advent of CD-ROM (see Chapter 8). This tends to be very visual, as most of it is Windows based. Content and presentation will determine its accessibility to visually impaired users, as will the individual's level of vision. Some partially sighted students choose to access Windows via a large monitor or with varying degrees of screen enlargement; others require no such adaptations. Some packages already incorporate options such as customized colours (from which a user can select as required) and the ability to change the size of the mouse pointer. As technology improves, an increasing number of speech and Braille users will be able to access the Windows environment with speech input/output systems – but this is not yet perfected. At the time of writing it is recommended that each package is evaluated in consultation with the student. If access to the package proves impossible, alternative ways of obtaining the information will need to be investigated.

Some courses involve considerable computer work. If this is the case, it is important to ensure that all essential packages can be accessed by the student before the course commences, that is, that any necessary adaptive technology is in place. This may involve some training for staff if no one on site is already familiar with the software.

If the packages used by the course are on a network, some of the adaptive technology can also be available via this system if a site licence is obtained. In this situation, technical support must be available from the institution's computer help desk (or equivalent) (see Chapter 8).

Equipment

If the course in question involves the use of equipment in a practical setting, some thought needs to be given to any adaptations that may be necessary, or changes in routine that will allow a visually impaired student to participate. Most of the suggestions for this have been mentioned earlier, for example enlarged or Braille labelling, the use of Hi Marks or Bump-ons, specific routines when using equipment, and assistance from other students or staff as appropriate.

Some manufacturers claim that all the machines they produce can be operated successfully by blind or partially sighted users. The machines are fitted with raised controls as standard which are arranged in a logical order in relation to their use. Other features include clear digital readouts and labelling, and, in some cases, auditory output. Experience with electrotherapy equipment has been relatively encouraging in this respect, but not all manufacturers work to the above specifications.

The use of models can be very helpful to visually impaired students and may replace diagrams in some instances. Examples of this could be models of the cell in human biology, molecular models in chemistry or anatomical models for medically based courses. Access to information is often enhanced, as the models can be explored by touch, which often improves understanding because they are three-dimensional representations of objects or structures rather than two-dimensional diagrams. In fact teaching aids of this type are used successfully by all students.

Teaching strategies

This section is intended to give some practical ideas for use in teaching situations. It is not possible to cover every scenario, due to the great variation in courses and teaching methods, but the principles are intended to be applied as appropriate.

When a visually impaired student has been identified as joining the course, staff should consider ways of increasing curriculum access by evaluating and modifying teaching strategies as necessary. It may be useful to designate a staff meeting to discuss ideas and to receive input from someone such as a current visually impaired student, the disabilities coordinator/learning support tutor and/or a member of RNIB's ESSN team.

Good communication is essential. One of the main ways that information about courses and general events is provided for all students is via noticeboards. Most importantly this includes timetables and day-to-day changes to the course. It is recommended that the general recommendations for signs (see Chapter 7) are followed when positioning noticeboards and posting information on them. They should be at a convenient height, well lit without glare and the student must be able to approach them closely enough to see the notices. The previously discussed issues of access to printed material should also be taken into account when producing information for visually impaired students. On discussion with the student, it may prove more helpful to provide individual copies of any notices in the preferred medium at the same time as they are published on the board.

Before the teaching begins

A book list should be available before the course begins to allow material to be made accessible, that is, transcribed on to tape or into Braille. It is also very useful to prioritize reading lists. This applies at any time before or during the course, as reading may be slower for someone with a visual impairment. Some people can only read for short periods of time before the onset of eye strain. Tape can be used to augment the text but this quite a slow method, requiring considerable concentration and practice, which does not permit efficient scanning of the material. It is helpful if some indication can be given of which material is to be prioritized; alternatively page numbers can be specified in texts rather than asking students to 'read Chapters 2–10'. This helps to reduce stress levels.

Lectures

Most students with visual impairments are unable to see at a distance, so any image or word that appears on a screen or black/white board will probably be inaccessible. Blind students cannot use these methods at all. Some partially sighted students make use of a monocular in class, but can only focus on a small area of the screen at once. This can be frustratingly slow and tedious and will probably be rejected as an efficient method to use given the speed at which many lecturers deliver their material.

Overhead transparencies

These were mentioned in the section on adaptation of learning materials, but there are some other points to add about their use in the teaching situation. Students should ideally be provided in advance with copies of each OHT to be used in the class. This enables simultaneous access to information by all students. It is helpful if the OHTs are numbered, as this prevents confusion and keeps them in the correct order. Consideration should be given to text size and quality, that is, can the student actually read it. If the text size is large already, there is often no need for extra enlargement. Typescript is preferable to handwriting, although some people do write clearly enough for it to be deciphered by many visually impaired students. Such issues should be discussed with each individual. As mentioned earlier, lower-case letters are easier to read; capitalization of text may make it inaccessible. If colour is used on the OHT, it needs to be remembered that the copies are usually in black and white – so referral to the colours during teaching – for example, 'look at the red line' – is to be discouraged.

When a lecturer refers to an OHT by using a pointer, the visually impaired student may not be able to see this, which could lead to lack of understanding. The use of terms such as 'this', 'that', 'here' and 'there' are also meaningless. It is difficult for the student if a lecturer writes on to an OHT during the lecture. Usually a little extra verbal description can negate any problems and may also facilitate learning among all the students in the group.

One important issue is the blacking out of rooms or reduction in lighting levels when using OHTs. This can seriously reduce the visually impaired student's access to the material, as it is not possible to view the photocopies provided. It can also make note taking very difficult for those who use print methods. It is not often necessary to reduce lighting levels in order to see the OHT, but if there is some reason for it the visually impaired student should be given the option of using task-specific lighting, such as a lamp, to allow full participation in the session.

Board work

Many lecturers still use the black/white board during lectures for jotting down points or for diagrams and so on. This method is usually inaccessible for visually impaired students and there are a number of strategies that can be adopted here. It is recommended that the lecturer should speak the words as they are being written up. If complex terms are used, these should be spelt. If diagrams or formulae are written on the board, the lecturer should provide pre-prepared paper copies for the students. If the board is used in an impromptu manner, verbal description is again very useful to supplement the graphics. Students should be assured that they will be able to look at the diagram more closely at the end of the session. Some students recruit fully sighted colleagues to take a copy of the material on the board for them. It is, however, not a strategy upon which teaching staff should rely as a substitute for producing accessible material. Staff have a duty to provide the curriculum to all students and the rights of those with different access needs should be respected.

Audio-visual teaching methods

The methods used to make these accessible have already been discussed in the earlier section on adaptation of learning materials. It is particularly important to ensure that visually impaired students have adequate access to these materials when they are to act as a focus or trigger for the teaching session, for example, for discussion in small groups. If this does not occur, some students will inevitably be excluded and will not be able to participate fully in the class.

Note taking

Visually impaired students use various note-taking methods. If they have copies of OHTs, it may be relatively easy to add notes to these as necessary. Some choose to hand write as their method of note taking, and often find the use of heavily lined paper, felt tip pens and highlighters helpful.

Many use tape recorders either as the sole note-taking method or to augment hand-written notes. These are usually set up at the front of the room in the interest of producing a reasonable recording. Students are advised to ask the lecturer's permission before recording the first lecture – as a matter of common courtesy. Most lecturers are cooperative but students may be faced with the need to negotiate with those who dislike being recorded.

The student may opt to dictate into a pocket memo during a lecture rather than recording the whole session. This could also usefully augment any written notes. Some students may use more technological equipment for note taking such as laptop computers with speech output or character enlargement, or Braille note takers.

Due to the diversity of students' entry behaviour when commencing any type of course, institutions often offer some form of study skills input at the beginning of courses. This will cover note-taking skills, but it may be useful to discuss the range of options mentioned above with the individual visually impaired student. If a study skills handbook is produced, this should be available to students before the commencement of the course, in the medium of choice.

Handouts

Many lecturers regularly use handouts. The same guidelines apply to making these accessible as to the provision of any paper-based material – (see above). If the handout is to be used in the class, it is important to note that it may take longer for a visually impaired person to read text (even when enlarged), to listen to something on audiotape or to read Braille than it does for a sighted individual to read the same amount of material. The handout should be available before the session to facilitate full participation.

If, due to the nature of the class, the material can only be made available during the session, some extra time should be allowed for any visually impaired students to read it (this also applies to students with different access needs such as those with the specific learning difficulty of dyslexia). Some students may find highlighter pens helpful to indicate the most important passages to return to during private study.

Practical classes

If the teaching session includes a practical element, it is useful to remember that some visually impaired people – especially those with field restriction – find it difficult to appreciate the whole picture in this type of setting. Ideally the following preparation should be made:

(1) Provide the student with all relevant material in advance, for example handouts, background reading and so on.
(2) Give full details of the content of the class in advance, for example, equipment to be used, video to be shown and so on.
(3) Prepare the room in advance. Ensure:
  (a) ordered arrangement of equipment;
  (b) good viewing potential;
  (c) consideration of lighting, colour, contrast, size and so on;
  (d) that the student has access to the room before the class if there is a particular set-up of equipment to be used by all students in the group.

Some of the following strategies have been found to be helpful in practical sessions:

(1) Increased verbal explanation of the technique, both before and during the demonstration and in the students' practice time.

(2) Encourage the student to adopt an appropriate position within the group in order to see and hear what is going on.

(3) If applicable, encourage the student to feel what is happening during the demonstration. Palpation is useful for all visually impaired students when learning a hands-on technique, and just feeling where equipment is positioned may facilitate understanding.

(4) Where appropriate, and after obtaining agreement, use the visually impaired student as a model, but afterwards provide an opportunity for that student to observe the technique being performed.

(5) After demonstration of the skill in its entirety as a fully integrated set of operations, the task should be broken down into its component parts. Each of these should be demonstrated, explained and analysed as necessary. Competence should be achieved in one component before moving on to the next.

(6) Give the opportunity for spaced, supervised practice to allow linkage of technique and understanding. 'Distributed practice', where shorter periods of activity are followed by intervals of rest (in which consolidation can take place), appears to produce better results than that from one longer unbroken period of practice (Curzon, 1985).

(7) Give detailed, accurate and unambiguous feedback about the student's performance. Feedback is important for any student and should contain praise as well as correction. This helps the student to close the gap between present achievement levels and the required standard.

(8) Encourage constant self-monitoring of procedures by the student where applicable. Suggest the use of the hands to supplement vision to check positioning and hazards (if appropriate). The latter is particularly important with regard to health and safety issues.

(9)   Where possible choose the simplest and most logical set-up. Encourage the student to be methodical in all practice, paying attention to points such as tidiness.
(10) Insist on regular practice outside of class time if appropriate.
(11) Encourage everyone to put equipment back in its identified place after use.

Many of these points are considered to be good practice for teaching in practical situations and so would benefit all students in the group.

Some visually impaired students find it helpful to dictate important points into a pocket memo during practical classes. It is then possible to review them in practice and private study periods.

Ideally, it is very useful to have an extra member of staff in the classroom to give support during student practice time. Depending on time and staff availability, it may be possible to provide follow-up tutorials or supervised practice sessions if these are felt to be necessary. Again, this may be useful for all students.

Depending on resources available, it may be possible to video practical techniques for the students to use in private study time. These could be impromptu videos of the practical sessions as they take place during the course, but there could be a variety of problems here such as lighting, sound (with a class of students present), not being able to film from the most advantageous position and so on. Taking these issues into account, it would probably be more successful if practical techniques could be filmed outside timetabled periods and the resulting videos then used to enhance resources for all students.

Verbal instructions

It is recommended that staff are as specific as possible when giving verbal instructions. Extra verbal description is often helpful for all students in a group and is a valuable tool to use in all teaching situations but particularly so if there are visually impaired students in the group. It is unhelpful to use vague phrases such as 'it's over there' or 'you do it like this'.

External lecturers

If a course is serviced by lecturers from outside the department or institution, it is useful to have a document available to send out which contains some of the above information. This will alert them to the fact that there are students in the group with different access needs and will allow time for any teaching materials to be produced in appropriate media.

Study skills

It is important that the student considers different study skills, preferably before the course begins. Much of the work done on today's current educational programmes is based around independent, student-centred learning. This often involves lead lectures followed by set reading, tutorials and seminars. The personal study periods may also introduce the student to the course material by the use of worksheets or study guides. The students may need to visit the library to obtain information rather than having it provided in set teaching times. Unless the student has had previous experience of undertaking academic work, it is likely that this approach will be unfamiliar. It is possible, therefore, that different study strategies and organizational skills will need to be adopted to cope with the amount of work to be undertaken.

The visually impaired student will usually take longer to work through text than will a student with full sight (the factors contributing to a slower reading speed were discussed earlier). The visually impaired student, therefore, will generally need to devote a greater amount of time to personal study than the other students on the course in order to get through an equivalent amount of material. This is a fact that the student should be encouraged to accept, and of which the teaching staff need to be aware.

It is useful for the student to have a personal timetable to follow, which helps to give a structure and a methodical approach to study periods. Within this, it is advisable to undertake short durations of concentrated study with built-in rests. Each phase of study could be of a different type, for example, a personal reader could read specific parts of the text, followed by a rest period. After 20–30 minutes, reading some text using the CCTV, followed by rest, then listening to material on tape or working in a group with some other students on the same course would be a good study strategy. The latter could be for discussion of specific points, going over material from worksheets or study guides, or, if appropriate, practising skills learnt in practical sessions during the day. It may be helpful to discuss the possible range of study strategies with individual students.

Readers

In the context of higher education, if a student receives funding, for example, from a DSA, the non-medical expenses portion of this can be used for payment of readers. In further education, provision of readers will depend on local procedures. Reading for a visually impaired student can take two forms: reading material on to tape for use in private study periods or spending a prescribed amount of time with the student reading specific items as requested.

Some institutions may already have a bank of voluntary readers available and a list should be given to the student so contact can be made. Alternatively, visually impaired students may recruit their own readers, often from among colleagues on their own course. It is a definite advantage if the reader is familiar with the subject; if not, considerable time can be wasted due to lack of familiarity with the material. Student readers can find the experience helpful, allowing review of material and possible opportunity for discussion. It is, however, important to guard against becoming distracted; the visually impaired student must lead the study session and make sure the appropriate material is covered.

As noted earlier, RNIB can provide a reading service and may arrange for items to be read on to tape for individual students. Training for readers can also be arranged. This can be useful for long-term requirements, but usually materials are needed immediately, so, if local readers are available, reading can be undertaken more quickly.

Cassette tape

Many students use cassette tapes for a percentage of their studying. This method requires concentration and needs practice. Memory plays a very important part here, as material cannot be scanned in the same way as printed text, which also slows the process down. Some equipment allows cassettes to be played at varying speeds and features a cue/review facility. Use of these features is a skill that requires practice. Cassettes occupy a large amount of space and so storage can be an issue. It is worth noting that if material is recorded at half speed and on four-track machines, this reduces the number of cassettes per book.

If a student records lectures, it is sometimes tempting listen to all of them again during the evenings. This is an inefficient way of using study time, which could be used more effectively by employing other study methods. Tapes can help the student to ensure that there are no gaps in notes taken; they can also be played again using a Walkman or desktop recorder while doing another activity. Specific lectures might be chosen for a repeat to summarize a subject after the student has undertaken further background reading.

Braille

A student may choose to use Braille as a study medium. If so, it is not recommended that students begin learning Braille at the commencement of the course because this could cause information overload. In some cases, however, a student may decide to learn Braille during the course, particularly if undertaking a language course where a different Braille code is used. This will depend on the individual student's abilities (see Chapter 8 for more information on Braille).

Students can use Braille note takers in class. The information can then be downloaded in ASCII text on to computer via a disk drive and accessed in a preferred medium (speech output, refreshable Braille display or printed out on a Braille embosser). As mentioned earlier, material can be provided on disk by staff in advance of teaching sessions to facilitate full participation. This will also reduce subsequent storage.

Screen-based study

Some students use screens for much of their study, such as CCTVs and enlarged text display produced by software packages. Again this method can be slower than reading standard text, as the enlargement can make scanning difficult, especially on the CCTV screen. Use of the equipment requires practice. On the computer screen, the parameters can be set, for example, to show only one line of text at a time and to scroll it at a specified rate. This can help to speed up reading, as can using a speech output system at the same time. It is however, important to remember the dangers of using a VDU screen of any sort for long periods.

Group work

Many students find studying in groups very helpful. This will depend on the situation; for example, if the students are sharing accommodation it is easy to get together. If the students live at home or in private rented accommodation, particularly at a distance from their peers, this method may require more organization. Some group work may take place in college if the timetable permits.

The choice of study methods falls to the individual student. It is, however, worth considering different ways of approaching the work within the specific environment and discussing options with each student. Having a range of study strategies available rather than being limited to one or two may help to reduce stress levels.

Accessing learning resources: libraries and media resource areas

It is important for visually impaired students to be able to access the learning resources provided by the institution, and many of these are often stored in the library. A useful strategy is for a specific member of staff to be identified with whom the student can make contact for particular requirements. Ideally, however, all of the library staff should be aware of students' differing access needs and how they can be of most assistance (Corlett and Cooper, 1992). This can be accomplished by training and awareness-raising programmes, which should involve a wide range of staff, not just the teaching staff.

It is useful for students to visit the library early in the course or even before it commences. This provides opportunities to become familiar with the environment, to identify the location of relevant books, journals and other resources and to meet the library staff. A tour of the library, in addition to that provided for all course participants, is useful. Signs and labels should be in large, clear text and Braille labelling and signing may be helpful to some students. The same points apply regarding signs as discussed in Chapter 7.

Some institutions provide equipment that enables visually impaired students to access texts in the library: CCTV, a scanner attached to a computer with screen enlargement or speech software installed, a Braille line and Braille embosser. Some of this equipment tends to be noisy (for example, embossers and synthesized speech), so it may need to be in a separate room.

It is good practice for some additional access arrangements to be available for items such as reference books or those on short-term loan. Visually impaired students should be able to borrow reference books overnight or short-term loans can be extended to make access more equitable. Some students have access to funding with which to purchase an occasional expensive reference book that may be very difficult or impossible to access in the library. This is particularly recommended if the book is an essential course text.

If a student has access to any funding, this can be used to pay for library assistance. This may involve, for example, some reading or identification of specific items and articles that may be difficult for the visually impaired student to retrieve. If no personal funding is available, the institution may be able to set up a volunteer system to enable the student to have better access to the library.

Course assessment procedures

The term 'assessment' covers a wide range of procedures that vary greatly depending on the course being undertaken and the institution in which they are taking place. This section will discuss some options that visually impaired students may request, but it may not cover every kind of assessment. It would be helpful for teaching staff to discuss individual preferences with the student in relation to the specific assessments for the course, and to apply the principles suggested here as appropriate.

It is important that preparation for any special arrangements decided upon should begin well in advance. In some institutions, such matters are discussed before the student accepts a place. Existing arrangements will vary depending on factors such as the examination boards in further education and the in-house organization of the institution and these need to be ascertained. Often, the student initiates the request for particular examination arrangements and may be able to make suggestions based on methods used previously. If, however, the student has no previous experience, possible options should be offered and discussed well before the assessment is to take place to enable the student to make an informed choice.

It is important to emphasize that these arrangements are introduced to remove the inequalities or barriers arising because of disability; they are not intended to give the student an advantage over other candidates. This should be remembered, as it safeguards the validity of the assessment and protects the student from allegations of receiving 'favourable treatment'. For these reasons, notification of examination modifications should be approved by the examinations officer (or equivalent) and be recorded in writing (Corlett and Cooper, 1992). The student should not be expected to fund any modifications or different arrangements.

Examinations

Examination papers

The examination papers should be prepared in the preferred medium after discussion with the individual student. The papers are generally in print and so the same principles apply regarding accessibility. Options include: standard print, enlarged print (with modified layout), tape and Braille. Some students prefer a combination for example, a print copy and a tape of the questions. If the student chooses print, a CCTV or magnifier may be required, or if the paper is read on to tape then a Walkman or tape recorder with earphones will be necessary. This equipment should be available from the institution or the student may choose to provide it.

If the paper involves long passages of text or has a large number of questions as in multiple-choice examinations, the student may prefer to use a reader. As this is an examination situation, the person should be a member of staff or someone familiar with subject-specific vocabulary and notation. The reader should not be someone who has a personal relationship with the student, who might be biased in their interpretation of the paper.

If the examination paper includes any graphics, these should also be produced in the student's preferred medium. If the student is a braillist, extra verbal description may be necessary, or the graphical information may need to be presented in a different form.

Answering examination papers

The student should decide on the preferred method of writing the examination, for which there are a number of options:

(1) Writing the answers in standard examination booklets with or without the use of a CCTV. Some students use thick felt-tip pens in order to be able to read the answers back. Heavily lined booklets may be helpful.
(2) Word processing – this may involve the examination taking place in a different room where computers are already in place or where the student could site personal equipment if this is used.
(3) A Braille user may require equipment such as a Perkins brailler or a personal computer with converted keyboard and refreshable Braille line (and possibly speech output) to write the examination. The answers could be produced in Braille, in which case the papers would need translation into text before being marked. If a computer is used, the answers could be printed out directly into text or produced on a Braille embosser.

(4) An amanuensis – here the student dictates the answer to someone who either writes, types or word processes the material. The answers can then be read back as required. As is the case with readers (mentioned earlier) the amanuensis should be someone familiar with the specific vocabulary and notation of the subject, but not someone who has a personal relationship with the student, who might be biased when reproducing the answers. If the student has never used an amanuensis before, it is essential that considerable practice is undertaken before the examination itself.

(5) Some papers involve a multiple-choice element which usually has a standard printed answer sheet marked by scanning into a computer. This is often inaccessible for visually impaired students. A useful strategy is for the student to indicate the answer to each question by writing the appropriate letter (that is a, b, c, d, sometimes e, and for papers that are negatively marked there may be a 'don't know' category) on a separately produced answer sheet. The responses are then transferred on to the standard sheet, usually by the member of staff invigilating the examination, ready for marking. These should be checked by a second, independent person before the answer sheet is submitted.

(6) Dictating answers on to a tape recorder – this may be an appropriate way of producing answers for some types of examination but, as with an amanuensis, practice is essential if the student has not previously used the method. If the answers are recorded on to tape, it will be necessary to arrange for them to be typed up in preparation for marking.

Timing

It is essential that visually impaired students are allowed extra time in written examinations which they can choose to use if necessary. This may vary between 25% and 100% additional time, depending on factors such as the type of examination, the student's method of writing the answers, the amount of text and so on. Some institutions do not set a time limit and the students take as long as they wish to complete the paper. It may not be easy to judge how much extra time should be given if no visually impaired student has taken the examination before. RNIB recommend at least 25% and there may be established institutional guidelines, but it is still recommended that particular requirements are discussed with the student. If eye strain is an issue, it may be necessary to incorporate some time for rest periods. If a time limit is set, it is recommended that the examination is started early so that all students finish at the same time.

Examinations involving extra time will have timetabling, rooming and staffing implications, dependent upon the number of examinations taking place simultaneously. It may be an advantage to timetable extra-time papers first and then to arrange the other papers around this framework (Corlett and Cooper, 1992). If a student is taking a number of examinations, for example, GCSEs that are controlled by different examination boards, the timetabling will need to be considered carefully if extra time is necessary in each examination.

Rooming

If possible, it is recommended that students who have extra time and/or use equipment to produce their answers are accommodated in a room other than the main examination room. Whichever room is allocated, it must be quiet and there should be appropriate facilities in the vicinity.

This allows completion of the paper without the disturbance of other students beginning or ending at a different time. Equipment can also be set up to the student's specifications, as this may take up considerable space. A student may for example wish to have a computer plus extra surface area for a CCTV, lamp, reading stand and for writing rough notes. If any of the students choose to have an amanuensis or to have the exam paper read aloud, being in a separate room avoids them being overheard or disturbing other students taking the examination.

Invigilation

Guidelines for invigilators are usually set by each institution, but there are some points that need to be considered if students are taking examinations in different rooms, having extra time and/or using equipment and assistants (an amanuensis or reader).

Timing. Invigilators need to know the modified times of the examination; for example, is it starting earlier or finishing later? It is also important to know how these changed times affect the periods when the student may or may not leave the examination room.

Facilities. If the examination is taking place in a different room (for example another classroom, a resource centre or a staff member's office), it is necessary to check where the nearest toilets are and where the student can obtain a drink during the examination (although very often students bring in their own drinks).

Equipment. If the student is using equipment, it needs to be set up before the examination begins. The invigilators may or may not be responsible for organizing this, but should at least check that the student has everything necessary before the examination begins. If the answers are being word processed it is important to ensure that there is no information relevant to the examination stored on the hard drive or any disks to be used. The students must also be reminded to save their work on a regular basis throughout the examination period.

It is possible that any equipment being used by a student could fail during the examination. The invigilators must know where to go to get replacements or technical help if this should occur.

Assistants. The invigilators need to be aware that extra people may be in the examination room and what their roles are. It may be useful to discuss, briefly, issues such as avoiding bias in the interpretation of the paper or the information the student gives in response to the questions on the paper. This will guard against giving the student an advantage over other candidates.

Practical examinations

As these assessments will be closely related to practical sessions that occur during the course, appropriate provision must be made regarding any equipment to be used, and the student should have the opportunity to check the layout of the room before the examination begins. Depending upon procedure, it may be decided, in discussion with the student, to allow extra time and/or to have assistance available (for example, a member of staff) to assist with accessing any visually inaccessible equipment or to indicate specific points or areas the student needs to consider.

In some cases, in practical assessment involving hands-on techniques or analysis of movement, a member of staff could act as a model if, in discussion with the student, this was felt to be helpful. For example, in our experience with physiotherapy students, some courses require a student to analyse a movement occurring on a video. If this is not accessible to a visually impaired student, the model could perform the movement and the student would then be able to use tactile methods in order to perform the assessment, rather than vision.

Coursework assessments

Not all assessment is carried out by examination. On many courses, substantive elements of the syllabus are assessed via coursework essays, laboratory reports or research project reports. It is important to decide on any different arrangements in discussion with the individual student. It may be useful to establish more flexible deadlines in some cases, and students may wish to present work for assessment in different formats.

If any work of this kind is word processed (which is often the case), it is essential that the student ensures the work is saved regularly and in a number of locations. All too often, students save large amounts of work on only one floppy disk and it can be totally lost if a computer crashes or the disk is corrupted. The recommendation is that all students avoid this extremely stressful situation by making back-up copies of all word-processed work.

In many cases the student is expected to carry out a great deal of background reading in order to produce items of coursework. As mentioned before, for visually impaired students it is helpful to be as specific as possible about the reading that needs to be done.

References

Barnard, S. and Hartigan, G. (1998) *Clinical Audit in Physiotherapy: From Theory into Practice*, Butterworth Heinemann, Oxford.

Corlett, S. and Cooper, D. (1992) *Students with Disabilities in Higher Education: A Guide for All Staff*, Skill, London.

Curzon L.B. (1985) *Teaching in Further Education: An Outline of Principles and Practice*, (3rd ed.), Cassell, London.

The total student experience

Being a student is more than attending lectures and completing assignments. For many young people it may be their first opportunity to move away from home and their local environment if they are going to university or to a new situation in further education. It is a chance to meet new people from different parts of the country and from different backgrounds and it is the ideal opportunity to participate in a wide range of social and cultural experiences. For visually impaired students who have attended boarding schools it may be a time of returning to the parental home on a longer-term basis and having to adjust to that situation.

For mature and/or part-time learners this can be a period of great change: meeting new groups of people, negotiating different environments and learning new study skills. Some students may have decided to leave paid employment to return to full-time or part-time study whereas others may have chosen to undertake a course in preference to being out of work.

It can be a period of great excitement and bewilderment and students will be required to take on new responsibilities. In this context it is important for visually impaired students to have the same opportunities to experience the whole of student life as their non-disabled peers.

Students spend varying amounts of time on their studies. For visually impaired learners this time is often far greater, for the reasons discussed in previous chapters. They will, however, still want to take part in social life and have access to other services offered by the university or college. The purpose of this chapter is to emphasize that the barriers that need to be dismantled in order for students to gain full access to the academic curriculum also need to be tackled in all other areas of student life.

Suggestions have already been given as to the ways in which the curriculum and teaching areas can be made more accessible. These access issues will also apply to the non-academic aspects of student life. The following service providers are examples of those that need to take account of these issues of access and indeed may be compelled to under the 1995 Disability Discrimination Act (see Chapter 3):

- Students' Unions
- affiliated clubs and societies – cultural or sporting
- medical services
- counselling services.

Colleges and universities need to address who is to take on the responsibility for considering these issues in such areas of student life, as it may not be within the remit of the coordinator for disabled students.

Grants and benefits

Money is of crucial significance for all students. Generally speaking, disabled people are some of the poorest in the UK (Barnes, 1991). Disabled individuals frequently experience a higher cost of living directly as a consequence of meeting the additional costs associated with impairment. They may also be receiving a lower income. These costs have been taken into account for disabled students in full-time higher education. Disabled students may qualify for the Disabled Students' Allowance (DSA). As from the 1998/99 academic year the DSA will no longer be income related and will continue to be in the form of a grant (Department for Education and Employment, 1997). The purpose of this allowance is to meet the specific costs associated with full-time higher education and it is split into three main components (the amounts given here are for 1998/99 but may change from year to year) (Skill, 1997a, 1997b; Skill and CRAC, 1997):

- Allowance for non-medical assistance – up to £10,000. This is the largest part of the grant and is available every year. This can be used for example, (a) to employ a reader, who might read directly to the student or on to tape; (b) to pay for assessments (such as low vision, technology or curriculum access), (c) for someone to help with mobility training around the campus or local area, (d) for assistance in the library, (e) for a support worker for students on work placements, (f) for payment for private transport to areas inaccessible by public services, especially if additional travel costs cannot be covered elsewhere within the grant.
- Equipment allowance – up to £3955. This is available for the duration of a student's course and may be used to purchase items of equipment to facilitate study. For visually impaired students this could include a computer that may be adapted to provide speech, Braille or large-print access.
- General allowance – up to £1315 annually. This may be used to top up the other components of the DSA in the event of more funds being required. It can be used to pay for services as necessary, for example, photocopying. Other possibilities for use of this money could be for the purchase of small items such as marker pens, cassette tapes or computer disks. The allowance may also be used to buy textbooks that are often in short supply in the library or that the student finds difficult to use under library conditions (that is, on short loan times or reference only).

Applications for mandatory awards and the DSA should be made to the LEA for students in England or Wales, to education and library boards in Northern Ireland, or in Scotland to the Student Award Agency for Scotland. For students undertaking health related courses, grants may be available through the Regional Health Authority (RHA).

DSAs are not available to students funded through their health authority. However, these students are usually eligible for very similar grants administered under regulations which shadow those for DSAs. These are not available to nurses studying under Project 2000. (Skill, 1997b.)

The management of the DSA will vary depending on the institution and on the individual student; the disability coordinator should be able to give advice on this. It will be helpful if a tutor more closely involved with the student's programme of study can act as a local source of support. The procedure for accessing the DSA may include one or both of the following options:

- The student may purchase services and/or equipment. Receipts must be produced, which are then sent to the funding authority and reimbursement should be approved.
- Alternatively the student can claim funding in advance by providing written quotations of equipment costs and/or estimates of service requirements (for example, number of reader hours). These quotations and estimates again need to be sent to the funding authority for approval.

At the time of writing, students who are studying part-time in higher education are not entitled to a mandatory grant, DSA or a student loan. They may, however, apply for a discretionary grant from the local authority. Smith (1997) states:

The government is also giving serious consideration to the Dearing recommendations that eligibility for DSAs be extended to part-time students, post graduate students and those people with disabilities who wish to acquire a second higher education qualification.

If these recommendations are implemented there will be an increase in the number of disabled students who will be able to benefit from this award.

Currently, postgraduate students may apply for the DSA if they are enrolled on a course that receives funding from the Post-Graduate Funding Council. An example is the Post Graduate Certificate in Education (PGCE), which is covered by the mandatory award scheme.

Additionally, graduate students on research council bursaries are usually eligible for very similar grants administered under regulations similar to those for DSAs. Students should contact the research councils for details (Skill, 1997b).

Students in further education may apply for a discretionary award from their LEA. The college can bid for funding from the Further Education Funding Council (FEFC) to meet the costs of disability, for example additional funding can be claimed for support workers or depreciation costs to which the student may be entitled following an assessment of need. The level of funding provided by the FEFC depends on the band in which the student falls as a result of this assessment. Further information can be obtained from FEFC Regional offices. RNIB's Employment and Student Support Network (ESSN) can be contacted for further information and advice. Students who do not receive funding from any other source may apply to RNIB for a small grant towards the purchase of equipment or services and support as a result of their disability.

Access and hardship funds

Institutions of further and higher education operate Access Funds. The government makes the Access Fund available to institutions in order to provide assistance to students who do not receive funding from any other source, especially those who 'suffer particular hardship' (Department for Education and Employment, 1997). Whilst this fund can be used to purchase a variety of support services, there are of course conditions attached to its allocation. Students other than those with disabilities are eligible to apply to this fund, and competition for resources is likely to be considerable. It is important therefore for the student to contact the disability coordinator or learning support tutor for further information and advice. The institution should ensure that all relevant documentation is accessible to visually impaired students and available in a range of media.

Some higher education institutions have specific hardship funds set aside for students, founded by wealthy alumni or fund-raising initiatives (Skill, 1997b).

Other sources of funding

It may be possible to obtain funding from a number of voluntary organizations and trusts. These are usually charities, or sections of large corporate organizations that have funds available that can be allocated for specific purposes. Applying for this type of funding involves a considerable amount of preparatory work and effort on the part of the student. This can prove to be a frustrating experience, as rejections are not uncommon. It would be advisable to apply to those organizations that declare a specific interest in relevant issues: education, visual impairment, disability and/or the area of study to be undertaken. Students should contact their local societies for the blind and other agencies such as Guide Dogs for the Blind Association (GDBA) to explore the possibilities of obtaining funding. There are several reference books and electronic databases listing grant-making trusts, including the INSPIRE database and a Skill information sheet (Skill, 1997b). RNIB (ESSN) can also provide a comprehensive list of grant-awarding organizations.

As Skill (1997b) point out:

> There will always, inevitably, be some students who cannot obtain adequate funding to cover the support they need. The institution needs to be clear whether, and to what extent, it can support these students. Some institutions make it clear that beyond general advice from the coordinator, support can only be provided to those with additional resources. Many institutions now have central budgets which are used to support students without their own funds. The more services which are delivered centrally, and the greater the accessibility of your institution's courses and other facilities, the less students will need to seek alternative sources of funding.

Benefits

Benefits do provide a significant source of income for many disabled students. If a student is in receipt of the mobility and/or care components of Disability Living Allowance (DLA) this should continue to be paid as long as needs remain the same.

Part-time students may be able to continue to claim Income Support and full-time students may be able to claim this benefit if, for example, they qualify for the Disability Premium (Skill, 1997b). The Disability Premium is an allowance that is paid to people who have a long-term incapacity and to people with disabilities (Disability on the Agenda, undated). It is recommended that appropriate advice is obtained, as the rules for claiming Income Support while a student are subject to change.

Incapacity Benefit is a contributory benefit for people medically unable to work and who satisfy the contribution conditions. Activity apart from work does not in itself affect entitlement but an education course could indicate a wider ability to perform certain work on completion (Disability on the Agenda, undated). This benefit may be reviewed when a student starts a course and, if it is withdrawn, its reinstatement is not guaranteed (Skill, 1997b).

If the disabled student lives in private rented accommodation or in the family home and is receiving housing benefit this may continue. It is not available for those living in institutional residences (Skill, 1997b).

Students who are claiming certain benefits may be restricted in the number of hours they are able to study. Again these rules are subject to change and the educational institution will be able to give advice at the time of application.

Disability on the Agenda (undated) provides a comprehensive list of benefits and definitions. For more information about benefits and eligibility contact:

- Skills's Information Service
- Benefit Enquiry Line
- Benefits Agency local offices
- Action for Blind People
- RNIB (Welfare Rights and Community Care Advocacy Service).

The Students' Union

The Students' Union is a constitutional organization for students, controlled by students. The central principle is that of student representation, so allowing negotiation of changes in all areas of college life. The whole union is made up of representatives at many different levels, including those from individual courses through to positions for students on college governing bodies.

The Students' Union provides many facilities, ranging from bars and coffee shops through to counselling services. In view of the fact that welfare is considered to be one of its most central roles, accessibility of all these services and facilities will be crucial for visually impaired students. Experience suggests that Students' Unions in universities tend to be more active than those in further education.

Students' Unions are affiliated to the National Union of Students (NUS), which provides extensive research facilities, welfare advice and training for all union representatives. The NUS also represents students at a national level. Part of student life includes participation in the election of officers to the Students' Union and so it is vital that the ballot system is accessible to all students. During their time at college, disabled students may wish to stand for election to the Students' Union but not necessarily for the post of disabilities officer. It is important to remember that disabled students have an interest in issues other than those associated with disability.

Freshers' or induction week

Freshers' or induction week is the time when first year students are introduced to college life. This may take place before the commencement of the academic year. There are usually, however, a number of students from other years available to show new students the ropes. This period is likely to include:

- formal registration and enrolment;
- introduction to courses and course tutors;
- conducted tours around the college site in order to become familiar with such facilities as the library;
- informal exploration of college site and facilities;
- more commonly in higher education, a Freshers' Fair to provide the opportunity to join various clubs and societies;
- opportunities to meet and socialize with other students and to make friends.

Any written information, including that provided by student-run clubs and societies as well as maps of the college site and the local area, should be available in a variety of accessible formats. If social and leisure activities are advertised on noticeboards, it should be remembered that these notices will probably be inaccessible to visually impaired students. A mechanism should therefore be in place to ensure that such information is communicated to everyone. It is not acceptable to rely on the assumption that there will always be somebody available to pass it on. Some students, however, may still choose to employ a personal assistant to overcome these barriers. The DSA could be used to pay for such services. In further education the provision of support workers may be organized through the college. As mentioned earlier, access to information is crucial during this introductory phase and it may be helpful for visually impaired students to receive in advance copies of any material usually provided in print. These copies should be available in accessible formats and prior discussion with the students may be necessary to establish individual preferences.

Some colleges operate a 'buddy' system. Buddies are usually from the second or third year and may be generally available to assist all new students. They can be linked to a particular course; alternatively students may be paired for a specific reason. An example of this could be to link a new visually impaired student with one who is already on the course. Some students may find this system useful whilst others could consider it restrictive.

In order to be more familiar with the environment and to avoid crowded situations, some visually impaired students may choose to visit the college and local area before the beginning of the term.

Accommodation

The type and standard of student accommodation, if available, is extremely variable. Some general issues, however, need to be considered in relation to offering appropriate facilities for visually impaired students:

- All documentation relating to the accommodation should be produced in a range of accessible formats. If notices giving information about health and safety matters (for example, details of fire exits, safe areas and building evacuation) are normally displayed on the wall, the content should be reproduced in other media to ensure accessibility for visually impaired residents.
- Visually impaired students have the same range of priorities as all other students when it comes to making decisions about where to live while undertaking a course of study. Choices may be restricted as to the location of accommodation and compromises may need to be made. For example, a visually impaired student may choose to live in a hall of residence at a considerable distance from the college because it offers rooms large enough to accommodate the extra desk space required for equipment. As a consequence of this choice other difficulties may be encountered, for example, in relation to transport facilities. If the person is a guide dog user, an area close to the accommodation will be required for relief and exercise.
- If the accommodation is a considerable distance away from the college and/or the student does not have assistive technology at home, the institution will need to be flexible in terms of providing adequate facilities and access to learning resources, for example, extended opening times for libraries and computer laboratories.
- Visually impaired students often require more space, as they may have a considerable amount of access equipment, such as a computer, CCTV and additional lighting. Extra storage space will also be necessary, particularly if a student uses tape, large print or Braille. Consideration must also be given to the needs of a guide dog: space for its basket, water and food bowls and any other requisite equipment.
- Some visually impaired students may require mobility training to help them to become familiar with the accommodation and its environs. Social Services may be able to offer assistance. Other helpful organizations include RNIB, GDBA, Action for Blind People and/or local societies for the blind. Some colleges and universities have personnel who are able to provide this service.

The disabilities coordinator or the learning support tutor can be contacted for further advice.

- If the accommodation provides self-catering and laundry facilities it will be important for these to be accessible to visually impaired students. An initial conducted tour of the area and facilities may need to be arranged.

Issues relating to accessing the environment are discussed in Chapter 7. It is important to take these into account in the context of accommodation.

Catering services

Self-service canteens often present problems for visually impaired students. Menus are commonly placed at a height well above eye level and may be hand written or in small print. This makes them inaccessible to most visually impaired students. Having to carry a plate of food, transfer it on to a tray and operate a drinks machine while managing books, bag and perhaps a cane or dog as well as negotiating other students, their chairs and bags can prove to be an impossible task. Canteens may be areas of uniformity – rows of tables and chairs with very few landmarks. Some visually impaired people may find this environment extremely disorientating.

If assistance is requested, it would be helpful for the catering staff to negotiate with each person exactly what is required. In any case the menu should be produced in an accessible format, and some students may ask for assistance with the serving of food, or carrying trays to tables. Guide dog owners carry health and safety certificates issued by the Department of the Environment to prove that the dogs are allowed into areas where food is served.

Guide dogs

Some visually impaired students may choose to have a guide dog as their means of accessing the environment. It is important, nevertheless, to remember that, however lovable, a guide dog is a working animal. It should not be distracted or petted when in harness. On no account should titbits of food be offered. It is always advisable to consult the owner at all times about how the dog should be treated. Dogs, like people, are susceptible to mood changes and can experience stress from being in a new environment. Some are sociable; others prefer to be left alone. Experience confirms, however, that the dog also provides a medium through which contacts and friendships may be made and often acts as an ice breaker. It should be remembered that, as part of the training process, the owner will have learnt to be firm about how others treat the dog. This could however be misunderstood by the general public and potential friends, who may withdraw if they feel they have been reprimanded for petting the dog at an inappropriate time.

Child care

Some visually impaired students may wish to take advantage of the college's child care or crèche facilities. Due to the general difficulties of accessing information, these students may be unaware of the facilities and services offered by the institution. It is important that any information about support services is made available in a range of media and that the procedures to be followed are clearly understood. If crèche or other facilities are not on the college site, it may be necessary to issue some visually impaired students with specific information and directions as to their location.

Counselling

Counselling can take various forms but is most commonly recognized as a one-to-one relationship between a client and someone who has received considerable formal training leading to membership of a professional body. It can be short or long term, lasting for six weeks or several years. Sessions vary in length but are usually between 45 minutes and one hour. Confidentiality is always maintained.

Counselling involves working with people to help them to understand and deal with problems that are often too complex to manage alone. The counsellor's role is to listen, provide support and assist the client to address particular issues. The aim of counselling is to enable the client to take a greater control over her or his life, by facilitating the development of self-awareness and problem-solving skills in relation to personal issues. The counsellor does not give directives but offers a psychologically safe and secure environment in which the client can explore, and ultimately gain a deeper insight into the workings of the self.

It is important to emphasize that, in common with non-disabled people, visually impaired clients come from a variety of social and cultural backgrounds. Equally, they may seek counselling for a variety of reasons, not necessarily associated with their visual impairment. These might include physical symptoms, anxiety, stress, loneliness or bereavement. In general, the student identifies a need to talk to someone about a problem that interferes with everyday activities and for which no solution has yet been found. She or he may describe being 'stuck' and experience feelings of frustration at being unable to deal with certain aspects of life.

> Often what emerges is a struggle over identity. The
> questions 'who am I'? and 'do I matter?' are particularly
> faced by people around the times of adolescence and
> major change. (Withers, 1996)

Inevitably, however, the life history presented by blind and partially sighted students will have been affected by their visual impairment, although the extent to which this has a bearing on the client's personal problems will vary from individual to individual. For some students, the presence of impairment could be a significant factor in their decision to seek counselling:

> People born with impairments may never have had their
> identities affirmed by being recognized as whole people.
> Those with acquired impairments (through accident,
> illness and age) may struggle to reconcile their new selves
> with their former non-disabled identities. (Withers, 1996)

Visually impaired students may have faced discrimination or have been subjected to verbal and/or physical abuse. Decisions about whether or not to enter into a long-term relationship and have children may be the cause of anguish. For the first time, clients may be painfully conscious of what they perceive to be significant differences between themselves and other students. The pressures of battling with access issues may be the cause of high stress levels (see Chapter 4).

Although visually impaired students may bring some of these issues to counselling, it would be inaccurate to state that every disabled client prefers to work with a disabled counsellor. In certain cases, however, this might be important, especially if the client's impairment is one of the principal reasons for seeking counselling help. It is estimated that few counsellors possess specialist knowledge of sight impairment (Royal National Institute for the Blind, 1997a) and this fact may well contribute to a reluctance on the part of some visually impaired people to seek professional assistance. Whether the impairment is congenital or acquired later in life, experience suggests that most visually impaired students have been socialized into the individual model of disability with all the negative consequences that such socialization brings. This process is extremely difficult to unlearn although there will be some clients who, because of exposure to the philosophy of the social model, have begun to challenge the tenets of the individual model (see Chapter 3).

If non-disabled counsellors are to be effective, therefore, it will be important for the counsellor to have an insight into the significance of both the primary and secondary barriers in the lives of disabled people. It may be helpful to participate in some form of awareness-raising programme and to become familiar with some disability-specific issues that might be encountered during counselling sessions. For example, in relation to visually impaired clients, it is crucial for counsellors to consider such topics as communication and to address ways in which methods might need to be adapted for people who are blind or partially sighted. Eye contact, upon which so many people rely to send and receive messages, may not represent an appropriate channel and counsellors need to remember this when talking to visually impaired clients.

Most colleges provide counselling services and it is important that these are as accessible to visually impaired students as they are to other students. Experience indicates that, although many visually impaired students are willing to discuss their problems on an informal basis with a designated tutor, some are reluctant to request formal counselling and encouragement to do so is sometimes needed. In such cases, the role of the counsellor needs to be explained and it is helpful to emphasize that to ask for counselling represents a sign of strength and not, as many students seem to believe, a sign of weakness (Royal National Institute for the Blind, 1997b). It may be appropriate to encourage students to practice communication and assertiveness techniques. Counsellors and/or visually impaired clients may find it useful to contact Action for Blind People and RNIB for further information and advice. RNIB's Voluntary Agencies Link Unit (VALU) can provide a list of local voluntary agencies for blind people, some of which offer counselling services. Additionally, it may be useful to contact impairment-specific societies for advice. Other sources of help include the Social Services department, the hospital's eye department and GP surgeries. The British Association for Counselling should be able to provide a full list of accredited counsellors, some of whom may be identified as having a specialist background in disability matters.

Assertiveness and self-advocacy

Assertiveness is associated with the ability to claim one's rights and is a continuum with passivity at one extreme and aggression at the other. Advocacy involves speaking and acting, persuasively and forcefully, on behalf of someone's rights and interests. This could be done by one person on behalf of another, or some people prefer to represent themselves: self-advocacy.

Although there is some variation in the way self-advocacy is defined by different groups, certain core components can be identified. Among these are:

- Being able to express thoughts and feelings, with assertiveness if necessary.
- Being able to make choices and decisions.
- Having clear knowledge and information about rights.
- Being able to make changes (Clare, 1990).

Effective advocacy and assertiveness techniques are closely linked with good communication skills and students may benefit from some training in these areas in order to manage potentially demanding situations.

Some of the issues faced by visually impaired students are different to those encountered by their peers. They may, for example, have to negotiate with lecturers and other staff who do not provide materials in the appropriate medium, or with support staff who are over-protective. It might be necessary to employ and supervise readers or other support workers. These situations will require the student to possess some level of assertiveness or self-advocacy skills when dealing with these service providers.

In further education colleges there may be self-advocacy groups whose remit includes elements of assertiveness training. The groups may also consider some of the issues addressed in Chapter 3. Any sessions offered by these groups in which these matters are considered may involve focus on individual students, preparation of portfolios and development of presentation and self-reflection techniques. For more details of this kind of group work see Clare (1990).

The Association of Blind and Partially Sighted Teachers and Students (ABAPSTAS), is a self-help organization. Among other things, it has an annual conference and often runs confidence-building and study skills workshops. Many visually impaired students derive a great deal of benefit from peer support, for example, from sharing information and advice. Many feel relieved that other students also experience problems related to visual impairment and gain confidence by talking things through with someone who has first-hand experience of disability.

Careers guidance

The Secretary of State has a duty to ensure that careers guidance and placing services are provided for all people attending schools and colleges and for those who have recently left the education system. The Careers Service is able to provide information, advice, guidance, referral and placing services to this client group. In contrast to the provision for non-disabled people, there is no age or time restriction for people with disabilities. They remain in the client group until they are settled in their career following education and/or training. These services are not available to students attending higher education, although universities offer careers advice as part of their general student services.

The Careers Service offers a more specific service to disabled people:

> To provide support or advocacy to enable clients at a disadvantage in the labour market to find suitable opportunities, and offer ongoing help after placement. (Disability on the agenda, undated)

To this end it is essential that visually impaired students have the same access to all information and facilities as those available to sighted students. This will involve provision of materials in appropriate media and speech, Braille or large-character access to electronically stored careers information.

There are many careers that are open to blind and partially sighted people (Jamison, 1995), and it should not be assumed that only certain stereotypical occupations such as music, physiotherapy and law are suitable. Visually impaired people work in a wide range of employment situations and many have achieved success in their chosen field. A significant number of these have been documented by RNIB and it is recommended that ESSN be contacted for further information (see also Chapter 9).

The aim of this chapter has been to consider the wider aspects of student life and to emphasize that the access needs of visually impaired students should be taken into account in the provision of the college's goods, facilities and services. Academic success can be achieved only if visually impaired students feel safe and secure in the college environment. It is important to enjoy social, cultural and personal activities and to be able to participate fully in the non-academic curriculum. It is also crucial that visually impaired students are able to establish their identity within the student cohort and that opportunities to form meaningful relationships are not restricted.

References

Barnes, C. (1991) *Disabled People in Britain and Discrimination*, Hurst and Company, London.

Clare, M. (1990) *Developing Self-Advocacy Skills with People with Disabilities and Learning Difficulties*, Further Education Unit, London.

Department for Education and Employment (1997) *Investing in the Future: Supporting Students in Higher Education. A Guide to the Financial Support Arrangements for Those Starting Higher Education in 1998/99*, DfEE, London.

Disability on the Agenda (undated) *Making Connections: A Guide for Agencies Helping Young People with Disabilities Make the Transition from School to Adulthood.*

Jamison, J. (1995) *Visually Impaired Candidates for Employment: A Survey of Further and Higher Institutions and Students*, NFER, Slough, UK.

Royal National Institute for the Blind (1997a) *Talking It Over: Some Suggestions for Help with Counselling*, RNIB, London.

Royal National Institute for the Blind (1997b) *Getting What You Want*, RNIB, London.

Skill (1997a) *Financial Assistance for Students with Disabilities in Higher Education*, Skill, London.

Skill (1997b) *The Co-ordinator's Handbook*, Skill, London.

Skill and CRAC, (1997) *Higher Education and Disability*, Hobsons, Cambridge.

Smith, A. (1997) Students: nothing to fear. *Disability Now*, December, p. 14.

Withers, S. (1996) The experience of counselling, in *Beyond Disability: Towards an Enabling Society* (ed. G. Hales), Sage. London, pp. 96–104.

Towards inclusive education: a strategic approach

Trends in tertiary education

Over the last decade or so, the number of people with learning difficulties and/or disabilities – including those with a visual impairment – entering post-school, mainstream educational programmes has risen dramatically. This is partly the consequence of the 1981 (Warnock) educational legislation (together with the relevant guidance and regulations) and the subsequent arrival of that generation in post-school education. Other legislation – for example, the Children Act (1989) and the Further and Higher Education Acts (1992) – has reinforced the principles of inclusivity, placing specific requirements upon educational establishments to consider the access needs of learners with disabilities and to provide appropriate facilities. Attitude change among disabled people themselves also accounts for their increased participation in mainstream, post-school education. Many have higher aspirations than before and are prepared to challenge the system. This determination has been reflected in their strenuous efforts to overcome the numerous barriers to entering mainstream institutions and has resulted in their participation in an increasingly wide variety of curricula. Alongside these struggles, the dedicated work of educational consultants (for example, Jean McGinty and Lesley Dee) and other voluntary organizations and agencies, such as Skill, in helping to raise awareness of disability and access issues must also be acknowledged. Predictions are that the growth in numbers of disabled students entering all levels of education is likely to continue, although it is anticipated that the rate will be less dramatic.

Further education

In general, the provision for students with learning difficulties and/or disabilities in further and continuing education has gradually improved. Most colleges are responding to the needs of a far wider range of students than was the case 15 years ago (McGinty and Fish, 1992).

> When provision for students with disabilities and learning difficulties was first introduced it was often low status and accommodated in annexes sometimes apart from the main college. However, attitudes have changed, work of quality has raised the status of provision and there has been steady progress in adapting college buildings and providing purpose-built facilities. It is now common for physical aspects to all further and continuing education to receive serious attention. (McGinty and Fish, 1992)

The concepts of teaching and learning have received increased attention from policy makers and providers and have undergone a redefinition to keep pace with the general climate of social, economic and political change. The Further Education Unit (FEU), which operated for many years, did much to improve the provision for disabled students. In recognition of the need to attract more disabled students and to provide a quality, needs-led service to such learners, colleges have responded by supplying flexible programmes designed to meet a variety of access needs. Thus 'block-release and day-release courses and twilight and night courses' are now commonly available and there is also 'a greater contribution in the community; for example, in day and residential centres of all kinds' (McGinty and Fish, 1992).

These changes in educational philosophy and practice within further and continuing education have had a significant impact upon the numbers of disabled students gaining access to sector courses. According to the first survey of English further education, there were 38,000 disabled students registered on full-time and part-time courses in 1985 (Stowell, 1987). A subsequent survey conducted between 1995 and 1996 revealed that:

> Across 272 colleges providing full data, 81,892 students are identified as having a learning difficulty and/or disability. Grossing this up to a national level implies that, for the further education sector as a whole in England, there are some 126,500 students with learning difficulties and/or disabilities which represents between 5.3% and 5.7% of the enrolled student population in November, 1995. (Further Education Funding Council, 1997a)

This figure is more than double that of a decade ago. The survey suggests that 'there are in excess of 4,400 students with a visual impairment (and without other impairments), itself close to a ten fold increase in the last decade' (Stowell, 1997). It is reported that 'the incidence of students with visual impairments is similar across most groups of colleges, but is much lower than average among students in art and design colleges and in agriculture and horticulture colleges' (Further Education Funding Council, 1997a). The survey identified 35.8% of institutions as providing Braille and taping services and 43.8% as offering specialist teaching and support for visually impaired students (Further Education Funding Council, 1997a).

In recognition of the general climate of constant change taking place within the further and continuing education sectors (McGinty and Fish, 1993) and the need to monitor progress, a Review Group initiated by the Further Education Funding Councils (FEFCs) led, in 1995, to the metamorphosis of the Further Education Unit (FEU) into the Further Education Development Agency (FEDA) which was 'set up to support further education' (Further Education

Development Agency, 1995). In its mission statement, the agency declares a commitment to ongoing staff training and development initiatives and to the promotion of equal opportunities across the further education sector. With specific reference to students with learning difficulties and/or disabilities, FEDA aims to 'improve access to and participation in further education' (Further Education Development Agency, 1995).

The Widening Participation Committee was set up by the FEFC in 1994 and focused on the educational and access needs of all socially disadvantaged and under-represented groups. Chaired by Helena Kennedy QC, its terms of reference were to identify areas of non-participation and poor-quality educational experiences in further education, and how participation could be widened and quality improved (Further Education Funding Council, 1997b, 1997c). The Committee's recommendations, published in June 1997, are wide-ranging and are underpinned by an inclusive educational philosophy that defines learning as a life-long process, the economic and social benefits of which are interdependent (Further Education Funding Council, 1997b). Participation in education 'must be widened, not simply increased' because national economic success is linked to 'maximizing the potential for all' (Further Education Funding Council, 1997b). The development of a national strategic approach to improving educational opportunities for everyone and the establishment of effective monitoring mechanisms are therefore regarded as crucial steps to realizing these ideals (Further Education Funding Council, 1997b). Although the Committee's recommendations do not focus specifically on the educational requirements of people with learning difficulties and/or disabilities, it is not unreasonable to assume that the needs of this group will be addressed by policy makers and educational providers in the future as reflected in the UK government's response (Department for Education and Employment, 1998a).

In 1995, the FEFC set up a second, more specific committee whose remit, according to its chairperson, John Tomlinson, was to 'examine current educational provision for those with learning difficulties and/or disabilities and say whether the new legal requirements of the Further and Higher Education Act (1992) were being satisfied and, if they were not in any respects, how that could be remedied' (Further Education Funding Council, 1996). The fundamental principle that underpinned the Committee's numerous recommendations to the FEFC was that of inclusivity. The practice of inclusivity is inextricably linked to improvements in the quality of service delivery, which, in turn, will guarantee wider participation in further education by disabled students. Quality standards cannot rise without appropriate funding to undertake activities such as strategic planning, data collection, comprehensive assessment of students' learning and access requirements, in-service staff-training and awareness-raising programmes, inter-departmental, and cross-college communication and collaboration with relevant external agencies (Further Education Funding Council, 1996). The FEFC have taken various steps towards implementing these recommendations, as first indicated in its press release (Further Education Funding Council, 1997d).

Higher education

In the past 15 years, the higher education sector has perhaps experienced even more significant changes than those that have affected further and continuing education. This period has witnessed the emergence of a continual, and sometimes heated, debate about the fundamental principles that underpin teaching practice. Traditionalist – and often elitist – views have been challenged by those whose concept of learning extends beyond the academic and whose primary concern is to increase participation by people from under-represented groups. Academic inequality, however, demonstrably exists:

> A sure indicator of this academic inequality is the emphasis upon 'transferable skills' within the new university sector, where specific subject areas assume less significance . . . 'they are looking for skills appropriate to any work-place – teamwork, communication and organizational skills' . . . In this context, the learner is held responsible for acquiring a range of social and life skills, nebulous in nature. (Corbett and McGinty, 1996)

As a consequence 'the old universities are relieved of so pressing a demand to respond to consumer needs while the new universities are overwhelmed with pressure for services' (Corbett and McGinty, 1996). In recognition that students require assistance with study skills and college life in general, a wide range of imaginative and innovative teaching approaches and methods have evolved in many institutions, some of which have become formalized projects that have attracted government funding (for example, the Enterprise in Higher Education Initiative). That such practices have reflected a radical redefinition of the concepts of teaching and learning has led, subsequently, to significant changes in the design and content of many course programmes. The features of these programmes include flexibility and adaptability and recognize and value students' prior learning and their potential contribution to *everyone's* educational experience (see Wailey, 1996).

Hurst (1996) states, however, that 'Disabled people have been rather neglected' and cites a number of reports on access which support this fact. With a remit to survey both the general provision for disabled students and the specific facilities available for students 'with a significant visual impairment', Patton (1993) reported that, of the 111 responses, only two of the 62 institutions that had a named person with responsibility for disabled students provided additional information and support for visually impaired students.

In 1992, the UK government (DfE) instructed the Higher Education Funding Councils (HEFCs) to take appropriate action to redress the balance. Whilst each Council's interpretation was different, all identified the need for positive action. For example, the Higher Education Funding Council for England (HEFCE) established a disability advisory group to advise it on disability matters. Myers and Parker (1996) describe the positive effect that the commitment of financial resources has had:

> The HEFCE special initiative funding offered in 1993–94 and 1994–95 across the sector to promote access to HE for students with disabilities and learning difficulties has very 'significantly raised the profile of disability' and progressed the policy and provision for students with disabilities in

many institutions. The special initiative funding was made available to institutions of HE with a proven track record of implementing work with students with disabilities who were invited to bid for funds to carry out research leading to the development of best practice.

For examples of projects that have led to the adoption of a strategic approach to service provision for students with disabilities and learning difficulties in higher education, see Hurst (1996), Cooper and Corlett (1996) and Myers and Parker (1996). For evaluation of these projects in terms of quality standards, see Corbett and McGinty (1996).

This increased focus on disability and participation in higher education is evident in statistics contained in the Dearing Report (Dearing, 1997). The report reveals that, of the 569,100 first-year UK students in 1996, 14,800 declared a disability, of whom 600 were blind or partially sighted. Visually impaired students comprise 4% of all known disabled full-time students and 5.2% of all known disabled part-time students. With reference to all undergraduates, the report estimates that 27,000 (2%) have declared a disability. According to the Labour Force survey, however, 7% of people between the ages of 18 and 30 declare a disability, which suggests that, whilst the numbers participating in undergraduate programmes has increased over the years, disabled people remain under-represented in higher education. Their percentage representation at postgraduate level is thought to be even lower than that at undergraduate level. In view of these findings, the Dearing Report contains various recommendations whose implementation would go some way to remedying the situation. In summary these are as follows:

(1) Higher Education Councils should provide funding for institutions to supply learning support for students with disabilities. Funding should be contingent upon the institution's ability to demonstrate widening participation and on its strategic development. Funding should be topsliced for initiatives designed to widen participation.
(2) Quality assurance issues should take priority in provision for disabled students, who should expect to receive a base level of

support in all institutions. Each institution should be required to engage in the process of standard setting and to produce audits of facilities and services. The Quality Assurance Agency for Higher Education will oversee this ongoing process.

(3) The UK government should extend the scope of the Disabled Students' Allowance (DSA) to be available, without a means test, to part-time and postgraduate students and to those who have become disabled and who wish to obtain a second, higher education qualification. To avoid the problems of diversity of policy and practice among LEAs, the award should be administered by a single authority.

(4) The budget allocated to universities for Access funds should be doubled and the criteria for application should be unified across all universities. Specifically, eligibility to apply should be extended to part-time students.

(5) The Institute for Learning and Teaching in Higher Education should include the learning needs of students with disabilities in its research programme accreditation and advisory activities. To comply with these recommendations, lecturers are likely to be required to demonstrate a minimum standard of competency.

Although it is disappointing that the Dearing Committee did not recommend the extension of the Disability Discrimination Act (DDA) to include higher education, the requirement that institutions should implement good practice is encouraging. Indeed, the government's response to the Committee's recommendations (Department for Education and Employment, 1998b) indicates that many of these will be adopted. As noted in Chapter 11, the government is addressing issues relating to the DSA which will go some way to alleviating the financial difficulties in which many disabled students find themselves.

Visually impaired students in further and higher education

In 1995, the National Foundation for Educational Research (NFER) undertook surveys of staff and visually impaired students in a comprehensive range of types and sizes of Further and Higher Education institutions. The objective of this research was 'to provide information on the numbers, characteristics and needs of visually impaired young people who will be seeking employment in the next two to three years' (Jamison, 1995). Two hundred and twenty further education colleges identified 1,947 visually impaired students as following a wide variety of non-degree programmes; 432 were identified by 42 universities as undertaking a total of 68 degree courses. Since the standard of record keeping varied between institutions, however, the accuracy of these figures may be questioned, although the researchers seem to be optimistic that the numbers may be even higher. Interestingly – and in common with some institutional staff – the researchers seem to identify the concept of student 'support' with the provision of specialized, high-tech equipment. They report that, of additional services offered to visually impaired students, those most frequently provided by institutions were adaptations of course materials and other IT facilities. Overall, these were considered to be adequate and included screen magnification software, speech and Braille output, CD-ROM and CCTVs. The researchers conclude, nevertheless, that visually impaired students would derive benefit from a central pool of up-to-date equipment and recommend that both students and staff should be alerted to the advantages of additional IT skills training.

A much more significant finding, however, was the wide diversity of approach in colleges and universities to meeting students' needs:

> . . . from, at one extreme, those who left it entirely to the students to approach them for requests for support, to those who made all possible efforts to assess needs and offer solutions. Special provision for VI students varied greatly from one institution to another as regards needs assessment, induction, mobility, counselling, learning support and careers advice. (Jamison, 1995)

The research suggests that, in general terms, some visually impaired students are receiving an adequate level of service provision. With the ever-increasing range of technical solutions to meet curriculum access problems, it is possible to be optimistic about the numbers of blind and partially sighted people likely to achieve success in post-school education. What emerges, however, is a clear impression that an *ad hoc* approach prevails and that institutions continue to place a considerable amount of responsibility upon individual visually impaired students for obtaining access to college services. The recommendations contained in reports produced by the Tomlinson (1996) and Kennedy (1997) Committees are worth revisiting.

The consumer perspective

In common with all customer groups disabled people are becoming increasingly knowledgeable and self-confident about consumer rights. The duties placed on funding councils by the Further and Higher Education Acts (1992) and the Disability Discrimination Act (1995) to take account of disabled students' needs reinforce their increasing expectations that all service providers – including colleges and universities – should make their facilities, goods and services universally accessible. As for all other service users, the requirements of disabled people should be met. The Charter for Higher Education (1993) emphasizes the rights of disabled students and the duty of institutions to respect those rights:

> Universities and colleges should explain their policies for providing access to students with disabilities or learning difficulties. They should tell you about any extra support that is available, such as extra staff or equipment, and any arrangements to cater for people with physical disabilities including access to buildings. (Department for Education, 1993)

The burgeoning amount of literature on disability and the information published by such agencies as Skill have also made a significant contribution to awareness-raising programmes designed for both students and college staff. (See, for example, Cooper, 1992; Corbett and Barton, 1992; Corlett and Cooper, 1992; Skill, 1993,

1997; Luker and Thompson, 1994; Skill and CRAC, 1996; Skill, 1997). The availability of the Disabled Students Allowance (DSA), although still subject to unacceptable restrictions, has been widely publicized and has done much to liberate those disabled students in full-time higher education who depend upon expensive equipment and support services in order to gain full access to the curriculum.

In spite of these positive influences, however, the progress towards dismantling many of the attitudinal, environmental and financial barriers faced by disabled students in all educational sectors remains painfully slow. Considerable experience supported by written evidence confirms that equal access to that enjoyed by their non-disabled peers continues to be denied to many disabled learners. (See, for example, Harrison, 1996; Gardiner, 1997; Gregory, 1997; Stowell, 1997.) The possible explanations for this are numerous but, it could be argued, some may be related to the general enterprise culture in which we now live and operate. Of course, there are positive aspects to such a culture: the economic benefits of investing in disabled people have been recognized by the UK government's New Deal (1997) initiative. Furthermore, competition tends to focus the minds of providers on such issues as customer needs and the quality of services offered. Whilst the positive effects on disabled people's educational experiences must be acknowledged, it can equally be argued that this enterprise culture nevertheless represents a significant challenge. Within the market-place ethos 'certain groups have always found difficulty in gaining access . . . and are vulnerable to market forces. Their needs may be different, difficult to meet and costly, generating insufficient income or profit' (McGinty and Fish, 1993). Other more specific reasons might include:

- inappropriate admission and transition procedures;
- crisis management of perceived 'problems';
- underdeveloped networking skills, both within the institution and with relevant external agencies;
- ideological tensions and pressures associated with the need to adapt to constant change, leading to staff insecurity and disharmony;

- ineffective college management information systems, resulting in poor planning and monitoring of services;
- inadequate cross-college human, physical and financial resources to provide essential learning support, appropriate curriculum and environmental access and ongoing staff development programmes in such subject areas as equal opportunities issues, disability, strategic planning, institutional audit, evaluation methods and quality control.

Meeting the challenge: an institutional approach

When considering ways of meeting these challenges and of improving the quality of services to disabled students, a formal, strategic approach should be adopted. In her FEDA report, Faraday (1996) recommends that 'Staff at both strategic planning and operational levels need to be proactive in liaising with other agencies' and suggests that colleges should:

- ensure early identification of particular requirements. Clear procedures need to be in place for referral for additional support requirements;
- develop whole-college approaches to supporting individual learners;
- identify and plan progression routes both through and beyond education ensuring that support is available at all stages.

It will, initially, be necessary to consider the quality of current practice and the level of provision. This may involve examining the structure and processes by which a service is offered and the college may wish to approach the task by conducting an audit.

The educational audit

The educational audit has been defined as:

. . . a practical approach to professional accountability within the educational service. It encompasses the systematic investigation, analysis and subsequent reporting of the performance, resources and systems of an educational unit. An educational unit may be a small section within an institution, a whole institution or a group of institutions within a Local Education Authority. Performance evaluation in education, carried out through the educational audit process embraces:

- all aspects of the activities of the authority, institution or unit under review;
- consideration of both effectiveness (i.e. quality, the relationship between expectations and outcomes) and efficiency (which covers relevant considerations of economy and the relationship between inputs and outcomes). (Further Education Unit, 1991)

It is important to emphasize that the audit process involves the comparison of a recognized set of quality standards with actual practice. It will, therefore, be important for all relevant personnel to agree such standards before conducting an audit exercise, since an objective evaluation of service provision cannot be made in their absence. Audits may fall into various categories. Barnard and Hartigan (1998) use the following classification:

Structure

- availability of high-tech equipment
- deployment of staff; staff skill mix
- training: budget; in-house versus external courses
- features of the working environment.

Process

- transition characteristics
- on-course monitoring and evaluation procedures
- time taken to gain access to specified equipment, e.g. photocopier
- staff appraisal systems.

Outcome

- student entry/exit patterns
- entry qualifications in relation to on-course performance
- outcome and use of specific teaching technique
- outcome and use of specific teaching approach or style.

Effective auditing requires the collaboration of a variety of college personnel – including senior management – and personnel from outside organizations and agencies who are selected to represent a range of legitimate interests. It is crucial that staff at all levels are committed to the principal of audit and that it is viewed as a positive and not a negative process. Anxieties are not uncommon and may exist due to the following factors:

- Inadequate financial resources.
- Pressures of work: audit is time consuming.
- Holding a recognized teaching qualification guarantees quality: audit is therefore unnecessary.
- Audit is a waste of time: recommendations may not, for various reasons, be implemented.
- Changes take place all too frequently: further change is unnecessary.
- Audit results may reveal poor practice, leading to possible job losses.

It is crucial that, if anxieties do exist, they are recognized and addressed before the commencement of the audit process. This will encourage involvement with its design and procedures from the outset, which, in turn, is likely to generate feelings of ownership, acceptance of the audit's findings and a commitment to implementing its recommendations and strategic plan (Further Education Unit, 1991; Barnard and Hartigan, 1998). It is particularly important for middle and senior college management to be supportive, especially those with budgetary control. In many cases, not only does the audit itself represent a costly exercise in terms of both human and financial resources, but the implementation of its recommendations often requires considerable financial outlay. An example of this might be the appointment of a new member of staff whose remit is to initiate change in college practices or the purchasing of external staff training programmes (Roy, 1998).

An integral part of the process of audit is the preliminary brainstorming exercise. McGinty and Fish (1993) recommend that the following questions should be posed:

- What is the principal purpose of the institution?
- On what conceptual framework is the institution's development based?
- What values are implicit or explicit in its policies?
- What should be the main priority in the institution's plan?
- What are the short-term and long-term objectives of its work?
- How do these objectives relate to the objectives of other further (and higher) education and training provision?

These authors continue:

> With the data provided by an audit, the answers to these questions should provide a basis on which to develop plans. The preparation of strategic and tactical development plans . . . and a business plan . . . should follow, setting out more detailed objectives and specifying what the college can offer.

At this stage, simultaneous consultation and discussion with personnel from other relevant organizations and funding authorities should take place to obtain information and ideas, determine the current level of expertise, and identify specific training and development needs.

Audit protocols

Once an appropriate topic has been selected and agreed, the audit process can begin. It is important to adopt a structured approach and to draw up an audit protocol that will ensure that tasks are kept on track, on time and that the audit process is completed.

Audit protocols are similar to research protocols and business plans in that they identify the aims and objectives, and the means by which these will be addressed. The protocol is also a statement of intent as to the reasons or need for the audit. In addition, it sets out the implications of undertaking such an audit, including costing, staff resources and a realistic time-scale. (Barnard and Hartigan, 1998)

Although it is not necessary for the protocol to be lengthy, it must be comprehensive and should be seen and agreed by all participants. It is a useful tool for keeping the project focused and on track. The timescale and all personnel involved in the audit process should be clearly identified so that everyone's commitment is recognized.

McGinty and Fish (1993) catalogue the stages of audit, providing a useful check-list:

- establishing priorities;
- setting quality standards;
- considering resource levels and management;
- identifying any 'specialisms' (to include the access needs of students with learning difficulties and disabilities);
- the development of cross-institutional strategic plans;
- providing staff training and development;
- delivering the programme (this might also be classified as delivering the goods and services and providing the facilities);
- evaluating current practice and provision (with modifications as appropriate).

It is worth repeating that the audit exercise should be regarded by everyone involved as a positive, crucial exercise, because it can facilitate the establishment of an agreed cross-institutional philosophy and indicate ways forward.

The pre-audit survey

The initial survey of any aspect of service delivery is sometimes described as an audit. Such preliminary surveys, however, focus on the level of existing provision and are not conducted in relation to a set of established quality criteria. They do not compare actual practice with any formulated standard. For the purposes of clarity, therefore, it is perhaps more accurate to describe them as pre-audit surveys (Barnard and Hartigan, 1998). Pre-audit surveys are, nevertheless, an important stage in the audit process 'because they identify the baseline at which to set standards which can then be used in a subsequent audit project' (Barnard and Hartigan, 1998). They can focus on structure, process or outcome. An example of a pre-audit survey might be an examination of the process of issuing portable equipment to visually impaired students, such as all types of cassette tape recorders. College staff want to identify exactly what the process and problems are before setting any standards and undertaking a formal audit. The following is an outline of the procedure:

Title

A survey of the process of issuing all types of cassette tape recorders by the learning support department.

Problem statement

Cassette tape recorders are issued indiscriminately by technical and support staff. The paperwork is currently inefficient and incomplete. No effective system exists for tracking or recalling cassette recorders that are not currently being used by students. The college budget for cassette tape recorders is not keeping pace with demand.

Aims and objectives

(1) To identify how many and what type of cassette tape recorders are being issued from the learning support department.
(2) To identify who is issuing them.
(3) To identify the reasons why the current logging system is not functioning satisfactorily.
(4) To investigate the present recall system.

Survey

Conduct a retrospective survey of cassette tape recorder issue, covering the period of the last six months, in order to:

(1) Identify the number and type of cassette tape recorders purchased by the college.
(2) Identify the number and type of cassette tape recorders held in college store.
(3) Survey the logging system to identify who has issued what type of cassette tape recorder and to whom.
(4) Survey the records to ascertain how many cassette tape recorders (noting which type) have been returned.
(5) Survey the records to ascertain how many cassette tape recorders should be recalled.

Audits of service provision to students with disabilities

Using the audit process outlined above, it should be possible to focus on issues related to disabled students. The following questions should be posed:

- Is there an identified policy on disability and what values does it reflect? Is there a disparity between policy statements, college ethos and current practice?
- What specific goods, facilities and services are currently available?
- Are these of high quality, fully accessible and cost effective?
- How is the quality of current practice monitored and evaluated, by whom and how often? What constitutes 'best practice'?
- Is the current resource allocation adequate to deliver a quality service?
- What additional human, physical and financial resources would be required to meet any identified improvements, developments and staff training requirements?

In relation to the above, more specific questions include:

- How are disabled people perceived? Are they perceived as 'problems'?
- What status do disability issues hold within the institution?
- Is there a named, full-time, permanent member of staff responsible for disabled students?
- Do disability statements and general policies on disability exist?
- Were such statements and policies drawn up by a representative group of staff and students, including people with disabilities?
- Is there an overall plan with identified aims and short-term and long-term objectives?
- Are disability statements and policies incorporated into the college's overall mission statement and its strategic plans?
- Are budget holders (for example, the estates department) sensitive to disability issues?
- Are adequate human, physical and financial resources allocated to meet all identified access needs throughout the institution?
- Are comprehensive disability policies developed as a continual process?
- Are disability statements and policies widely publicized (internally and externally) and available in all media?
- Are these policies translated into general practice and owned by all staff?
- What monitoring mechanisms exist to ensure staff compliance with these policies?
- Are feedback mechanisms in place and are such policies regularly reviewed by a representative group including disabled students?
- Are statements of current limitations and future intention to improve and develop facilities and services regularly drawn up and widely publicized to present and prospective disabled staff and students?
- Is there an overall equal opportunities statement, officer and committee?
- Is there a committee for staff and students with disabilities?
- Does a representative from that committee sit on the equal opportunities committee?

- Do all staff receive in-service training and support on disability and equal opportunities issues, including the DDA and other relevant legislation relating to equal opportunities?
- To what extent does liaison take place inter-departmentally and between the institution and relevant external agencies and organizations concerned with disability, including schools, specialist colleges, Careers and Social Services Departments and the Employment Service?
- Is there a cross-college system of quality monitoring and information exchange which incorporates disability issues and which has the support of management?

If institutions are to adopt a strategic approach to disability-related services, it will be essential to obtain relevant data that reflect current levels of provision. This will provide a framework within which more specific plans can be made; these can then be modified and refined as the ongoing process of consultation and review with staff and students takes place.

As noted above, the audit can take many forms and can be used to focus on specific areas of provision. With reference to disabled students, it may be subdivided into the following areas:

- curriculum access
- technology and access systems
- environmental access
- support services (including library)
- staff training and development
- institutional (including philosophy and equal opportunities issues and structures).

The audit may also be considered in terms of the phases of a disabled student's experience (see Faraday, 1996):

- pre-entry
- on entry
- on programme
- on exit.

All of these areas have received attention in other chapters, which have provided specific examples of best practice. It is axiomatic that, given the declaration of, and a genuine commitment to, widening participation and a truly inclusive philosophy, the institution's provision for *all* students will, necessarily, be of a high quality. It follows, therefore, that services and facilities available to students with disabilities will be accessible.

To take three specific examples:

(1) It has been recommended that the institution's buildings and its immediate external environment should be constructed on the 'design for all' principle (see Chapter 7). This necessitates giving consideration to the access requirements of all those who live and work within it. If the design features of each corridor in a building are identical, if all the walls, doors and floors of the same building are in similar shades of light grey, with poor lighting and irregularly placed steps, the effect is disorientating – and depressing – for *everyone*.

(2) *Everyone's* learning experience will be adversely affected if tutors are required to work in difficult circumstances. If they are employed on short, fixed-term contracts, or on a part-time basis for one evening per week, opportunities to gather data relating to college policy and practices are likely to be limited. This will make the dissemination of crucial course-related information impossible, which, in turn, will place a strain on staff–student relationships because of the mismatch between expectations and staff capabilities. If there is no time to become familiar with all students' individual needs and the roles of other colleagues, to network and to establish supportive cooperative relationships, feelings of isolation and frustration are almost inevitable. The situation will be compounded if lack of funds is given as the reason for poor teaching resources and a working environment that is not conducive to learning, for example, a Nissen hut with poor heating and lighting. If staff development opportunities are non-existent due to lack of finances or participation is denied simply as a consequence of ignorance of their availability, this may lead to a complete breakdown in tutor–student relationships. The ultimate

collapse of the course could result due either to the resignation of the member of staff and/or to a significant number of students leaving the course.

(3) If the handouts produced by staff are hand-drawn diagrams, labelled in small scribble using light-coloured ink, photocopied on a machine that needs a replacement toner cartridge and issued to students as a casual afterthought two days following the lecture, *everyone's* learning experience will be impoverished.

The audit process and service provision for visually impaired students

Although institutional staff need to be closely involved in the audit process, it is recommended that, with reference to disability in general, the expertise available through external agencies is sought. With specific reference to service provision for people with a visual impairment, personnel from RNIB have considerable experience and this agency may be a useful first contact point for further advice and guidance. RNIB's Employment and Student Support Network (ESSN) and the Joint Mobility Unit (JMU) have, for several years, undertaken many kinds of audit: environmental, curriculum access, training needs analysis, and technology provision. As part of the audit service, a detailed report is compiled following the college visit. This is a comprehensive document which draws on a wide range of information supplied by the college, including its in-house documentation, interviews with staff and students and a tour of the relevant sites, which is synthesized to produce an overview of service provision upon which the college can reflect. The report also contains a catalogue of current provision, identifies areas of mismatch between current practice and established standards and makes recommendations on possible future developments. Following the production of such a report, a further visit is offered at which college staff have opportunities to discuss possible methods of implementing the report's recommendations. It is important to note that audit reports are also informed by general information relating to the support of students with learning difficulties and disabilities, especially that obtained from relevant government, FEFC and HEFC publications. Roy (1998) considers that the inculcation of such material into the audit report is crucial because it might otherwise be overlooked by staff. Furthermore, the importance and relevance of its advice and guidance are emphasized. These documents do not, however, contain explicit and specific guidelines on how learning support systems ought to be developed within the mainstream college structure. Given the current variation in college structures, therefore, opportunities to be creative are numerous. The audit report represents a tailored response to an individual college's requirements at a specific point in time and it can help to highlight these opportunities.

> Students with disabilities can only be given inclusive
> learning opportunities if their systems of support are woven
> into the fabric of institutional mechanisms. This comes
> from awareness of the institution's structures and forms of
> internal communication on the one hand and current
> SLDD guidance resources on the other. (Roy, 1998)

In view of the many advice and guidance documents and reports available (see, for example, Further Education Unit, 1992, 1993, 1994; Faraday, 1996) and recommendations from such bodies as the Tomlinson, Kennedy and Dearing Committees, the need for external audit services such as that offered by RNIB is becoming increasingly apparent:

> Evidence from all parts of further education confirms that
> unless senior management is knowledgeable, committed
> and energetic in the pursuit of creating a good service for
> students with learning difficulties (and disabilities) the
> work and dedication of middle management and teachers
> is diminished or frustrated. (Further Education Funding
> Council, 1996)

Indeed, experience confirms that many institutions place considerable value on the audit report. Roy (1998) observes that:

The pressure on some F/HE institutions which sometimes triggers an audit is a response to the regular reports sent by government agencies to F/HE principals about the need to integrate students with learning difficulties and disabilities, linked, in many cases, with F/HE funding mechanisms. There is also legislative pressure: principals must adhere to the Disability Discrimination Act (1995) and produce disability statements and so on.

That institutions value the audit report is confirmed by evidence that staff use the record of current provision as a basis on which to make future plans in the light of the recommendations received (Roy, 1998). If those plans include the development of current provision or the introduction of additional goods and facilities for visually impaired students, it is likely that staff training will be requested. The Report of the Learning Difficulties and/or Disabilities Committee emphasizes the importance of staff training in the promotion of inclusive learning opportunities (Further Education Funding Council, 1996), and experience indicates that staff derive considerable benefit from participating in these sessions. RNIB's ESSN is able to offer a full range of staff-training/awareness-raising and consultancy services and colleges are encouraged to contact the information officer for further information.

Marketing and publicity

Given that colleges are being urged by the government and the funding councils to undertake market research and to target, specifically, under-represented customer groups, it would be encouraging to see institutions taking positive action to address issues of inclusivity. It is recommended, therefore, that all educational institutions should develop marketing and publicity strategies. In an increasingly competitive market, it is crucial for the college to advertise its services and courses, as well as its support structures, to potential students with disabilities. Such people must feel welcome and confident that they will be able to participate fully in college life. In order to translate principles into practice, it is suggested (adapted from Warwick, 1990) that colleges should:

- develop a marketing and publicity policy that includes the careful scrutiny of publicity for discriminatory attitudes and practices, which might be reflected in language or visual imagery;
- develop publicity materials that, visually and verbally, positively seek to attract students with disabilities;
- promote equal opportunities in all college publications;
- liaise with schools and other relevant institutions and organizations to introduce disabled students to the availability of educational and vocational programmes on offer and which might have been considered as unsuitable or inaccessible;
- offer taster courses including study skills programmes designed to meet the specific needs of disabled students;
- organize open days that address the access requirements of disabled people;
- use non-traditional role models to encourage disabled people to take an interest in joining the college community;
- design and aim some materials at disabled students and target this group specifically;
- liaise with adult education providers, social and careers services and voluntary organizations, including local voluntary societies to establish good communication channels and to develop an ongoing relationship.

The importance of undertaking relevant investigations and developing good networks cannot be over-emphasized. Colleges should research their local market of visually impaired people by requiring staff to visit schools and other establishments to ascertain the trends in students' preferences and to discuss with individuals the services on offer. Being involved in auditing various aspects of service provision should enable college representatives to provide a realistic and up-to-date presentation of the college's facilities and of what can, and what cannot, currently be provided to meet the requirements of disabled students.

Responding to consumer needs

If institutions are to take the access requirements of disabled students seriously, such students must be perceived as consumers, with equal rights and status to all other customers. Inextricably linked with an institution's response to consumer needs are concepts such as performance indicators, accountability, enhancement, the assessment of quality provision, quality assurance and 'fitness for purpose' (Corbett and McGinty, 1996). The adoption of such concepts will necessarily result in the establishment of a formal structure within which staff can respond to disability issues with a planned approach instead of dealing with 'a problem' on an *ad hoc*, crisis-management basis. Involvement in a continual process of critical evaluation and review of policy and practice will result in the adoption of institution-wide strategic plans, which, in turn, will ensure that future practice takes account of everyone's rights. Ideally, this process should not be confined to the academic curriculum but must include the social and cultural aspects of student life (see Chapter 11).

There are, of course, many institutions that have demonstrated attempts to open doors to disabled students. In the further education sector, Lancaster and Morecambe College has been praised for its innovative approach to disabled people, both staff and students. The ethos is accurately described as 'inclusive', college resources have been put into providing curriculum access and staff training, and the physical environment is built on the 'design for all' principle (The Staff College, 1994). In the higher education sector, the University of East London declares its commitment to promoting equal opportunities for all under-represented groups and provides a wide range of support services to disabled students (Wolfendale and Corbett 1996). Every effort is made to provide the curriculum in accessible media and disabled students benefit from the services offered by RNIB's Resource Centre and the HEFCE-funded Access Centre, both of which are located on the Stratford campus.

Experience suggests, nevertheless, that the contents of a college's mission statement and the verbal commitment expressed by many staff to access issues do not always translate into practical application. In the final analysis, there always seems to be a reluctance to commit scarce resources to what is, covertly, still regarded as a low-priority consumer group. It seems that a radical change in an institution's value system is required for budget holders to commit scarce resources to improving the quality of provision for disabled students. Many more attitudinal, physical and financial barriers to education must be broken down if claims to offer equal access and opportunity to disabled learners are to be taken seriously.

References

Barnard, S. and Hartigan, G. (1998) *Clinical Audit in Physiotherapy: From Theory into Practice*, Butterworth Heinemann, Oxford.

Cooper, D. (1992) *Transitions – TVEI and Special Educational Needs: A Literature Review*, Skill, London.

Cooper, D. and Corlett, S. (1996) An overview of current provision, in *Opening Doors: Learning Support in Higher Education* (eds, S. Wolfendale and J. Corbett), Cassell, London and New York, pp. 145–57.

Corbett, J. and Barton, L. (1992) *Facing Challenges: The Changing Perspectives of Special Needs Co-ordinators*, Skill, London.

Corbett, J. and McGinty, J. (1996) Responding to consumer needs: working towards a quality service, in *Opening Doors: Learning Support in Higher Education* (eds S. Wolfendale and J. Corbett), Cassell, London and New York, pp. 84–100.

Corlett, S. and Cooper, D. (1992) *Students with Disabilities in Higher Education: A Guide for All Staff*, Skill, London.

Dearing, R. (1997) *Higher Education in a Learning Society: Committee Report*, HMSO, London.

Department for Education (1993) *Higher Quality and Choice: The Charter for Higher Education*, Crown, London.

Department for Education and Employment (1998a) *The Learning Age: Further Education for the New Millennium* (Response to the Kennedy Report), DfEE, London.

Department for Education and Employment (1998b) *The Learning Age: Higher Education for the 21st Century* (Response to the Dearing Report), DfEE, London.

Faraday, S. (1996) *Assessing the Impact: Provision for Learners with Learning Difficulties and Disabilities,* Developing FE: FEDA Report, Vol. 1, No. 3, FEDA, London.

Further Education Development Agency (1995) *Leading to Success: Development and Innovation for Further Education,* FEDA, London.

Further Education Funding Council (1996) *Inclusive Learning: Principles and Recommendations,* FEFC, Coventry.

Further Education Funding Council (1997a) *Mapping Provision: The Provision of and Participation in Further Education by Students with Learning Difficulties and/or Disabilities,* FEFC, Coventry.

Further Education Funding Council (1997b) *Learning Works: Widening Participation in Further Education,* FEFC, Coventry.

Further Education Funding Council (1997c) *Pathways to Success: The Widening Participation Committee Emerging Conclusions,* FEFC, Coventry.

Further Education Funding Council (1997d) FEFC press release, July.

Further Education Unit (1991) *Towards an Educational Audit,* FEU, London.

Further Education Unit (1992) *Supporting Learning: Promoting Equity and Participation, Part 1: A Model for Colleges,* FEU, London.

Further Education Unit (1993) *Supporting Learning: Promoting Equity and Participation, Part 2: Practical Guidance for Colleges,* FEU, London.

Further Education Unit (1994) *Supporting Learning: Promoting Equity and Participation, Part 3: Assessing Learning Support Needs,* FEU, London.

Gardiner, J. (1997) Colleges are still reluctant to woo disabled students. *Disability Times,* April, 3.

Gregory, H. (1997) Sample the student life. *Disability Now,* June, 10.

Harrison, J. (1996) Accessing further education: views and experiences of FE students with learning difficulties and/or disabilities. *British Journal of Special Education,* **23** (4), 187–96.

Hurst, A. (1996) Equal opportunities and access: developments in policy and provision, in *Opening Doors: Learning Support in Higher Education* (eds S. Wolfendale and J. Corbett), Cassell, London and New York, pp. 129–44.

Jamison, J. (1995) *Visually Impaired Candidates for Employment: A Survey of Further and Higher Education Institutions,* NFER Slough, UK.

Luker, K. and Thompson, L. (1994) *Developing an Approach: Provision for Disabled Students in Higher Education*, University of Surrey and Skill, London.

McGinty, J. and Fish, J. (1992) *Learning Support for Young People in Transition: Leaving School for Further Education and Work*, Open University Press, Buckingham and Philadelphia.

McGinty, J. and Fish, J. (1993) *Further Education in the Market Place: Equity, Opportunity, and Individual Learning*, Routledge, London.

Myers, L. and Parker, V. (1996) Extending the role of the co-ordinator for disabled students, in *Opening Doors: Learning Support in Higher Education* (eds S. Wolfendale and J. Corbett), Cassell, London and New York, pp. 66–83.

Patton, B. (1993) *RNIB Student Support Service: Provision in Higher Education*, RNIB, London.

Roy, A. (1998) Personal communication.

Skill (1993) *Further and Higher Education Acts, 1992*, Skill, London.

Skill (1997) *The Coordinator's Handbook*, Skill, London.

Skill and CRAC (1996) *Higher Education and Disability; A Guide to Higher Education for People with Disabilities*, Hobsons, Cambridge.

The Staff College (1994) Beyond ramps and rhetoric: new challenges and issues in learning difficulties. *Innovations in FE*, Issue 1, Autumn, The Staff College, Bristol.

Stowell, R. (1987) *Catching Up? Provision for Students with Special Educational Needs in Further and Higher Education*, National Bureau for Handicapped Students, London.

Stowell, R. (1997) Mapping provision: the provision of and participation in further education by students with learning difficulties and/or disabilities, The Further Education Funding Council, 1997: A Review. *New Beacon*, **81** (954), 26.

Wailey, T. (1996) 'Developing the reflective learner: learning development entitlement and AP(E)L, in *Opening Doors: Learning Support in Higher Education* (eds S. Wolfendale and J. Corbett), Cassell, London and New York, pp. 31–48.

Warwick, J. (1990) *Planning Human Resource Development Through Equal Opportunities (Gender): A Handbook*, FEU, Shaftesbury, UK

Wolfendale, S. and Corbett, J. (eds.) (1996) *Opening Doors: Learning Support in Higher Education*, Cassell, London and New York.

Suggested reading

Department for Education and Employment (1995) *Labour Market Information for Further Education Colleges*, DfEE, Sheffield, UK.

Dryden, G. (1994) Developments in student support. *Visability*, Spring, 8–9.

Hurst, A. (1993) *RNIB Student Support Service and Higher Education: A Consultancy Report*, RNIB, London.

Remmington, B. (1993) *RNIB Student Support Service: Consultancy Package for Further Education*, RNIB, London.

Royal National Institute for the Blind (1993) *See It Right: New Approaches to Information for Blind and Partially Sighted People*, RNIB, London.

Appendix A:
The eye – anatomy and physiology in brief

Anatomical structures of the eye

(See Figure A.1)

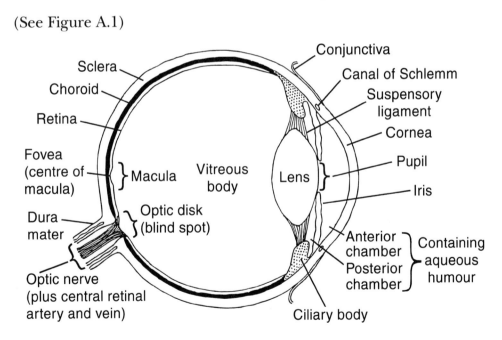

Figure A.1 Diagrammatic representation of structures making up the eye.

Eyeball

Almost spherical structure; 2.5 cm in diameter. Eyes face forwards; suspended in fat in protective orbit of skull.

Eyelids

Additional protection for eye; blink reflex distributes tear film and facilitates removal of foreign particles. Comprised of skin, fibrous tissue and muscle. Eyelashes arise from margins. Upper lids raised by levator palpebrae superioris (third cranial nerve supply). Lesions cause drooping lid: ptosis. Entropion: inward turning. Ectropion: outward turning.

Conjunctiva

Surface lining of lids. Wet mucous membrane folding back on eye as sac covering sclera; unfolds forwards, blending with cornea. Susceptible to atmospheric dryness: inflammation.

Lacrimal gland

In upper temporal segment of orbit. Produces lubricating tear film. Excess tears drain through tiny holes in eyelids; thence to ducts on nasal borders of eyelids, draining into nose.

Sclera

Outer covering of eye. Gristle-like substance comprising white fibrous tissue containing collagen. Front portion seen as 'whites of eyes'. Assists in maintaining eye's shape. Red when inflamed. Junction with cornea: limbus.

Cornea

Front aperture of sclera through which eye is examined. 'Window of eye'. Transparent convex tissue permits transmission of light to lens and retina. Specialized refractive surface facilitates focusing mechanism. Disturbance of cellular arrangement causes opacity and scattering of light. Blink reflex eliminates debris: maintains corneal clarity; also dependent on internal pump to ensure semi-hydration. Oedema: failure of pump. Dysfunction: cloudy appearance. Arcus senilis: white band around circumference: natural consequence of ageing.

Anterior and posterior segments of eye

Separated by lens. Iris divides anterior segment into anterior and posterior chambers. Aqueous humour flows through both chambers to fill anterior segment; posterior segment contains vitreous body.

Aqueous humour

Fills anterior segment. Thin, transparent fluid secreted at regular rate by ciliary body. Flows from behind iris in posterior chamber through pupil to area between cornea and iris in anterior chamber. Aqueous humour carries nutrients to and waste products from specialized tissues, draining through trabecular meshwork into canal of Schlemm, at iris–cornea angle, then to episcleral veins. Formation and dispersal of aqueous humour occurs at an equal rate, maintaining intra-ocular pressure of 12–20 mm Hg. Interference of flow increases pressure which may lead to glaucoma.

Uveal tract

Middle vascular layer: pigmented part of eye; receives nutrients from rich blood supply. Includes:

Iris

Visible, anterior portion; behind cornea. Eye colour determined by pigment levels: hereditary. Capillaries contribute to production of aqueous humour. Pupil: centre; black spot contrasted against colourful background. Muscle sphincter encircling aperture rim regulates light entering eye: enlarges in poor light (due to dilator pupillae); constricts in bright light (due to sphincter pupillae). Involuntary muscles controlled by parasympathetic nervous system. Drugs artificially dilate/constrict. Pupil abnormalities: size discrepancies. Aniridia is absence of iris possibly causing photophobia; nystagmus; glaucoma. Iris extends posteriorly into:

Ciliary body

Circular enlargement of muscle tissue. Fibres of suspensory ligament originate from inner surface and converge at periphery of lens. Ciliary body controls shape and focal length of lens. Produces aqueous humour.

Choroid

Backward continuation of uveal tract containing pigment and rich vascular network. Lines inner aspect of sclera; feeds deep surface of retina. Uveitis: inflammation.

Lens

Bi-concave oval disc, behind iris. Layered inner viscous matrix surrounded by thin outer elastic capsule. Focuses light on to retina. Undergoes shape changes when focusing on near/distant objects: ciliary muscles alter tension of suspensory ligament to which lens is attached. Elastic fibres in lens capsule facilitate process. Contraction of ciliary muscle: relaxation of suspensory ligament and outer lens capsule: lens becomes more spherical. Increase in convexity permits focusing on near objects. Successful focusing contingent upon ability of lens to change focal length: 'accommodation'. Elastic properties reduce with age. Presbyopia: inability to focus on near objects. Nutrients: from aqueous humour. Loss of transparency: cataract.

Retina

Inner layer of eye. Name derived from cobweb-like appearance of blood vessels: 'net'/'cobweb'. Thickest posteriorly, lines three-quarters of eyeball, from back to ora serrata (border between ciliary body and choroid). Outgrowth of optic vesicle in brain; regarded as part of central nervous system with light-sensitive cells; undertakes information processing. Visual information relayed from ganglion cells to brain via optic nerve. Three layers of neurones: ganglion cells, bipolar cells, light-sensitive rods and cones: photo-receptors at back of retina, behind blood vessel meshwork. Light rays must pass through meshwork and other nerve and supporting cells before reaching rods and cones. Rods and cones lie adjacent to outer pigment layer of cells at back of retina (25 million rods; 7 million cones). Generally positioned alongside each other although peripheral parts of retina are more densely populated by rods. The cones are concentrated at centre of retina: in macula. Fovea centralis: centre of macula, containing mostly cones. Rods specialized for perception of light and movement; associated with dark adaptation and night/scotopic vision. Insensitive to colour, respond to shades of grey. Cones concerned with photopic/daylight vision and form/colour perception. Macula, particularly fovea centralis: perception of fine detail.

Chemical process of converting light into nerve impulses. Retinal pigments bleached by bright light, stimulating nerve. This is a cyclical process with time being necessary to allow photo-chemicals to return to normal state. Bleached area: reduced sensitivity to stimuli; surrounding region has increased sensitivity producing after image. When the image is positive, it represents continued firing of retina and optic nerve after cessation of original stimulus; when negative, this signifies reduced sensitivity of stimulated cells, partially caused by bleaching of photo-pigments. Retinal disease/damage: severe visual impairment.

Vitreous body

Soft, transparent, jelly-like inert substance; low metabolic rate. Occupies posterior segment of eye, in cavity between retina and lens. Assists in maintenance of eye's shape. A healthy eye possesses 'floaters' caused by vitreous cells. Stare at a clear sky: small particles float across vision. Vitreous defect: increases floaters: visual disturbance. Low metabolic rate jeopardizes resolution of diseases if they occur. Detaches as part of ageing process without causing visual impairment. Simultaneous retinal detachment precipitates visual disorder.

Optic nerve and visual pathway

(See Figures A.2 and A.3.) Ganglion cell fibres of retina travel towards light-insensitive optic disc: 'blind spot'. Optic disc marks commencement of optic nerve (second cranial), along whose fibres (axons) impulses from rods and cones travel to brain. Optic nerve fibres pass backwards to optic chiasma: nasal retinal fibres decussate;

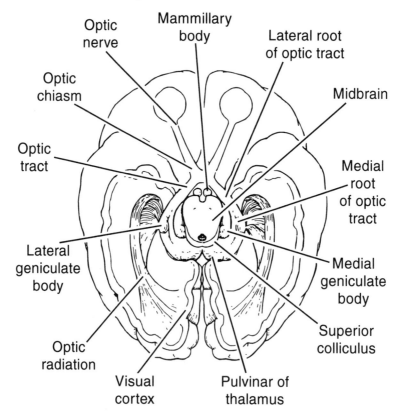

Figure A.2 Diagram showing the visual pathways as seen from the under aspect of the brain.

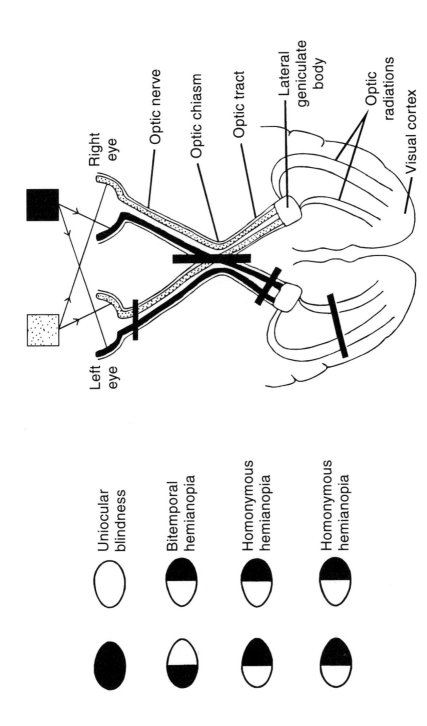

Figure A.3 Visual field defects. Diagram to show visual pathways to the brain and the visual field defects caused by damage to different sites.

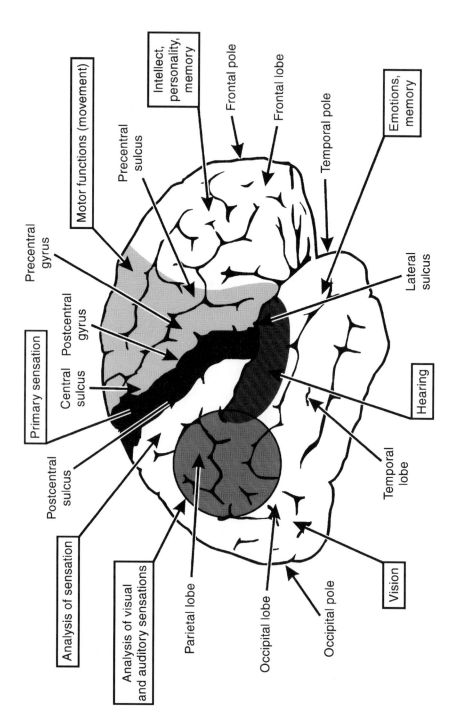

Figure A.4 The cerebral hemisphere and its subdivisions into lobes, principal sulci on the lateral surface and principal functions of certain regions of the cerebrum.

temporal fibres remain uncrossed. Right optic tract carries fibres from right halves of both retinae; each half of retina receives impulses from opposite half of field of vision. Right optic tract, therefore, represents left half of visual field. From optic chiasma, optic tract passes backwards to: superior colliculus – centre for visual reflexes – and lateral geniculate body, where new relay of fibres travels backwards as optic radiation carrying temporal fibres from same eye and nasal fibres from contralateral eye (see Figs A.2 and A.3). Optic radiation terminates in visual cortex of occipital lobe of brain, an area corresponding to back of head. Relatively large cerebral area, signifying importance of vision in humans (see Figure A.4). Decoding of visual stimuli occurs, producing an intelligible picture. Psychological interpretation of visual image occurs in another cerebral area.

Eye movements

(See Figure A.5.) The image from an object of regard must fall simultaneously on the fovea of each retina for unimpaired vision. Eyes must be aligned and move together. In conjugate gaze, eyes move to sides and vertically; in disjugate gaze, they converge towards an approaching object or diverge in response to a receding object.

Eyeball moves inwards, outwards, upwards and downwards. Six extrinsic eye muscles: cranial nerve supply. Lateral and medial recti rotate eyeball – outwards and inwards, respectively – around a vertical axis; superior and inferior recti move it upwards and downwards. Superior oblique pulls eyeball downwards, outwards and rotates it inwards; inferior oblique pulls eyeball outwards and upwards. Precise coordination of eye movements is crucial in the meaningful interpretation of retinal images by the brain as one coherent picture.

Laws

Sherrington's: reciprocal relationship between prime mover / agonist and antagonist: when agonist contracts, antagonist relaxes.

Hering's: when one muscle contracts, its contralateral synergist also

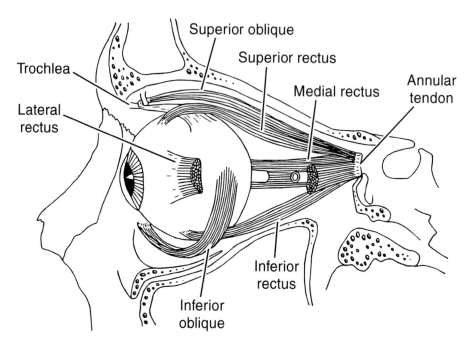

Figure A.5 Muscles of the left orbit (lateral aspect).

contracts, e.g.: when right medial rectus contracts, left lateral rectus does likewise while reciprocal relaxation occurs in right lateral rectus and left medial rectus. Eyes will move smoothly to the left.

Control of eye movements

Cerebral centres: permitting eyes to move upwards, downwards, left and right and rotate clockwise or anticlockwise. Four movements: saccadic, smooth pursuit, vergence, vestibular. Saccadic: controlled by frontal cerebral cortex; rapid involuntary (subconscious) jumps/driftings of eye as observer attempts to fix gaze on stationary object. Function: to prevent sensory adaptation. Absence: fading of image. Occur in opposite direction to smooth pursuit eye movements upon which they are superimposed. Smooth pursuit movements: controlled by occipital cerebral cortex; occur when moving object is followed/tracked or when object remains stationary and the head is slowly rotated. Vergence permits focusing of an object as its distance from observer varies or when gaze shifts between two objects at different distances. Vestibular (involuntary) movements compensate for changes in head posture and maintain alignment of eyes. 'Doll's head' (involuntary) movements direct eyes to right when head is quickly moved to left. Reflex may be overridden voluntarily. Cerebellum controls smooth movements of eyes.

Characteristics of normal vision

Central vision (most noticeable if affected): macula (fovea). Cones: object/person discrimination: reading small print; facial detail. Field vision: (less noticeable if affected): rods: twilight conditions. Defects pass unrecognised. Field: background for central vision. (See Figure A.6.)

Shape of each field: 'recumbent pear with the bulbous end pointing to the lateral side' (McKenzie, Chawla and Gordon, 1986). Each eye views world from different perspective; fusion of views produces binocular vision: perception of depth/ distance. Semi-lunar portion, at temporal aspect of each field, seen only by eye of same side.

Refraction and focusing

Eye's task: to produce retinal image capable of interpretation. Contingent upon past experience of world. Recognition of environmental components: dependent upon visual clarity: object in focus. (See Figure A.7.)

Traditional analogy: eye/camera. Light rays refracted on passing through cornea and lens: converge on fovea. Retinal image inverted; decoded at occipital cerebral area. Degree of refraction depends upon angle at which rays hit cornea/lens. Lens accommodation ensures clarity of perception. Ciliary muscles: alter focal length. Near objects: contraction: relaxation of suspensory

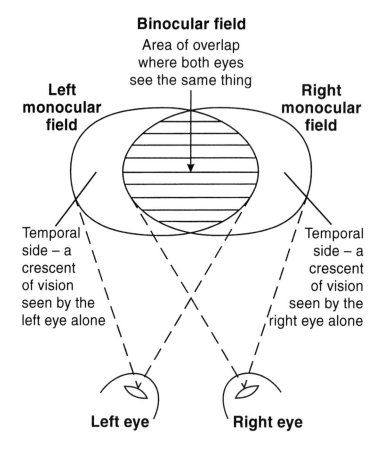

Figure A.6 Diagram to show the visual fields of each eye and their area of overlap.

ligament: lens becomes spherical: increase in convexity: decrease in focal length. Distant objects: relaxation: increase tension of suspensory ligament: lens flattens: decrease in convexity: increase in focal length. Accommodation for near objects: lens takes account that light rays strike cornea at a more acute angle than if object were more distant. Muscular control facilitates focusing mechanism. Presbyopia: accommodation difficulties due to hardening of lens with age.

Binocular vision gives wider visual field than possible with monocular vision. Eyes: 6.3 cm apart: this disparity of retinal image facilitates depth/distance perception: stereoscopic vision.

Normal

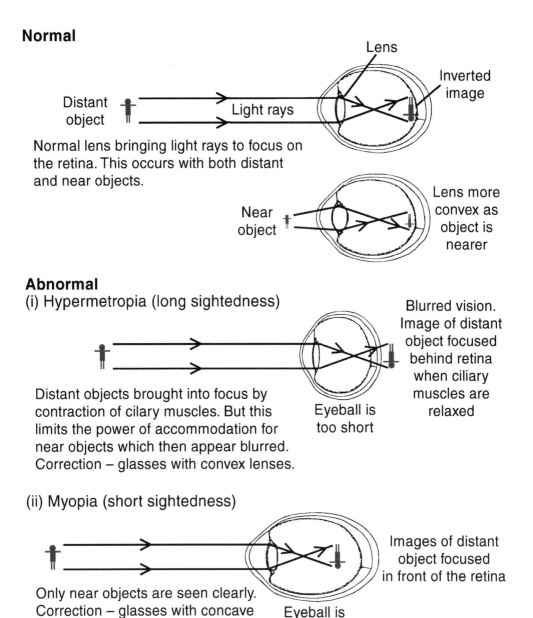

Lens

Inverted image

Distant object — Light rays

Normal lens bringing light rays to focus on the retina. This occurs with both distant and near objects.

Near object

Lens more convex as object is nearer

Abnormal

(i) Hypermetropia (long sightedness)

Blurred vision. Image of distant object focused behind retina when ciliary muscles are relaxed

Distant objects brought into focus by contraction of cilary muscles. But this limits the power of accommodation for near objects which then appear blurred. Correction – glasses with convex lenses.

Eyeball is too short

(ii) Myopia (short sightedness)

Images of distant object focused in front of the retina

Only near objects are seen clearly. Correction – glasses with concave lenses.

Eyeball is too long

Figure A.7 The lens and its action. A convex lens, as in the eye, will form a real, inverted, small image of an object on the retina. This inverted image is then interpreted by the brain into the picture that we see.

Development of vision

Development of normal vision contingent upon: anatomical/ physiological development of eyes, visual pathways and cerebral visual areas and appropriate sensory feedback: adequate stimulation and sensory reward (e.g. mother/child interaction).

Visual function

Form sense

Acuity: determined by smallest retinal image whose form can be appreciated by observer. Develops during first 6 months, normal vision attained by 3 years. Visual field quadrants appear to be reduced in infants but this is thought to be functional and perceptual in origin rather than constituting a physiological defect. Contrast sensitivity: ability to differentiate between light and dark. Established: 3 months.

Light sense

Light/dark differentiation: 6–8 weeks; only tested in absence of form sense.

Colour sense

Wavelength distinction: 5 months.

Binocular vision

Neonates: presence of blink reflex; peripheral retina developed. When head tilted: eyes remain straight with horizon. Slow horizontal tracking possible. Fixation reflex enables binocular vision. Established: 3–4 weeks. Macula developed: saccadic re-fixation movements and vertical tracking. 6–8 weeks: presence of defensive blink; head turning to stare at light source.

3 months: vertical/horizontal tracking movements established; convergence/divergence in response to approaching/receding objects. Re-fixation reflex: alternate object focusing without head movement.

6 months: fusion reflex developed. Permits coordination of convergence/divergence reflexes with accommodative reflex for binocular vision. Infant reaches for objects. Stereopsis developing.

8–10 months: crawling: response to depth/distance cues.

12 months: movement of objects observed/selected; recognition of familiar objects/people at 6 metres: establishment of visual acuity. Voluntary movement of eyes in one sweep.

2 years: vision well developed. Up to 2 years: image fusion and development of binocular vision possible. Presence of uncorrected squint (strabismus) at or after 2 years, learning of image fusion impossible: focusing done by alternate eyes. Defective bilateral vision in both eyes under 2 years: development of permanent nystagmus: oscillation of eyes or impairment of fixation reflex.

5 years: critical stage in establishment of eyesight. Although mechanisms developed, disease/injury of part of mechanism is detrimental. By 8 years: risks lower due to maturity of function: prognosis good if problem occurs and is addressed.

Motor development and development of hearing, listening, and communication

Beyond remit of this text but knowledge helpful in considering issues of visual impairment.

Bibliography

Disabled Living Foundation (1991) *Visual Handicap: A Distance Learning Pack for Physiotherapists, Occupational Therapists and Other Health Care Professionals*, DLF, London.

Humphreys, G.W. and Riddoch, M.J. (1987) *To See but Not to See: A Case Study of Visual Agnosia*, Lawrence Eribaum Association, London.

Sheridan, M.D. (1975) *Children's Developmental Progress: From Birth to Five Years the Stycar Sequences*, NFER Publishing, Windsor, Berkshire, UK.

Reference

McKenzie, G.J., Chawla, H.B. and Gordon, D. (1986) *The Special Senses*, 2nd edn, Churchill Livingstone, Singapore.

Suggested reading

Jose, R.T. (ed.) (1989) *Understanding Low Vision*, 2nd edn, American Foundation for the Blind, New York.

Levitt, S. (ed.) (1989) *Paediatric Developmental Therapy*, Blackwell Scientific Publications, Oxford.

Vander, A.J., Sherman, J.H., and Luciano, D.S. (1994) *Human Physiology: The Mechanisms of Body Function*, 6th edn, McGraw-Hill, New York.

Some common conditions affecting the external tissues of the eye

Eyelids

Problems: malformation; malposition; inflammation. Ectropion: over-exposure of eye. Entropion: corneal damage due to scraping of eyelashes over eye.

Ptosis: lid droops to upper pupil margin; congenital/acquired. Untreated congenital cases: development of binocular vision threatened due to obscuring of part of visual field. Sudden onset: lesion of nervous system. Insidious onset: ageing process.

Cysts and ulcers

Acute/chronic inflammation.

Stye

Infection of eyelash root. Blepharitis: affecting more than one root.

Conjunctivitis

Acute/chronic inflammation of conjunctiva: gritty sensation on eye movements; excessive watering and photophobia.

Dry eye

May be known as: keratitis sicca; keratoconjunctivitis sicca (KCS); xerophthalmia. Cause: insufficient production of tears due to: deterioration of lacrimal tissue; dysfunction of the Meibomian gland destabilizing the tear film; or blockage of secretary ducts of lacrimal gland. Usually age related; women more frequently affected. May be associated with glaucoma, systemic glandular disorders and rheumatoid arthritis. Increase in mucus strands: contamination. If material cannot be dispersed, blinking assists. Symptoms include irritation/burning; sensation of 'foreign body' in eye; mucus discharge; blurred vision; pain on blinking. Treatment options: avoidance of dry/warm atmospheres; regular blinking; eye drops; ointment; hormone replacement therapy; antihistamines; surgery to close tear drainage ducts.

Some common conditions affecting the internal structures of the eye

Aniridia

Rare congenital disorder: incomplete formation of iris: muscles that constrict/dilate pupil are absent, leaving a thick collar of tissue around outer edge. 'Black iris': enlarged pupil. Causes: hereditary (autosomal dominant/recessive) and unknown. May be associated with kidney tumour (Wilms') and chromosomal/ eye disorders. Increased sensitivity to light; lens clouding. Treatment: regular monitoring; treatment of associated symptoms/disorders.

Keratitis

Corneal inflammation: cause: bacterial/viral/fungal organisms. Non-infective keratitis: associated with over-exposure to ultraviolet rays and overwearing of contact lenses. Can cause oedema; lack of oxygen (hypoxia) in superficial tissue layers. Misty vision remains long after removal of lenses. Can cause corneal damage: appearance of a tear across cornea with jagged edges. Treatment: antibiotics (if infected). If corneal scarring occurs (widespread): transplant may be necessary.

Iritis

Causes: infection; allergic response; injury.

Cyclitis, choroiditis and pan uveitis

Cyclitis: involvement of ciliary body. Choroiditis: involvement of choroid. Pan uveitis: incrimination of uveal tract: iris, ciliary body, choroid. Spasm of iris and ciliary muscle, with photophobia and visual impairment if adhesion between iris and lens. Variable pain, less in choroiditis. Treatment: antibiotics and/or anti-inflammatory. Uveal tract inflammation: associated with glaucoma.

Refractive errors

(See Figure A.7.) Minor image-focusing problems, corrected by prescription of lenses.

Presbyopia

Decreased lens flexibility, associated with ageing. Problems of accommodation.

Hypermetropia

Cause: short eyeball; retina situated in front of normal focal point. Lens capable of accommodating to compensate in youth: eyestrain and fatigue. Convex lenses facilitate near-object focusing.

Myopia

Short sight. Eyes may appear large (exophthalmos). Cause: may be genetic; long eyeball, or steeply curved cornea. Light rays are focused in front of retina, which lies behind normal focal point. Near objects seen clearly; distant objects blurred. Near-object focusing possible with inhibition of accommodation reflex of lens. Concave lenses: minimize ocular stress. May stabilize when growth process is completed.

Mild degree myopia. Up to 3.0 D (dioptres; lens focusing power).

Moderate degree myopia. Between 3.0 D and 6.0 D.

High degree myopia. From 6.0 D correction and above. Sometimes termed 'progressive/pathological myopia': gradual elongation of eyeball; sometimes results in retinal detachment.

Treatment. Corrective lenses (glasses and/or contact lenses); laser surgery: photo-refractive keratotomy (PRK). Suitable for mild or moderate myopia. Many complications.

Astigmatism

Cause: flattening of eyeball in vertical/horizontal/oblique axis. Accurate focusing impossible because eye is not a perfect sphere. Blurred vision: near/distant objects. Lens unable to accommodate: fatigue. Treatment: lenses with appropriate curvatures along two meridians.

Cataract

Myths: (a) skin over eyes; (b) material fallen from brain over pupils like a waterfall: (hence name). Cataract: lens disorder or opacity: one of three principal causes of visual impairment (along with glaucoma and macular degeneration). Accounts for 23% of causes of blindness in England (Trevor-Roper, 1986) and 'for at least 50% of cases of blindness worldwide' (Vaughan, Asbury and Riordan-Eva, 1992). Varieties: acquired/congenital.

Acquired

Associated with degenerative cell changes in ageing. Cause of lens opacities: over-exposure to infrared and ultraviolet rays both emitted by sun, former emitted by electric heaters. Steroid treatment for rheumatoid arthritis/arthropathies: lens opacities may develop. Secondary to eye trauma, intra-ocular inflammation and metabolic disturbances as in diabetes. Poor oxygen supply to lens.

Congenital

Associated with rubella (German measles) during pregnancy: intra-uterine infection. Also associated with hypocalcaemia and Down's syndrome.

Signs

Single or multiple lens opacities, sited in nucleus or periphery. Bilateral. White opacity in pupil. Gradual yellowing of lens. Failure to transmit light to retina results in misty central vision with distortion at edges of objects. Colours: increasingly dull.

If cataract in front layers of lens: glare; photophobia (may need tinted lenses). If in back layers: problems of near vision, as cataract coincides with focal point of lens when fully accommodated.

When cataract formed: progression not inevitable. May remain small: no symptoms. Congenital cataracts: range from opaque lens to occasional dots. If severe: macular fixation never develops unless early treatment. (Light must reach retina in early life or it will not learn to see.) Symptoms: ocular nystagmus; squint (strabismus), which develops due to impoverished visual stimulation; results in a form of amblyopia (impaired visual function). May account for problems of depth/distance perception. Possible retinal involvement with reduction in visual field and impaired night vision.

General symptoms: difficulty in perception of detail, especially at a distance: world may appear indistinct: objects too small to be discerned accurately. May be concurrent with good macular function.

Treatment

Lens opacification: irreversible tissue change: material must be removed. Method: dependent upon age and size of opacity: the degree to which its presence interferes with performance of daily activities. Below 35 years: inappropriate to remove entire lens since this leads to the detrimental escape of vitreous fluid (Trevor-Roper, 1986). Surgery for younger person: colloquially described as 'needling': aspiration of opaque lens material through a wide bore needle following tearing away of anterior lens capsule (Trevor-Roper, 1986). Above 35 years: removal of both anterior lens capsule and hardened nucleus; incision through upper edge of cornea necessary. Both procedures: 'extracapsular extraction'. Intracapsular extraction: removal of entire lens: lifted out of eye with forceps or cryoprobe. Eye without lens: aphakic.

Following surgery, necessary to replace intraocular lens with thick external convex lenses: regular wearing of spectacles or contact lenses essential. Trevor-Roper (1986): vivid description of some problems associated with wearing of cataract spectacles and suggests that an acrylic lens implant is a more satisfactory alternative although permanent damage to eye is sustained in approximately 10% of cases, due to oedema of the cornea or macula RNIB (1995a). Corneal oedema is one of side effects experienced by some wearers of contact lenses (usually of the soft variety): 'hazy' world. Oedema remains long after removal of lens.

Glaucoma

Any state where intra-ocular pressure rises above normal. Due to blockage to aqueous circulation at any point in its journey from ciliary body through pupil to drainage angle of anterior chamber. Rise in intra-ocular pressure. Varieties: acute: 'closed angle'; chronic:

'simple' or 'openangle' glaucoma. May be primary or secondary complication to other disorders. Acquired: disease of later life; congenital: malformation of drainage angle of anterior chamber. Tension increase: 'ox-like' eyes of neonate: buphthalmos. Trevor-Roper (1986): glaucomas account for 13% of causes of blindness in England. A variety of glaucoma affects approximately 2% of UK individuals aged over 40 years (Royal National Institute for the Blind, 1995b). Risk factors: hereditary; African race; myopia; diabetes.

Acute glaucoma

Dramatic; severe, boring eye pain due to rapid rise in intra-ocular pressure. Predisposing factors as follows. Eye's shape: anterior chamber may prove be too shallow to permit unimpeded pupil dilatation, associated with small, hypermetropic eye. Shallow anterior chamber exists: drainage angle formed by gutter between front of iris and cornea is narrow. Narrowing, caused by channel blockage: associated with ageing. Thickening lens may compound problem by pushing iris forward into narrow gutter. Critical situation: during natural pupil dilatation: iris drawn backwards against lens thus impeding aqueous humour's flow through pupil: 'pupil block'. Pressure in posterior chamber rises. In attempt to escape down canal of Schlemm, aqueous humour succeeds only in driving peripheral part of iris up against cornea: complete fluid blockage behind it, as in mid-pupil dilatation. The already narrow drainage angle becomes closed: 'closed-angle' glaucoma.

Precipitating factors: pupil dilatation: emotional stress, coping with deteriorating lighting conditions, pupil-dilator drugs.
Signs/symptoms: intense, intractable pain, headache, nausea, with general constitutional upset. Eye: red, congested, hard, tense: pupil appears vertically oval, in permanent dilated state and fixed to light. Visual disturbance: depends on severity of condition: misty/blurred due to corneal oedema. This causes break-up of white light into constituent colours: objects seen in coloured 'halo' rings. Alternatively: light perception only or complete blindness may occur.

Because relentless rise in intra-ocular pressure would eventually

destroy sensitive retina or optic nerve due to deprivation of blood
supply, acute attack: emergency: hospital admission necessary.
Emotional trauma may trigger attack in other eye. Treatment: aims:
reduce raised pressure by drops or oral preparations; to maintain
patency of drainage system to prevent subsequent attack. If treatment
fails: enucleation (removal of eyeball): artificial replacement is fitted
when appropriate.

Recurrent, subacute variety of closed-angle glaucoma: commonly
found in tropical climates, particularly among West Indian women
(Cullinan, 1986). In subacute attacks, where mild signs/symptoms,
treatment aims: to control factors associated with pupil dilatation.
Pupil constrictor drops, good lighting conditions may prevent onset
of full-blown attack.

Chronic 'open-angle' glaucoma

Not a milder version of acute/subacute varieties. It is a distinct
disease of the elderly. Insidious onset: irreversible changes in optic
nerve: sight loss.

Increased intra-ocular pressure caused by clogging up of filter
(trabeculum) through which aqueous fluid drains from canal of
Schlemm into main circulation. With age: sclerosis of tiny pores in
trabeculum which normally regulate rate of fluid drainage, resulting
in obstruction of aqueous humour; consequent rise in intra-ocular
tension. Optic nerve death due to increased pressure and impairment
of blood supply; retinal symptoms.

Signs/symptoms: gradual increase in intra-ocular tension;
progressive reduction in visual field. Visual impairment undetected
initially; gradually affects functional activities. Eye feels hard; appears
normal.

Treatment to reduce intra-ocular pressure. Immediate attention
needed in acute cases. Drops or oral preparations; laser/surgical
treatment; trabeculectomy: relieves drainage problem; sclerotomy:
cutting of small strip of sclera at upper corneal edge and removal of
part of root of iris, making a hole through which aqueous can drain
freely (Trevor-Roper, 1986). Repeat surgery sometimes necessary.

Some common conditions affecting the retina and choroid

Exudative retinitis: Coats' disease

Progressive retinal capillary abnormality; affects (usually male) children and young adults. Usual onset: 10 years. One eye only. Gradual progression. Cause: unknown. Retinal capillary dilation/malformation/leakage. Threat of superficial haemorrhaging/leakage due to increased size of capillaries. Complications: strabismus (squint); retinal detachment. Deterioration in central/peripheral vision. Treatment: laser; surgery by light (photocoagulation) or cold (cryotherapy). Condition may resolve spontaneously.

Macular degeneration/dystrophy

An hereditary, progressive, degenerative disease of macula: may be juvenile (see below) or age related.

Age-related macular degeneration/dystrophy

This accounts for 27% of causes of blindness in England (Trevor-Roper, 1986) and is 'the leading cause of acquired *legal blindness* in people of 60 years of age' (Small, 1994). 'It is a matter of some doubt whether the changes seen in the degenerative macular diseases of old age are different in kind from the normal ageing process or merely more rapid and florid extensions of it' (Cullinan, 1986).

Insidious onset affecting both eyes. 10–15% of people with degenerative changes leading to reduction/loss of macular function in one eye will eventually have bilateral symptoms.

Devitalization of nerve cells due to reduction of blood supply. With age, retinal pigment cells manufacture deposits in macula, from small, discrete patches to larger continuous areas: drusen:

detectable only through ophthalmoscope. Normal for some to be present in the ageing eye. Lie beneath layer of retinal pigment cells. If they increase in size and number, drusen effectively separate pigment cells from their nutritional bed: loss of retinal function. In many cases, the combination of large amounts of white disciform debris, grouping of pigment cells and considerable haemorrhage from devitalized blood vessels signifies severity of disease.

If degenerative changes affect macula of one eye only: no visual impairment: contralateral eye compensates for functional reduction. Eventually: both eyes involved. Signs/symptoms: inability to perceive fine detail. Blurred vision; objects distorted; central vision affected. Dark mass may appear, obliterating objects placed directly before eyes whereas those within field are clearly detected. Total blindness unlikely. Appearance of swollen and bloodshot eye; ophthalmoscopic examination: degenerative signs described above.

Little effective treatment. Visual appliances. Utilization of remaining visual field (Cullinan, 1986).

Detached retina

Layers of retina in contact although a potential space exists between them. Detachment: separation of layers: not true detachment.

Primary

Tear in neuro-retina permits vitreous fluid to fill potential space and separate it from pigment layer. Cause: violent shaking of head or severe head trauma. At risk: elongated, myopic eye (retina thinner than usual) (Trevor-Roper, 1986). Other cause: following cataract extraction. 25% chance of second eye becoming affected.

Secondary

Traction on neuro-retina: tumours; retinal degeneration: diabetes. Signs/symptoms: neuro-retinal cells lose specialized function;

gradually replaced by fibrous tissue. Retina more vulnerable to tears: typical retinal response of flashing lights in visual field. 'Floating opacities' may appear (Trevor-Roper, 1986). Death of cells: 'a dark curtain coming over' eyes. Curtain may be perceived as if ascending 'if the detachment started above – corresponding to the lower visual field' (Trevor-Roper, 1986). If tear spreads to include macula: abrupt loss of central vision. 'There is no pain, only panic.'

Signalling signs/symptoms treated as emergency. Examination of contralateral eye. Aim: prevent further damage by sealing rupture: laser; cryotherapy; surgical repair of retinal hole (possible provided retina is still in place; poor prognosis if considerable separation of layers). Visual impairment may be present but, left untreated, complete detachment: blindness. Re-detachment may be precipitated by physical activities. Advice: for all at-risk individuals: bed rest. Post-surgery: rest to avoid re-detachment (RNIB, 1995c).

Juvenile macular dystrophies, Best's disease, Bull's eye maculopathy and Stargardt's macular dystrophy

Cause associated with genetic abnormality of pigment loss or accumulation of abnormal protein. Early onset, progress rapid. Central vision affected. Treatment: genetic counselling. Symptoms determined by variety.

Cone dystrophy

Photophobia; day blindness; reduction in visual clarity and colour vision.

Albinism

Hereditary condition characterized by pigmentary deficiency which may affect skin, hair and eyes, or confined to one tissue. Ocular albinism: eyes (bilateral) affected. Iris: appears translucent/pinkish due to pigment deficiency: haemoglobin only remaining substance (Trevor-Roper, 1986). Equated with underdeveloped macula: poor central vision. ocular nystagmus, squint (strabismus), severe photophobia. Usually person is partially sighted; blindness rare. Photophobia: prominent: exposure to moderately bright light may precipitate severe eye pain. Treatment: tinted lenses. Associated linguistic problems have been noted.

Retinitis pigmentosa (RP)

Umbrella term. Not inflammatory but progressive, degenerative disease; genetically determined group of diseases in some of which a disorder of lipid metabolism has been incriminated. '. . . carriers of the gene may show depression of the electrical retinal responses before the retinal pigmentation becomes apparent' (Trevor-Roper, 1986). Believed to commence in adolescence, but may be diagnosed earlier. RP: most frequent cause of field loss amongst retinal dystrophies.

Ophthalmoscopic examination reveals retinal changes: begin peripherally, eventually affecting entire retina. Thinning of retinal blood vessel walls cause blood leakage. Scattered areas of black pigmentation which increase in size and number as disease progresses. Death of optic disc cells.

Gradual reduction in peripheral field predisposing collisions with objects, and people, lying outside visual range: 'tunnel vision'. Symptoms also of being surrounded by ring of white cloud which clears progressively as centre of field is reached. Manoeuvring of eyes may facilitate focusing on objects. Possible unawareness of field loss, due to compensatory cerebral mechanisms. Retinal periphery initially attacked: destruction of rods: night blindness. Red-tinted glasses counteract photophobia; facilitate pupil dilation. Treatment: genetic counselling.

Retinoblastoma

Retina is viciously and ruthlessly attacked by progressively enlarging malignant tumour. Often bilateral. Disease of infancy, affecting 1 in 25,000 babies. 10% of cases hereditary; remaining are sporadic (Coakes and Holmes Sellors, 1985).

Pupil appears white, due to tumour lying behind it. Squint.

Distress: painful and inflamed eye. Secondary closed-angle glaucoma due to enlarging tumour, which can spread to optic nerve and brain; may cause death.

Treatment

If tumour fills eyeball: enucleation. Alternatively: radiotherapy or cryotherapy.

Some retinal vascular conditions

Diabetic retinopathy

Complication of diabetes mellitus. In West, represents most common cause of 'new sight loss in middle age' (Cullinan, 1986); also principal cause of blindness in people under 65 (Coakes and Holmes Sellors, 1985). Lens and retina usually involved but other structures may be affected.

Diabetes mellitus: disease of pancreatic insulin-producing cells affecting approximately 2% people in UK (Royal National Institute for the Blind, 1995d). Insulin crucial in regulation of blood-sugar levels. Insufficient insulin: high blood sugar levels: hyperglycaemia; problems with metabolizing starches (carbohydrates), proteins and fats. General weakening of blood vessels; premature ageing. Tendency to leak contents into tissues. Capillaries particularly affected. Signs and symptoms: include excessive hunger, thirst and urination; poor wound healing and lethargy. Treatment: dictated by time of onset and severity of disease. Insulin and/or dietary control prescribed (Jose, 1989.)

Visual complications: begin years after onset. Lens loses power of accommodation. Blood vessel changes/leakage: retinal dysfunction. Sudden obliteration of capillaries causes death of cells due to ischaemia; other areas become hypoxic due to gradual capillary blockage. In response: retinal tissue creates new vessels: these are impaired and rupture due to associated high blood pressure. Leakage of contents affects vitreous body. Cyclical sequence: continual haemorrhage culminating in fibrosis of area, increased traction on neuro-retina and possible eventual retinal detachment.

Two varieties:

Proliferative

Associated with younger, insulin-dependent individuals in whom disease has been present for 10–15 years. Gradual haemorrhages of weak peripheral retinal vessels but more particularly with extensive bleeding into vitreous body and formation of fibrous tissue, leading to retinal detachment and glaucoma. Variable signs/symptoms: from patchy visual field to complete irreversible blindness.

Background/simple

In elderly not receiving insulin treatment. Small, discrete, scattered retinal haemorrhages; leakage of plasma: retinal oedema. Fats from leaked plasma deposited around damaged vessels: 'dot and blot' appearance under ophthalmoscope. Macula involvement: central visual loss; low risk of eventual blindness.

Treatment

Maintenance of insulin–sugar balance; injection therapy, dietary control. Laser treatment to leaking capillaries to reduce haemorrhage and prevent new vessel formation.

Retinopathy of prematurity (retrolental fibroplasia)

Formation of fibrous tissue behind lens. Cause: premature babies exposed to inappropriate oxygen levels during incubation.

In premature infants, retinal periphery still avascular. Blood vessels particularly sensitive to oxygen levels: constrict if levels become excessive. Reversible if environment returns to normal but permanent damage if oxygen levels remain high. Formation of new vessels with overlay of fibrous tissue in response to constriction of others: development of fibrovascular membrane behind lens, which contracts: bilateral retinal detachment: blindness.

Personal experience suggests additional features: poor orientation sense, especially in large open spaces; little difficulty when moving from one point to another in confined areas; proprioceptive difficulties; poor conceptualization of geographical relationships. Tentative conjecture: neurological damage. Treatment: none effective. Emphasis on prevention through vigilant monitoring of oxygen levels administered during incubation.

Conditions affecting the vitreous body

Vitreous body may be involved in congenital abnormalities; injury; infection; degeneration; diabetic retinopathy; retinal detachment (Small, 1994).

Syneresis

Contraction/liquefaction of vitreous gel with ageing; detachment from retina at 60 years plus. May occur earlier in myopes and as complication to other retinal conditions. Symptoms include: flashes of light (traction on retina); floaters (possible cause: haemorrhage); muscae volitantes (flying insects – these have the appearance of flying insects, hence the name) affect vision. Very disabling. Complication: retinal detachment. Treatment: monitoring; possible vitreotomy.

Neurological conditions

(See Figure A.3.) Conditions where visual impairment associated with neurological damage/disease.

Optic nerve

From retinae, visual impulses travel along optic nerve to cerebral visual cortex (visual pathway). Any part may be affected. Partial decussation of nerve fibres: diagnostic implications. Causes: stroke;

trauma; tumour. Symptoms consequent upon damage/disease at various points. If damage before optic chiasm: monocular visual loss. Damage at optic chiasm: bi-temporal hemianopia/hemianopsia (both temporal components of visual field affected); in nerve tracts (rare) or optic radiation (common): homonymous hemianopia/hemianopsia: (nasal half of visual field in one eye; temporal half of visual field in other eye). Other types of field loss due to disease of trauma to optic nerve: absolute (retina blind to light); relative (loss of colour and form sense); congruent (identical effects bilaterally); incongruent (dissimilar effects in each field). Eye remains healthy. Treatment: management of medical condition diagnosed.

Papilloedema

Swelling of optic nerve head. May lead to transient/permanent visual impairment/loss.

Optic nerve atrophy

Most common single cause of visual impairment in childhood: accounts for 20% of children with registered sight loss. Causes include: hereditary; injury; meningitis; tumour; hydrocephalus. Symptoms dependent upon site of lesion and may include reduction in visual acuity; specific field loss; poor colour vision. Object recognition unaffected as vision remains normal in unaffected areas of field (Humphreys and Riddoch, 1987). Monocular sight loss: person not diagnosed as partially sighted. No effective treatment. Condition usually stabilizes.

Leber's optic atrophy/neuropathy

Atypical presentation.

Other cranial nerves

Lesions of the third, fourth, sixth cranial nerves cause muscle paralysis: gaze palsy (Bannister, 1979). Diplopia: third cranial nerve.

Perceptual conditions

Upside-down/back-to-front retinal messages depend upon healthy cerebral function for their interpretation. (Source for following: Disabled Living Foundation, 1991. See also Humphreys and Riddoch, 1987.)

Visual agnosia

Recognition disorder; unaffected eyesight. When objects are placed before an individual they can be seen, described and drawn accurately but cannot be named due to visual recognition failure. If objects are touched, recognition successful: failure not simply one of assigning name to given item. Possible causes: (1) inability to determine overall shape of object or how its component parts relate to overall shape; (2) cognitive: failure to remember specific shapes or visual characteristics of objects; (3) failure to appreciate use to which specific objects might be put, even though their familiarity is acknowledged.

Prosopagnosis

Recognition disorder specific to faces. Possible causes: (1) perceptual: inability to distinguish between particular features; (2) impairment of knowledge of face: face is recognized as familiar but it cannot be contextualized. Common experience.

Disorders of depth perception

Difficulties: appreciation/interpretation of environmental monocular/binocular cues: perspective, occlusion, motion parallax, stereopsis. Riddoch (in Disabled Living Foundation, 1991) refers to reports by Holmes and Horrax (1919) and Riddoch (1917) concerning individuals whose impairment is complete but whose eyesight is unaffected. Appearance of severe visual disability: collide with objects perceived as further away than they are. Interpretative failure of what is seen.

Optic ataxia

Problem of reaching out for objects or undertaking skilled movements requiring good manual dexterity/precision. Tactile exploratory techniques used as coping strategies to overcome problems. Misreaching occurs when using visual input; fine finger/thumb movements skilfully undertaken when sight excluded.

Apraxia

Visuo–motor disorder. Intact muscle power/function and sensory input but inability to perform purposeful movements. Such movements can be undertaken without vision: suggests difficulty in linking certain appropriate actions with specific signals.

Spatial disorders

Unilateral neglect

Common disorder; individual appears to ignore space on opposite side to cerebral lesion.

Neglect associated with disorders of attention

Unaffected sight but person visually attracted by some striking object in environment that effectively prevents perception of other things. Distracters: bright colours. Similar problem: person unable to scan both left and right sides of printed page, visual fixation on one side.

Some common eye conditions in developing countries

Although classification criteria vary, estimates suggest there are approximately 42 million visually impaired people throughout the world. 80% of blind people live in developing countries: approximately 20 million in Asia; approximately 6 million in Africa. Clustered in disadvantaged rural and urban areas. Risk of blindness is 10–40 times higher than in developed regions of Europe and USA. Leading causes include: cataract; trachoma; leprosy; onchocerciasis (river blindness); xerophthalmia (vitamin A deficiency); age-related macular degeneration; chronic glaucoma; diabetic retinopathy; keratitis; retinal detachment; inherited retinal disorders; measles; malnutrition. WHO estimates 80% of cases are avoidable (Vaughan, Asbury and Riordan-Eva, 1992).

Trachoma

Most notable single cause of preventable visual impairment in developing countries. 'About 360 million people have trachoma, most of them in Africa, the Middle East and Asia' (Vaughan, Asbury and Riordan-Eva, 1992). Poverty: spread of infectious disease in overcrowded communities. The micro-organism is carried by flies, transmitted to both eyes. Attacks conjunctiva and cornea in childhood, causing eventual corneal scarring due to chronic inflammation. Treatment: antibiotics; improvement in living conditions: hygiene.

Onchocerciasis (river blindness)

'. . . disease affects about 30 million people in Africa and Central America and is a major cause of blindness' (Vaughan, Asbury and Riordan-Eva, 1992). Black or jinja fly: lives by rivers, plays host to *Onchocerca volvulus* worm, which migrates to human body. Signs and symptoms: micro-organisms spread beneath skin; skin nodules may be present. Infection of cornea: appears as 'snowflake' infiltrations;

obstructs vision (Trevor-Roper, 1986). It can cause keratitis; iritis; uveitis; retinitis; retinal degeneration; development of optic nerve atrophy. Treatment: nodulectomy; antibiotics; topical steroid therapy.

Miscellaneous conditions

Coloboma

Absent portion of a structure: eyelid; iris; lens; choroid; optic disc. Cause: hereditary: imperfect closure of foetal cleft, usually closed by birth date. Protective closure of eyelids. Signs/symptoms: depend upon size of gap and structure affected. Eye may be small: microphthalmos. Complications: neurological; retinal detachment.

Nystagmus

Symptom associated with: corneal opacities, albinism, congenital cataract, retinopathy, optic nerve atrophy. May be of idiopathic origin. Two types: ocular and labyrinthine-cerebellar.

Ocular

Most common. Development associated with infant who, because of visual deficiency, fails to focus on surrounding objects and obtain macula image clarity. Regular pendular movements of eyeball in horizontal or (rarely) vertical direction. Movements exaggerated during certain activities e.g. looking to side. When focusing attempted, eyes often wobble: involuntary oscillatory movement sometimes perceptible to person. Disconcerting: image, wobbles, eluding fixation; tiredness and stress exacerbates problem. Often accompanied by involuntary head movements.

Labyrinthine-cerebellar

Eye movements: slow driftings of eyeball in one direction, followed by faster jumps in opposite direction. Eye usually drifts towards side of lesion, and specific variety of nystagmus is labelled according to direction of jerky correcting phase of movement cycle. Symptoms exaggerated when individual is looking in opposite direction. If unilateral: brainstem damage. If bilateral: demyelinating diseases such as multiple sclerosis.

Thyroid eye disease

(TED, dysthyroid ophthalmopathy, Basedow's disease, endocrine exophthalmos, Graves' disease, thyrotoxic/thyrotrophic exophthalmos). Exophthalmos: forward protrusion of eyes. Second most common glandular disorder. Cause: genetic: associated with autoimmune conditions; hyperthyroidism. 10%-15% cases: no thyroid involvement. Retraction of eyelids; weakness of ocular muscles; inflammation due to drying of over-exposed cornea causing grittiness; swelling of tissues behind eye may lead to squint and double vision; reduced/absent eye movement; corneal and optic nerve damage; possible loss of vision. Treatment: eye drops; ointment; steroid therapy; radiotherapy; surgery to eyelids/muscles.

Usher's syndrome

Congenital condition: deafness followed by RP, which usually appears before 20 years of age. Occurs in about 7% of the born deaf population. Cause: little understood. No known medical treatment. Major cause of deafblindness in adult population.

Marfan's syndrome (arachnodactyly)

Rare inherited syndrome characterized by increased length of long bones, developmental anomalies of joints and internal organs. Visual impairment common. May cause: bilateral lens dislocation; refractive errors due to megalocornea; cataract; uveal coloboma; secondary glaucoma. 'Incomplete expression' of syndrome often seen (Vaughan, Asbury and Riordan-Eva, 1992). Treatment: of lens/cataract as appropriate.

References

Bannister, R. (1979) *Brain's Clinical Neurology*, 5th edn, Oxford University Press, Oxford.

Coakes, R.L. and Holmes Sellors, P.J. (1985) *An Outline of Opthalmology*, John Wright & Sons, Bristol.

Cullinan, T. (1986) *Visual Disability in the Elderly*, Croom Helm, London and Sydney.

Disabled Living Foundation (1991) *Visual Handicap: A Distance Learning Pack for Physiotherapists, Occupational Therapists and Other Health Care Professionals*, DLF, London.

Holmes, G. and Horax, G. (1919) Disturbances of spatial orientation and visual attention with a loss of stereoscopic vision. *Archives of Neurology and Psychiatry* **1** pp. 385–407.

Humphreys, G.W. and Riddoch, J.M. (1987) *To See but Not to See: A Case Study of Visual Agnosia*, Lawrence Eribaum Association, London.

Jose, R.T. (ed.) (1989) *Understanding Low Vision*, 2nd edn, American Foundation for the Blind, New York.

Riddoch, G. (1917) Dissociation of visual perceptions due to occipital injuries with especial reference to appreciation of movement. *Brain* **40** pp. 15–57.

Royal National Institute for the Blind (1995a) *Understanding Cataracts*, RNIB and RCO, London.

Royal National Institute for the Blind (1995b) *Understanding Glaucoma*, RNIB, RCO and IGA, London.

Royal National Institute for the Blind (1995c) *Understanding Retinal Detachment*, RNIB and RCO, London.

Royal National Institute for the Blind (1995d) *Understanding Diabetic Retinopathy*, RNIB and RCO, London.

Small, R. (1994) *The Clinical Handbook of Ophthalmology*, Pantheon Publishing, Carnforth, UK.

Trevor-Roper, P.D. (1986) *Lecture Notes on Ophthalmology*, 7th edn, Blackwell Scientific Publications, Oxford.

Vaughan, D.G., Asbury, T. and Riordan-Eva, P. (1992) *General Ophthalmology*, 13th edn, Prentice Hall International, London.

Suggested reading

Kanski, J.J. (1990) *Synopsis of Ophthalmology*, 6th edn, Wright, London.

Millodot, M. (1993) *Dictionary of Optometry*, 3rd edn, Butterworth-Heinemann, Oxford.

Snell, R.S. and Lemp, M.A. (1989) *Clinical Anatomy of the Eye*, Blackwell Scientific Publications, Oxford.

Glossary

Abduct/abduction – to turn away from the mid-line as when the eye rotates outwards.

Accommodation – ability of the lens to alter its shape (increased convexity) in order to focus the rays of light from a near object.

Achromatic – without colour.

Achromatopsia – total colour blindness.

Adaptation – (1) the process by which a sensory organ (e.g. the eye) adjusts to its environmental conditions; (2) the change in sensitivity to continuous sensory stimulation.

Adduct/adduction – to turn towards the mid-line as when the eye rotates inwards.

Aetiology – the cause or origin of a disease.

Afferent – impulses transmitted from the periphery towards the centre of the body.

After-image – the persistence of visual sensation after the removal of the original stimulus.

Agnosia – inability to recognize the significance of sensory stimuli, e.g. familiar objects/people, although the receptors in the sensory pathway remain intact.

Agonist – the muscle that initiates the movement: the 'prime mover'.

Albinism – a congenital disorder characterized by an absence of pigment in the skin, hair, iris, retina and choroid. Symptoms include nystagmus, poor visual acuity and photophobia.

Amaurosis – partial or total sight loss, thought to be due to a lesion somewhere within the visual pathway, but not within the eye itself.

The term is sometimes used as a synonym for blindness without a known organic cause.

Ambient sound – existing sound.

Amblyopia – failure of development of vision, resulting from a situation where a clear image is not presented to the retina. Symptoms include low visual acuity that is not correctable by optical measures. No detectable lesion of the eye.

Aniridia – complete or almost complete absence of the iris of the eye.

Anisocoria – unequal pupil size.

Anisopia – unequal vision in the two eyes.

Anomia – loss of ability to name an object.

Anophthalmia/anophthalmos – congenital absence of one or both eyes.

Anosognia – inability to perceive a defect in one half of the body.

Antagonist – reciprocal muscle to the agonist: relaxes to permit the movement of the agonist.

Anterior – in front of; as when one structure is anatomically positioned in front of another.

Anterior segment – cornea, anterior chamber, iris, pupil and lens.

APEL – Assessment/Accreditation of Prior Experiential Learning (uncertificated).

Aphakia – absence of a lens of the eye, due either to a congenital disorder or to surgical removal of the lens consequent upon a cataract.

APL – Assessment/Accreditation of Prior Learning (certificated).

Apraxia – inability to perform skilled and useful movements despite having intact power and sensation.

Arcus senilis – a greyish line or ring caused by the infiltration of fatty material during middle or old age in the periphery of the cornea, separated from its edge by a clear zone.

Asthenopia – eye fatigue/strain.

Astigmatism – a condition giving rise to a refractive error, possibly caused by distortion of the normal spherical shape of the eye.

Atrophy – reduction in size, as in muscle bulk.

Atrophy, optic – degeneration of the optic nerve fibres, characterized by a pale optic disc. Symptoms include reduced visual acuity, reduced visual fields or both.

ATW – Access To Work scheme. Employment Service programme designed to help disabled people to overcome employment-related barriers.

A:V – ratio of thickness of arteries to veins; usually 2:3.

BA – Benefits Agency.

Binocular – pertaining to both eyes.

Binocular vision – the simultaneous use of both eyes so as to produce one coherent mental image.

Bi-temporal hemianopia/hemianopsia – loss of both lateral visual fields.

Blepharitis – inflammation of the eyelids.

Blindness – (1) inability to see. (2) absence or severe impairment of vision such that one is unable to perform any work for which eyesight is essential (National Assistance Act, 1948).

Blind spot – normal defect in the visual field where the optic nerve enters the eye.

Braille – embossed script, invented by Louis Braille in 1824. A system of printing comprising the use of raised dots in six-cell units, configurations of which represent letters of the alphabet or symbolize parts of or entire words. Interpretation of these symbols is traditionally done by using the fingertips, although they can be read visually.

Bulbar – refers to the eyeball.

Buphthalmos – enlargement of the eye as in congenital glaucoma.

BV – binocular vision.

Canal of Schlemm – canal encircling the eye close to the trabecular meshwork, into which aqueous humour drains via the trabecular meshwork and thence to the scleral veins.

Canthus – angle at either end of the opening between the eyelids.

Cataract – partial or complete loss of transparency of the lens of the eye. The condition has several causes, congenital and acquired, and the principal symptom reduction in vision, which is described as 'cloudy' or 'misty'.

CATS – Credit Accumulation and Transfer Scheme.

CCTV – closed circuit television.

C.D. – ratio of optic cup to optic disc. Normal: <0.5 (not too deeply cupped). >0.5 with deep cupping is indicative of glaucoma.

CD-ROM – compact disk – read only memory.

Chemosis – oedema of the conjunctiva.

Choroiditis – inflammation of the choroid.

Chroma – colour.

Chromatic vision – colour vision.

Circumpapillary – around the optic disc.

C/O – complaining of.

Coloboma – congenital absence of part of the eyelid, iris, choroid or retina.

Colour sense – the appreciation of all colours of the spectrum.

Commotio – pigmentary disturbance of the retina after blunt trauma.

Contrast sensitivity – the ability to discriminate between light and dark.

Convergence – (1) movement of the eyes turning inwards or towards each other; (2) characteristic of a pencil of light rays directed towards a real image point.

Convergence test (Conv.) – assessment of the two medial muscles of each eye. A pen is held at 1/3 m and moved towards the nose.

Corectopia – displacement of the pupil from its normal central position.

Cover test (CT) – records the eye position when the person is looking straight ahead. Approximate size of the squint is recorded: min; sl; sl+; mod; mkd (marked); RDS (right divergent squint); LCS (left convergent squint).

CRAC – Careers Research Advisory Centre

Cylinder – cylindrical lens used to correct astigmatism.

Δ – symbol used to denote the word 'diagnosis'.

Dacryocystitis – inflammation of the lacrimal (tear) sac.

DDA – Disability Discrimination Act.

DEA – Disability Employment Adviser.

Decussation – crossing of nerve fibres passing through the mid-sagittal plane of the central nervous system and connecting with structures on the opposite side. Partial decussation occurs at the optic chiasma.

DfEE – Department for Education and Employment.

Diabetic retinopathy – a condition in which there is a prolific growth of new blood vessels with haemorrhages occurring in the retina. This is a complication of the more generalised condition of diabetes mellitus.

Dioptre – the unit measurement of the refracting power of the lens, used to measure the power of spectacle lenses, being the reciprocal of its focal length measured in metres.

Diplopia – a condition in which a single object is seen as two rather than one: double vision. It may be due to images not stimulating corresponding retinal areas.

Disability – any restriction or loss of ability to perform an activity in the manner considered normal for an individual (WHO; not generally used by disabled people).

DLA – Disability Living Allowance.

DoH – Department of Health.

DOS – Disk Operating System.

Drusen – degenerative products of retinal pigment epithelium appearing as yellow spots in the macula.

DSA – Disabled Students Allowance.

DSS – Department of Social Security.

DWA – Disability Working Allowance.

Dystrophy – a non-inflammatory, developmental, metabolic or nutritional disorder.

Eccentric viewing – the eye is encouraged to move so that the image falls on an active part of the retina, ideally close to the macula. It may be necessary to look below or to the right of the target.

Echo-location – the phenomenon whereby the brain picks up differences in the time self-generated sound leaves the traveller and the time at which it arrives back at the ears.

Ectropion – outward turning of the lower eyelid.

Emmetrope – a person who has no refractive errors and therefore does not need corrective lenses or glasses.

Emmetropia – normal refractive power of the eye.

Enopthalmos – abnormal retraction of eye into the orbit.

Entropion – inward turning of the lower eyelid.

Enucleation – removal of an eye from its socket.

Epiphora – watering of the eye; excessive production of tears.

ES – Employment Service.

Evisceration – removal of the eyeball from within the sclera.

Exophthalmos – abnormal protrusion of the eyeball from the orbit, usually caused by some form of endocrine disturbance, muscle dysfunction or orbital injury.

FEDA – Further Education Development Agency.

FEFC – Further Education Funding Council.

FEU – Further Education Unit. (Now FEDA; see above.)

Field, visual – the extent of space in which objects are visible to an eye in a given position.

Focus – the point at which rays of light converge after passing through a convex lens to form a real image, or diverge after passing through a concave lens.

Fundus – interior of a hollow organ, such as the eye.

Gestalt – the identification and recognition of people, objects, sound, and other sensory phenomena by the conversion of the random stimuli into form, shape or pattern.

Glare – a condition in which the observer perceives either discomfort and/or exhibits a reduction in performance levels in specific visual tests: visual acuity or contrast sensitivity. This is produced by the presence of a relatively bright lightsource within the visual field.

Glaucoma – a condition characterized by a raised or unstable intraocular pressure which cannot be sustained without damage to the eye's structure or impairment of its function. Varieties are: 'closed' and 'open' angle; primary or secondary. Symptoms include severe pain and reduction in the visual field.

Globe – the eyeball.

GROW – Gateway to Reaching Opportunities for Work.

Haemophthalmia – an effusion of blood into the eye.

Handicap – a disadvantage or the restriction imposed by impairment or disability preventing the fulfilment of a role that is normal for that individual (WHO; Not generally used by disabled people).

Haptic – the zone of a scleral contact lens which rests on the conjunctiva.

HEFC – Higher Education Funding Council.

Heliophobia – the fear of exposure to bright sunlight.

Hemeralopia – day blindness.

Hemiachromatopsia – loss of colour appreciation in one half of the visual field.

Heteronymous hemianopia/hemianopsia – loss of vision in opposite halves of the visual fields of both eyes.

Heterotropia – see strabismus.

HM – hand movements.

Homonymous hemianopia/hemianopsia – loss of vision in the same halves of the visual fields of both eyes.

Hordeolum – external stye.

HPC – history of present condition.

Hypermetrope – a person who has long sight.

Hypermetropia – a refractive error in which distant objects are focused behind the retina: longsightedness. The near vision is blurred.

Hypertrophy – increase in size, as in muscle fibres.

Hyphaema – the presence of blood in the anterior chamber of the eye.

Hypopyon – pus in the anterior chamber of the eye associated with infectious diseases of the cornea.

Hypotony – decreased intraocular pressure.

IB – Incapacity Benefit.

ILF – Independent Living Fund.

Impairment – any loss or abnormality of anatomical, physiological or psychological function (WHO: not generally used by disabled people).

Inferior – below; lower than, as when one structure is anatomically positioned below another.

Iridectomy – the surgical removal of part of the iris.

Irideremia – absence of all or part of the iris; total absence is termed 'aniridia'.

Iridotomy – creation of a small opening in the base of the iris.

Iris bombe – a condition of the eye in which the iris bulges forwards towards the cornea.

Iritis – inflammation of the iris.

Irrigation – the process of washing or cleansing of a wound or hollow organ (the eye) with a continuous stream of water or saline solution.

IS – Income Support.

JSA – Job Seeker's Allowance.

Keeler chart – standard chart used to assess a person's ability to read different print sizes.

Keratitis – inflammation of the cornea, usually caused by infection; sometimes due to trauma or disease.

Keratoconus – a progressive condition of the cornea in which it loses its approximately spherical curvature and becomes conical in shape.

Keratopathy – disease of the cornea.

Keratoprosthesis – plastic corneal implant.

LA – Local Authority.

Lacrimal – relating to the tears.

Lagophthalmos – delayed/incomplete eyelid closure, due to paralysis of the seventh cranial nerve.

Laser – an intense luminous source of monochromatic light. Acronym for 'light amplification by stimulated emission of radiation'.

Lateral – away from the mid-line of the body.

LE – left eye.

LEA – Local Education Authority.

Learning agreement – specified additional support identified by the college when a disabled person first moves into further education.

Light sense – the appreciation of light from dark.

Mac – macula area.

Macular degeneration – a condition of gradual painless loss of central vision, associated with the ageing process.

Macular vision – the central area of greatest visual acuity/clarity.

Medial – towards the mid-line of the body.

Megalophthalmos – an inherited condition, occurring only in males, in which the eye is abnormally large.

Meibomian glands – found at margins of eyelids; secrete oily substance which stabilises tear film and helps to make closed eyelids airtight.

Melanosis oculi – abnormal pigmentation of the eye.

Metamorphopsia – an anomaly of visual perception in which objects appear to be distorted in shape or larger (marcropsia) or smaller (micropsia) than their actual size. The cause is a displacement of the visual receptors as a consequence of inflammation, tumour, retinal detachment, or due to some disturbance in the central nervous system, e.g. migraine.

Microphthalmos – a developmental condition in which the eye is abnormally small.

Migraine – a condition giving rise to symptoms of intense pain, vertigo, nausea, photophobia and other visual distortions.

Monocular vision – vision using one eye only.

Moon – embossed script; invented by Dr. William Moon in 1845. Tactile reading system based on a simplified form of the Roman alphabet. Easier to learn and read than Braille. No contractions used: bulkier than Braille.

Muscae volitantes – opacities (floaters) that float before vision in the healthy eye.

Myopia – a refractive error in which the images of distant objects are focused in front of the retina: shortsightedness. The distance vision is blurred.

NAD – no abnormality detected / nothing abnormal discovered.

NFAC – National Federation of Access Centres.

NFER – National Foundation for Educational Research.

NI – National Insurance.

Null point – a head position that minimizes eye movements in nystagmus.

Nystagmus – regular, repetitive, involuntary oscillation of the eyes. The direction, amplitude and frequency of movements are irregular. The condition can be induced, acquired or congenital.

OCR – optical character recognition.

Oculus/oculi – the eye(s).

O/E – on examination.

Oedema – swelling caused by the presence of an excessive amount of fluid in and/or around the cells/tissues of the body.

OM (1) ocular movements; (2) orientation and mobility.

Ophthalmoplegia – paralysis of the extraocular muscles (EOM) or pupil.

Ophthalmoscope – an instrument that enables the clinician to view the various interior parts of the eye.

Ophthalmoscopy – a term used to describe the method of examining the interior of the eye using an ophthalmoscope.

Optic – pertaining to light or to vision.

Optic ataxia – inability to link action to the appropriate part of space.

Optic atrophy – atrophy of the optic disc due to degeneration of the optic nerve fibres and tract.

Optic neuritis – inflammation of the optic nerve.

Optical dispensing – the act of issuing an optical appliance that corrects, remedies or relieves defects of vision. (International Optometric and Optical League).

Optometer – an instrument for measuring the refractive state of the eye.

Optotype – the test type used for measuring visual acuity.

Ora serrata – the serrated anterior border of the retina.

Orbit – a rigid bony cavity in the skull which contains and protects the eyeball and all its associated structures.

Orthoptics – the study, diagnosis and non-operative treatment of anomalies of binocular vision, including squint.

PACT – Placing Assessment and Counselling Team, (Employment Service).

Palsy – synonym for 'paralysis'; a term regularly used to imply partial paralysis or paresis.

Panophthalmitis – inflammation of all the structures of the eye.

Papilla – a term used to describe any small elevation shaped like a nipple.

Papilloedema – non-inflammatory oedema of the optic nerve and disc, usually due to an increase in intracranial pressure.

Paresis – partial or slight paralysis.

Partial sight – substantial and permanent disability by congenitally defective vision of a substantial and permanently handicapping character (National Assistance Act, 1948).

PCT – prism cover test.

Percept – the complete mental image of an object, obtained in response to sensory stimuli.

Perception – the process of becoming aware of objects, qualities, or relations by way of the sense organs.

Perimeter – an instrument used to measure peripheral (field) vision.

Perimetry – the determination of the extent of the visual field, usually for the purposes of detecting anomalies within the visual pathway; assessment of peripheral visual fields.

Perspective – perceptual attribution of the third dimension in space or in graphic representation on a plane, as in a drawing.

Phakic – an eye possessing its crystalline lens or an intra-ocular lens implant.

Photic – pertaining to light or to the production of light.

Photophobia – hypersensitivity to bright light; abnormal fear or intolerance of bright light.

Photopic vision – daytime vision.

Photopsia – hallucinatory perceptions, such as sparks, lights or colours, arising in the absence of light stimuli and observed when the eyes are closed. They may be associated with diseases of the retina, optic nerve or brain. They may be a symptom of migraine.

PL – perceives light.

PMH – past medical history.

Polyopia – a condition in which more than one image of a single object is perceived. The condition is characterized by symptoms of double vision or multiple vision.

Posterior – behind; as when one structure is anatomically positioned behind another.

Posterior chamber – small space posterior to the iris.

Presbyope – a person who has short sight.

Presbyopia – a refractive condition, gradual in onset, in which the accommodative ability of the (lens of the) eye becomes unsatisfactory for near vision without the use of corrective plus lenses (called the addition). The lens loses its elasticity and ability to accommodate due to the general process of ageing.

Prognosis – the prediction of the probable course of a condition, and the likely outcome of events, based on all the relevant factors of a particular case.

Proprioception – the awareness of the body's position in space and of the relationship of one part to another; awareness of posture, balance, or position.

Proprioceptor – a specialized sensory nerve ending that monitors internal changes in the body brought about by movement and muscular activity. Proprioceptors located in muscles and tendons transmit information utilized in the coordination of muscular activity.

Proptosis – forward protrusion of the eyeball.

Prosopagnosis – inability to recognise faces.

Prosthesis (ocular) – an artificial eye or ocular implant.

Pseudo- – a prefix meaning false or spurious.

Ptosis – drooping of the upper eyelid.

Pupils NDC – the pupils' reaction to light: D, direct light (pupil constricts to direct light); C, consensual (pupil constricts when opposite eye is illuminated); N, pupils constrict as objects are moved towards the nose.

RE – right eye.

Reflection – return or bending of light by a surface such that it continues to travel in the same direction.

Reflex – an involuntary response to a stimulus.

Refraction – (1) the change in direction of the path of light as it passes obliquely from one medium to another having a different index of refraction; (2) the process of measuring and correcting the refractive error of the eyes.

REM – rapid eye movements.

Resection – a surgical procedure, used to correct strabismus, in which a portion of extra-ocular muscle is removed (usually at its insertion) and the muscle is reattached, at or near the original site of insertion. The objective of the procedure is to shorten the muscle.

Retina – the light-receptive, innermost tissue of the eye.

Retinal detachment – a condition in which detachment of the retina from the choroid occurs, either in small areas of tears or holes or over a wider area.

Retinitis – inflammation of the retina.

Retinitis pigmentosa – a chronic, hereditary, degenerative condition of the retina. Principal symptoms include night blindness and loss of field and colour vision.

Retinoblastoma – a malignant tumour of the retina.

Retinopathy of prematurity (retrolental fibroplasia) – a condition in which a fibrous strand forms behind the lens. The cause is

over-exposure to oxygen, associated with the care of premature
babies.

Retinopathy – disease of the retina.

Retinoscope – an instrument for determining the refractive state of
the eye.

Retrobulbar – behind the eyeball.

RAM – random access memory.

ROM – read only memory.

Rx (1) – a symbol that indicates all details of the prescription of the
lenses prescribed to correct a refractive error.

Rx (2) – a symbol used as an abbreviation for the word 'treatment'.

Saccades – rapid eye movements.

SAD – seasonal affective disorder.

Sarcoma – malignant tumour formed by the proliferation of cells.

Sclerotomy – excision of a piece of sclera to permit escape of
aqueous.

Scotoma – an area of visual impairment or loss within the normal
visual field.

Scotopic vision – night vision, associated with the function of the rods.

SDA – Severe Disability Allowance.

See – (1) to perceive by the eye; (2) to discern; (3) to note; to
understand.

Self-generated sound – sound that is deliberately created and utilized
to facilitate the process of mobility.

SEN – special educational needs.

Sensation – the conscious response to the effect of a stimulus exciting
any sense organ.

SG – Sheridan Gardiner test (single letter).

Shadow – a darkened area from which rays from a source of light are
excluded.

Sight – the special sense by which the colour, form, position, shape,
etc. of objects is perceived when light from these objects impinges
upon the retina of the eye.

SLDD – severe learning difficulties and/or disabilities.

Sound signatures – unique characteristics of particular sounds.

Sn – Snellen chart reading.

Snellen chart – standard chart to test visual acuity.

Sphere – a lens used to correct hypermetropia (plus sphere) or myopia (minus sphere).

SPS – Supported Placement Scheme.

SSD – Social Services Department.

Stargardt's disease – hereditary retinal dystrophy, usually commencing between 8 and 14 years; loss of central vision and macular degeneration.

Statement – describes the specific special educational provision that a young person should receive at school to meet identified educational needs as a consequence of disability.

Steady eye strategy (SES) – the eye is kept steady and reading material is moved across the newly established line of (eccentric) vision.

Stereopsis – direct awareness of depth due to retinal disparity; binocular depth perception.

Stereoscope – an instrument that allows targets to be presented independently to the two eyes.

Stigmatism – the condition of an optical system in which light from a point source forms an image, which is also a point, as distinguished from astigmatism.

Stimulus – any agent or environmental change that provokes a response.

Strabismus (squint) – (1) a condition in which the lines of light of the two eyes are not directed towards the same fixation point when the subject is actively fixating on an object.
(2) deviation of the normally parallel visual axes: the two eyes are not directed at the same object.

Stroboscope – an instrument that produces brief flashes of illumination at a variable frequency.

Superior – above; higher than, as when one structure is anatomically positioned above another.

Suppression – the process by which the brain inhibits part or the whole of the retinal image of one eye when both eyes are simultaneously stimulated. The objective is to avoid diplopia and results in the ability to ignore a second (double) image.

Symeblepharon – adhesion of the eyelid to the eyeball.

Synapse – the junction where one nerve impulse is transmitted from one neurone to another.

Syndrome – the aggregation of signs and symptoms associated with a disease or condition.

Synechia – adhesion of the iris to the cornea or the lens.

Synergist – a muscle which prevents unwanted movements associated with the action of the agonist.

Tachistoscope – an instrument that presents visual stimuli for a brief and variable period of time.

Tarsorrhaphy – union of the opposing margins of the upper and lower eyelids.

TEC – Training and Enterprise Council.

Telescope – an optical instrument for magnifying the apparent size of distant objects.

TFW – Training for Work.

Theory – an explanation of the manner in which a phenomenon occurs, has occurred or will occur.

Threshold – the value of a stimulus that just produces a response.

Tonometer – an instrument used to measure intraocular pressure.

Torsion – rotation of the eye about an antero-posterior axis.

Trachoma – a chronic, bilateral, contagious infection of the conjunctiva caused by one of the TRIC viruses.

Transition plan – a comprehensive plan for the transition period, produced at the first annual review after a disabled person's fourteenth birthday. Can be created for any period of transition from one period of life to another.

Trichiasis – irritation of the cornea by the eyelashes.

Tunnel vision – reduction in the peripheral part of the visual field, leaving a small area of central vision.

UCAS – University and Colleges Admissions System.

Ulcer – a localized lesion of the skin or a mucous layer in which the superficial epithelium is destroyed and deeper tissues are exposed.

Ultraviolet – radiant energy of wavelengths smaller than those at the violet end of the visible spectrum; invisible to the naked eye.

Vision – the appreciation of differences in the external world, such as form, colour, shape, position, etc., resulting from stimulation of the retina by light.

Visual acuity – clarity or sharpness of vision, as when a lens is in focus to produce a visual image.

Visual field – the area of vision of each eye working alone, focused on a fixed point.

Visual neglect – the visual field on one side is ignored.

WEA – Workers Education Association.

Wink – the rapid, voluntary closing and opening of one eye.

Xerophthalmia – a condition in which opacity with ulceration of the cornea results from vitamin A deficiency.

Personnel associated with the management of visual impairment in Britain

The following information has been supplied by the British College of Optometrists (DLF, 1991) and the Royal National Institute for the Blind's (undated) *Low Vision Training Pack*, Compiled by D. Davis and R. Wilson.

Dispensing opticians (D.O.) are registered with the General Optical Council only if they are qualified to fit and supply spectacles, contact lenses and other optical appliances. They are not qualified to undertake eye examinations. They are employed in general practice or in hospital eye departments.

Ophthalmologists or ophthalmic surgeons are medically qualified, registered with the General Medical Council and specialize in eye disorders and their management and treatment. They may prescribe corrective lenses although they do not generally fit and supply spectacles and contact lenses. They diagnose and treat all defects and diseases of the eye by prescribing drugs and other types of medical care including surgery. They usually work in eye hospitals or hospital eye departments.

Ophthalmic medical practitioners are doctors, registered with the General Medical Council, who have chosen to specialize in eyes and eye care. They are qualified to undertake eye examinations in the National Health Service, identify abnormal eye conditions and prescribe corrective lenses and other optical appliances. They generally work in conjunction with dispensing opticians.

Optometrists (ophthalmic opticians) (O.O.) are registered with the General Optical Council. They are employed in general practice or in hospital eye departments. They are qualified to examine eyes, to identify defects of vision and signs of disease or abnormality in the eyes. They prescribe, fit and supply spectacles, contact lenses and other visual appliances to correct defects of sight. They provide advice on eye care, both generally and with specific reference to occupational and recreational needs and also with particular regard to problems of clients with reduced vision.

Orthoptists usually work under the direction of ophthalmologists in the National Health Service. They are engaged in the investigation and treatment of various abnormalities of binocular vision such as squints and diplopia. In cases where control of a squint or relief from other eye symptoms can be achieved by exercises designed to develop or restore normal binocular visual function, the orthoptist plans and implements this therapy.

Rehabilitation workers are usually employed by the local authority to undertake rehabilitation work with blind and partially sighted people. They may specialize in orientation and mobility (OM) or technical skills.

Principal sources

Disabled Living Foundation (1991) *Visual Handicap: A Distance Learning Pack for Physiotherapists, Occupational Therapists and Other Health Care Professionals*, DLF, London.

Millodot, M. (1993) *Dictionary of Optometry*, 3rd edn, Butterworth-Heinemann, London.

Royal National Institute for the Blind (undated) *Low Vision Training Pack*, RNIB, London.

Small, R. (1994) *The Clinical Handbook of Ophthalmology*, Pantheon Publishing, Lancashire and New York.

World Health Organisation (1980) *International Classification of Impairments, Disabilities and Handicaps: A Manual of Classification Relating to the Consequence of Disease*, WHO, Geneva, and HMSO, London.

Useful addresses

Abbeyfield Society
Abbeyfield House
53 Victoria Street
St Albans
Hertfordshire AL1 3UW
Tel: 01727-857536

Access Ability
The Norton Park Centre
57 Albion Road
Edinburgh EH7 5QI
Tel: 0131-475-2300

Access Committee for England
12 City Forum
250 City Road
London EC1V 8AF
Tel: 0171-250-0008
Fax: 0171-250-0212

Access to Information and
    Reading Services (AIRS)
Gateshead Central Library
Prince Consort Road
Gateshead NE8 4LN
Tel: 0191-477-3478
Fax: 0191-477-7454

Action for Blind People
14–16 Verney Road
London SE16 3DZ
Tel: 0171-732-8771
Fax: 0171-639-0948

Action Trust for Blind and
    Disabled People
Mr Ian Barclay
West London Resource Centre
    for the Blind
Holy Innocents Church
Paddenswick Road
London W6 0UB
Tel: 0181-563-2922

ADA Reading Service
c/o Mrs Artus
6 Dalewood Rise
Laverstock
Salisbury
Wiltshire SP1 1SF
Tel: 01722-326987

Advisory Centre for
    Education
18 Victoria Park Square

London E2 9PB
Tel: 0171-980-4596

Age Concern England
Astral House
1268 London Road
London SW6 4EJ
Tel: 0181-679-8000

AHEAD (Ireland)
Newman House
86 St Stephen's Green
Dublin 2
Republic of Ireland
Tel: +353-1-475-2386
Fax: +353-1-475-2387

Alliance for Inclusive Education
Micheline Mason
Unit 2
Ground Floor
70 South Lambeth Road
London SW8 1RL
Tel: 0171-735-5277

Alms House Association
Billingbear Lodge
Wokingham
Berkshire RG11 5RU
Tel: 01344-452922

AlphaVision Ltd
North's Estate
Piddington
High Wycombe
Buckinghamshire HP14 3BE
Tel: 01494-883838
Fax: 01491-881211

American Foundation for the
   Blind
15 West 16th Street
New York, NY 10011
USA
Tel: +1-212-620-2020
Fax: +1-212-727-7418

Association for the Development
   of Life Skills and
   Independence of the Visually
   Impaired
Chris Clarke
The West of England School
Topsham Road
Countess Wear
Exeter
Devon EX2 6HA
Tel: 01392-454200

Association for the Education
   and Welfare of the Visually
   Handicapped
Mrs J. Stone, Hon. Secretary
4 Stockdale Place
Westfield Road
Edgbaston
Birmingham B15 3XH
Tel: 0121-454-7053

Association of Blind and Partially
   Sighted Teachers and Students
   (ABAPSTAS)
Nick Clarke, contact officer
BM Box 6727
London WC1V 6XX
Tel: 01484-517954

Association of Blind Asians (ABA)
322 Upper Street
London N1 2XQ
Tel: 0171-226-1950
Fax: 0171-226-1950

Association of Blind Chartered
  Physiotherapists
Mrs Ann Weatherley, Secretary
7 Benningholme Road
Edgeware
Middlesex HA8 9HF
Tel: 0181-906-2175

Association of Blind Piano Tuners
Mr A.F. Spencer Bolland, Hon.
  Secretary
24 Fairlawn Grove
Chiswick
London W4 5EH
Tel: 0181-995-0295
Fax: 0181-742-2396

Association of Carers
29 Chilworth Mews
London W2 3RG
Tel: 0171-724-7776

Association of Charity Officers
c/o RICS Benevolent Fund Ltd
2nd Floor
Tavistock House North
Tavistock Square
London WC1H 9RJ
Tel: 0181-387-0578

Association of Disabled
  Professionals (ADP)

Sue Maynard Campbell,
  Chairperson
170 Benton Hill
Horbury
Wakefield
West Yorkshire WF4 5HW
Tel/Fax: 01924-283253

Association of Visually
  Handicapped Office Workers
  (AVHOW)
Catherine Carter, Secretary
16 Ravensmede Way
Chiswick High Road
London W4 1TD
Tel: 0181-995-0050

Association of Visually
  Handicapped Telephonists
Martyn Wilson, Chairperson
34A The Broadway
Woodford Green
Essex TG8 0HQ
Tel: 0171-441-6698 (daytime)

BBC Radio Collection
Marketing Co-ordinator
BBC Enterprises
Room A2100
80 Wood Lane
London W12 0TT
Tel: 0181-743-5588

Behçet's Syndrome Society
B.M. Seaman, Chairperson
3 Church Close
Lambourne
Newbury

Berkshire RG16 7PU
Tel: 01488-71116
Fax: 01488-73482

Benefits Agency Benefits Enquiry
Line
Freephone: 0800-882200

Benefits Agency Distribution and
Storage Centre
Heywood Stores
PO Box 50
Heywood
Lancashire OL10 2GF

Birmingham Royal Institution for
the Blind (BRIB)
48 Court Oak Road
Harborne
Birmingham B17 9TG
Tel: 0121-428-5000
Fax: 0121-428-5008

Blind Business Association Ltd
(BBA)
George Carratt,
Chairperson
20 Althorpe Road
Harrow
Middlesex HA1 4RA
Tel/Fax: 0181-427-3052

Blind in Business Trust
Lintas House
15–19 New Fetter Lane
London EC4A 1AP
Tel: 0171-931-5674/5
Fax: 0171-931-5637

British Association for
Counselling
1 Regent Place
Rugby
Warwickshire CV21 2PJ
Tel: 01788-578328

British Blind Sport
Maurice J. Bright, Chief Executive
67 Albert Street
Rugby
Warwickshire CV21 2SN
Tel: 01788-536142
Fax: 01788-536676

British Broadcasting Corporation
Publications
PO Box 234
London SE1 3TH

British Broadcasting Support
Services
PO Box 7
London W3 6XJ

British Computer Association of
the Blind
Derek Naysmith, Secretary
BCM Box 950
London
Tel: 01203-562946
Mobile: 0370-500385

British Computer Society
Disability Group
Geoff Busby, Chairperson
EASAMS Ltd

Room 126
Great Baddow
Essex CM2 2HN
Tel: 01245-242950
Fax: 01245-478317

British Council for the
  Prevention of Blindness
  (BCPB)
Rachael Carr-Hill
12 Harcourt Street
London W1H 1DS
Tel: 0171-724-3716

British Council for Rehabilitation
  of the Disabled
Unit 12
City Forum
250 City Road
London, EC13 8AF
Tel: 0171-250-3222

British Council of
  Organisations of Disabled
  People (BCODP)
Richard Wood, Chief Executive
Litchurch Plaza
Litchurch Lane
Derby DE24 8AA
Tel: 01332-295551
Fax: 01332-295580

British Diabetic Association
10 Queen Ann Street
London W1M 0BD
Tel: 0171-323-1531
Fax: 0171-637-3644

British Dyslexia Association
  (BDA)
98 London Road
Reading
Berkshire RG1 5AU
Tel: 01889-662667
Fax: 01889-351927

British Journal of Visual
  Impairment
108 High Street
Hurstpierpoint
West Sussex BN6 9PX
Tel: 01273-834321
Fax: 01273-833050

British Orthoptic Society (BOS)
Avril Sharnock, Hon. Secretary
Tavistock House North
Tavistock Square
London WC1H 9HX
Tel: 0171-387-7992
Fax: 0171-383-2584

British Red Cross
9 Grosvenor Crescent
London SW1X 7EE
Tel: 0171-235-5454

British Retinitis Pigmentosa
  Society
Lynda Cantor MBE
Pond House
Lillingstone Dayrell
Buckingham MK18 5AS
Tel: 01280-860363
Fax: 01280-860515

British Wireless for the Blind
Fund
Gabriel House
34 New Road
Chatham
Kent ME4 4QR
Tel: 01634-832501
Fax: 01634-817485

Brook Street
Clarence House
134 Hatfield Road
St Albans
Hertfordshire AL1 4JB
Tel: 01727-841187

Cadwell Recording Services for
the Blind
17 Trusthams
Broadwindsor
Beaminster
Dorset DT8 3QB
Tel: 01308-868500/868465

Calibre Library for Blind and
Print Disabled
New Road
Weston
Aylesbury
Buckinghamshire HP22 5XQ
Tel: 01296-432339
Fax: 01296-392599

Camsight
167 Green End Road
Oakington
Cambridge CA4 1RW

Tel: 01223-220033
Fax: 01223-426672

Care and Repair
Castle House
Kirtley Drive
Nottingham NG7 1LD
Tel: 01159-744091

Carers National Association
20–25 Glasshouse Yard
London EC1A 4JS
Tel: 0345-573369 (advice line)
0171-490-8818 (administration)

Carematch
Residential Care Consortium
Computer Service
286 Camden Road
London N7 0BJ
Tel: 0171-609-9966

Cecelia Charity for the Blind
61 West Smithfield
London EC1A 9EA
Tel: 0171-606-5711

Centre for Accessible
Environments
Nutmeg House
60 Gainsford Street
London SE1 2NY
Tel: 0171-357-8182
Fax: 0171-357-8183

Centre for Studies on Inclusive
Education (CSIE)

1 Redland Close
Elm Lane
Redland
Bristol BS6 6UE
Tel: 0117-923-8450
Fax: 0117-923-8460

Centre for Policy on Ageing
25 Ironmonger Row
London EC1
Tel: 0171-253-1787

CHANGE
Phillippa Bragman,
   Co-ordinator
First Floor
69–85 Old Street
London EC1V 9HY
Tel: 0171-490-2668
Fax: 0171-490-3981

CHARGE Association
   Family Support
   Group
115 Boundary Road
Colliers Wood
London SW19 2DE
Tel: 0181-540-2142

Charterhouse Partnership
Jean Brading and John Curtis,
   Directors
Morrell House
98 Curtain Road
London EC2A 3AA
Tel: 0171-613-4956
Fax: 0171-739-5482

Chest, Heart and Stroke
   Association
Tavistock House North
Tavistock Square
London, WC1H 9JE
Tel: 0171-387-3102

Chest, Heart and Stroke
   (Scotland)
65 North Castle Street
Edinburgh EN2 3LT
Tel: 0345-720720

Chester-care
Sidings Road
Low Moor Estate
Kirkby-in-Ashfield
Nottinghamshire
   NG7 7JZ
Tel: 01623-757955
Fax: 01623-722582

Children in Scotland
   (Special Needs
   Forum)
Princess House
5 Shandwick Place
Edinburgh EH1 4RG
Tel: 0131-228-8484
Fax: 0131-228-8585

Chivers Press Publishers
Windsor Bridge Road
Bath
Avon BA2 3AX
Tel: 01225-335336
Fax: 01225-310771

Circle of Guide Dog
  Owners
Mrs Christine Parker
116 Potters Lane
Send
Woking
Droylsden
Surrey GU23 7AL
Tel: 01483-770361

Clarke and Smith
Melbourne House
Melbourne Road
Wallington
Surrey SM6 8SD
Tel: 0181-669-4411

Clerics Group
Revd C.W.M. Bracegirdle
The Rectory
Parsonage Close
Salford M5 3GT
Tel: 0161-872-0800

Cobolt Systems Ltd
The Old Mill House
Mill Road
Reedham
Norwich
Norfolk NR13 3HA
Tel: 01493-700172
Fax: 01493-701037

Community Service Volunteers
  (CSV)
237 Pentonville Road
London N1 9NJ

Tel: 0171-278-6601
Fax: 0171-833-0149

Committee of Vice-Chancellors
  and Principals of the
  Universities of the United
  Kingdom (CVCP)
Woburn House
20 Tavistock Square
London WC1H 9HQ
Tel: 0171-419-4111
Fax: 0171-388-8649

Concept Systems
204–206 Queens Road
Beeston
Nottingham NG9 2BD
Tel: 0115-925-5988
Fax: 0115-925-8588

Confederation of Tape
  Information Services (COTIS)
Project Office
67 High Street
Tarporley
Cheshire CW6 0DP
Tel: 01829-733351
Fax: 01829-732408

Contact-a-Family
170 Tottenham Court Road
London W1P 0HA
Tel: 0171-383-3555
Fax: 0171-383-0259

COST 219 UK Group
Dr John Gill

1 The Grange
85 High Street
Iver
Buckinghamshire SL0 9PN
Fax: 0171-388-7747

Counsel and Care for the
  Elderly
Lower Ground Floor
Twyman House
16 Bonny Street
London NW1 9PG
Tel: 0171-485-1566

Coverdale Organisation
Claire Finlow, contact
St James's Court
Wilderspool Causeway
Warrington
Cheshire WA4 6PS
Tel: 01925-570962

Crossroads Care Attendant
  Schemes
94A Coton Road
Rugby
Warwickshire CV21 4LN

Cruse
Cruse House
126 Sheen Road
Richmond
Surrey TW9 1UR
Tel: 0181-332-7227

Department for Education and
  Employment (DfEE)

Sanctuary Buildings
Great Smith Street
London SW1P 3PT
Tel: 0171-925-5000

Department for Education and
  Employment (DfEE)
Publications Centre
PO Box 6927
London E3 3NZ
Tel: 0171-510-0510

Department of Health (DoH)
Richmond House
94 Whitehall
London, SW1A 2NS
Tel: 0171-972-2000

Department of Health
Social Services Inspectorate SC6
Wellington House
133–135 Waterloo Road
London SE1 8UG
Tel: 0171-972-2000

Department of Transport
2 Marsham Street
London SW1P 3EB
Mobility Unit
Room S10/21
Tel: 0171-276-5257
Orange Badge Unit
Room C10/02
Tel: 0171-276-6291

Deutsche Blindenstudienanstalt
D3550 Marburg 1

AM Schlag 8
Germany
Tel: +49-0-6421-6060

DIAL UK (National
  Association of Disablement
  Information and Advice
  Lines)
Park Lodge
St Catherine's Hospital
Tickhill Road
Doncaster
South Yorkshire DN4 8QN
Tel: 01302-310123
Fax: 01302-310404

Disability Access Rights
  Advice Service
  (DARAS)
Unit 303
The Chandlery
Westminster Bridge Road
London SE1 7QY
Tel: 0345-585445
Fax: 0345-585446

Disability Action (Northern
  Ireland)
2 Annadale Avenue
Belfast B17 3UR
Tel: 01232-491011
Fax: 01232-491627

Disability Advice and Welfare
  Network
64–66 Bickerstaffe Street
St Helens

Merseyside WA10 2DH
Tel: 01744-451215

Disability Alliance
  Educational and Research
  Association
1st Floor East
Universal House
88–94 Wentworth Street
London E1 7SA
Tel: 0171-247-8776
Rights advice line
  (Monday and
  Wednesday 2–4 p.m.)
0171-247-8763

Disability Casebook
Hobsons Publishing plc
FREEPOST
175–179 St John Street
London EC1V 4RP
Tel: 0171-336-6633

Disability Discrimination Act
  Information Line
0345-622633
Disability Employment Adviser
  (DEA)
Contact at local Jobcentre

Disability Information Trust
Mary Marlborough Centre
Nuffield Orthopaedic Centre
Headington
Oxford OX3 7LD
Tel: 01865-227952

Disability on the Agenda
DDA Information
FREEPOST MIDO2164
Stratford-upon-Avon
Warwickshire CV37 9BR
Tel: 0345-622688

Disability Now Magazine
6 Market Road
Holloway
London N7 9PW
Tel: 0171-636-5020 (editorial)
     0171-383-4575 (circulation)

Disability Resource Team (DRT)
Office 2
Pallmark House
11 Amwell End
Ware
Hertfordshire SG12 9HP
Tel: 01920-466005

Disability Scotland
Princes House
5 Shandwick Place
Edinburgh EH2 4RG
Tel: 0131-229-8632
Fax: 0131-229-5168

Disability Wales/Anabledd
   Cymru
Llys lfor
Crescent Road
Caerphilly CF83 1XL
Tel: 01222-887325
Fax: 01222-888702

Disability West Midlands
Moseley Hall Hospital
Birmingham
West Midlands B13 8JL
Tel: 0121-449-1225

Disabled Graduate
   Careers Information
   Service
Skill
336 Brixton Road
London SW9 7AA
Tel: 0171-274-0565

Disabled Information Service
   Westminster
10 Warwick Row
London SW1
Tel: 0171-630-5994

Disabled Living Foundation
   (DLF)
380–384 Harrow Road
London W9 2HU
Tel: 0171-289-6111
Fax: 0171-266-2922

Disabled Persons Railcard Office
PO Box 1YT
Newcastle upon Tyne
NE99 1YT

Disablement Income Group
   (DIG)
Unit 5
Archway Business Centre
19–23 Wedmor Street

London N19 4RZ
Tel: 0171-263-3981

Dis-forum
dis-forum@mailbase.ac.uk

Dixey of Wigmore Street
19 Wigmore Street
London W1H 9LA
Tel: 0171-491-2713

Dolphin Computer Access Ltd
Unit 96c
Blackpole Trading Estate West
Worcester WR3 8TU
Tel: 01905-754577
Fax: 01905-754559

Dorton College of Further
   Education (RLSB)
Wildernesse Avenue
Seal
Sevenoaks
Kent TN15 0ED
Tel: 01732-764123
Fax: 01732-761055

Dorton House School (RLSB)
Dorton IT Support Centre
Seal
Sevenoaks
Kent TN15 0EB
Tel: 01732-761477
Fax: 01732-763363

Dragon Systems (UK) Ltd
Millbank

Stoke Road
Bishops Cleeve
Cheltenham
Gloucestershire GL52 4RW
Tel: 01242-678575
Fax: 01242-678301

Dyslexia Institute
133 Gresham Road
Staines
Middlesex TW18 2AJ
Tel: 01784-463851
Fax: 01784-460747

Dyspraxia Foundation
8 West Alley
Hitchin
Hertfordshire SG5 1EG
Tel: 01462-454986
Fax: 01462-455052

Dystonia Society
Weddel House
13–14 West Smithfield
London EC1A 9HY
Tel: 0171-329-0797
Fax: 0171-329-0689

Electricity Association
30 Millbank
London SW1P 4RD
Tel: 0171-344-5700
Fax: 0171-963-5959

Electronic Aids for the Blind
   (EAB)
Suite 4b

73–75 High Street
Chislehurst
Kent BR7 5AG
Tel: 0181-295-3636
Fax: 0181-295-3737

Electronic Services for the Blind
28 Crofton Avenue
Orpington
Kent BR6 8DU
Tel: 01689-855-651

Employers Forum on Disability
Sue Scott-Parker, contact
Nutmeg House
60 Gainsford Street
London SE1 2NY
Tel: 0171-403-3020
Fax: 0171-403-0404

Enable
6th Floor
7 Buchanan Street
Glasgow G1 3HL

Eyecare Information Service
  (EIS)
PO Box 3597
London SE1 6DY
Tel: 0171-357-7730
Fax: 0171-357-7155

Eyeline
c/o Janet Wallace
22 Whitaker Lane
Prestwick
Manchester M25 5FX
Tel: 0161-872-1234

Family Fund
PO Box 50
York YO1 1UY
Tel: 01904-621115

Family Welfare
  Association
501/505 Kingsland Road
Dalston
London E8 4AU
Tel: 0171-254-6251
Fax: 0171-249-5443

Fast-Track Management Training
  Scheme
16 Fitzroy Square
London W1P 5HQ
Tel: 0171-387-9571

Fingatip Labels
Unit 26A
Lenton Business Centre
Lenton Boulevard
Nottingham NG7 2BY
Tel: 0115-942-0941

Foundation for Communication
  for the Disabled
Beacon House
Pyrfind Road
West Byfleet
Surrey KT14 6LD
Tel: 01932-336912
Fax: 01932-336513

Further Education Development
  Agency (FEDA)

Head Office
Dumbarton House
68 Oxford Street
London W1
Tel: 0171-436-0020
Fax: 0171-436-0349

Further Education Development
  Agency (FEDA)
Publications Department
FEDA
Mendip Centre
Blagdon
Bristol BS18 6RG
Tel: 01761-462503
Fax: 01761-463140

Further Education Funding
  Council (England) (FEFC)
Cheylesmore House
Quinton Road
Coventry CV1 2WT
Tel: 01203-863207

Further Education Funding
  Council (Scotland)
St Andrew's House
Regent Road
Edinburgh EH1 3DG
Tel: 0131-556-8400

Further Education Funding
  Council (Wales)
Linden Court
The Orchards
Ty Glass Avenue
Llanishen

Cardiff CF4 5DZ
Tel: 01222-761861

Gardner's Trust for the Blind
61 West Smithfield
London EC1A 9EA
Tel: 0171-606-5711
Fax: 0171-600-3094

Gift of Thomas Pocklington
5 Castle Row
Horticultural Place
Chiswick
London W4 4JQ
Tel: 0181-995-0880
Fax: 0181-987-9965

Greater London Association of
  Disabled People (GLAD)
336 Brixton Road
London SW9 7AA
Tel: 0171-346-5800
Fax: 0171-274-7840

Greater London Fund for the
  Blind
12 Whitehorse Mews
37 Westminster Bridge Road
London SE1 7QD
Tel: 0171-620-2066
Fax: 0171-620-2016

Greater Manchester Coalition of
  Disabled People
Carisbrooke
Wenlock Way
Gorton

Manchester M12 5LF
Tel: 0161-273-5153

Guide Dogs for the Blind
  Association (GDBA)
Hillfields
Burghfield Common
Reading
Berkshire RG7 3YG
Tel: 0118-983-5555
Fax: 0118-983-5433

Guide Dogs for the Blind
  Holidays
Shap Road
Kendall
Cumbria LA9 6NZ
Tel: 01539-735080
Fax: 01539-735567

Hadley School for the
  Blind
700 Elm Street
Winnetka IL 60093-0299
USA
Tel: +1-708-466-8111

Hagger Electronics
Unit 22, Business West
Avenue One
Letchworth
Herts SG6 2HB
Tel: 01462 677331
Fax: 01462 675016

Health Education Authority
Hamilton House

Mabledon Place
London WC1H 9TC
Tel: 0171-383-3833

Health Publications Unit
Heywood Stores
No. 2 Site
Manchester Road
Heywood
Lancashire OL10 2PZ

Help the Aged
Head Office
St James Walk
London EC1R 0BE
Tel: 0171-253-0253
Fax: 0171-250-4474

Hemiahelp
Hilary Latham
166 Boundaries Road
London SW12 8HG
Tel: 0181-672-3179

Henshaw's College
Bogs Lane
Starbeck
Harrogate
North Yorkshire HG1 4ED
Tel: 01423-886451
Fax: 01423-885095

Henshaw's Society for the Blind
John Derby House
88–92 Talbot Road
Old Trafford
Manchester M16 0GS

Tel: 0161-872-1234
Fax: 0161-848-9889

Higher Education Funding
  Council for England
  (HEFCE)
Northavon House
Coldharbour Lane
Bristol BS16 1QD
Tel: 0117-931-7317
Fax: 0117-931-7203

Higher Education Funding
  Council for Wales / Cyngor
  Cyllido Cymru
Lambourne House
Cardiff Business Park
Llanishen
Cardiff CF4 5GL
Tel: 01222-761861
Fax: 01222-763163

Hobson's Casebook for Graduates
  with Disabilities
Tel: 0171-336-6633

Holiday Care Service
2nd Floor
Imperial House
Victoria Road
Horley
Surrey RH6 7PZ
Tel: 01293-774535
Fax: 01293-784647

Horizon CCTV
11–12 Lowman Units

Tiverton Business Park
Devon EX16 6SD
Tel: 01844-254172
Fax: 01844-253114

Horticultural Therapy
1 Goulds Ground
Vallis Way
Frome
Somerset BA11 3DW
Tel: 01373-464782

Illuminating Engineering Society
York House
Westminster Bridge Road
London SE1

Innovations in Information
National Information Forum
British Telecommunications
Burne House
Post point 10/10
Bell Street
London NW1 5BZ

Insurable
Simon Newman, Project Manager
Workable
Saffron Cottage
Halstock
Dorset BA22 9SN
Tel: 01935-891999

In Touch Programme for People
  with a Visual Impairment
Room 7075
BBC Radio 4

BBC Broadcasting House
London W1A 1AA
Tel: 0171-580-4444

International Glaucoma
  Association (IGA)
c/o Mrs B. Wright
King's College Hospital
Denmark Hill
Camberwell
London SE5 9RS
Tel: 0171-274-6222
Fax: 0171-737-3265

Irish National Council for the
  Blind
10 Lower Hatch Street
Dublin 2
Republc of Ireland
Tel: +353-176-1018

Irish National League of the
  Blind
35 Gardiner Place
Dublin 1
Republc of Ireland
Tel: +353-174-2792

Isis Publishing Ltd
7 Centremead
Osney Mead
Oxford OX2 0ES
Tel: 01865-250333
Fax: 01865-790358

Jessica Kingsley Publishers Ltd
116 Pentonville Road

London N1 9JB
Tel: 0171-833-2307

Jewish Care
Stuart Young House
221 Golders Green Road
London NW11 9DQ
Tel: 0181-458-3282
Fax: 0181-455-7185

Job Covenant Scheme
Judy Skillington, contact
Tel: 0171-931-5675

Keep Able Ltd
Fleming Close
Park Farm
Wellingborough
Northamptonshire
NN8 3UF
Tel: 01933-679426
Fax: 01933-401403

King's Fund Centre
126 Albert Street
London NW1 7NF
Tel: 0171-267-6111

Laurence-Moon-Bardet-Biedl
  Society
Diana Parker, Secretary
Spring Grove
Loudhams
Wood Lane
Chalfont St Giles
Buckinghamshire HP8 4AR
Tel: 01494-764924

LEAD Scotland (Linking
   Education and Disability)
Queen Margaret College
Clerwood Terrace
Edinburgh EH12 8TS
Tel: 0131-317-3439
Fax: 0131-339-7198

Learning Direct
Freephone: 0800-100900

Learning From Experience Trust
   (LET)
Anglia Polytechnic University
Victoria Road South
Chelmsford
Essex CM1 1LL
Tel/Fax: 01245-348779

Lebers Optic Neuropathy
   Trust
Theresa Hanscome
13 Palmer Road
Maidstone
Kent ME16 0DL
Tel: 01622-751025

Legable
Mike Moulds, Centre
   Manager
Workable
The Innovation Centre
Whiteknights
Reading
Berkshire RG6 6BX
Tel: 0118-925-2912
Fax: 0118-986-7767

Library Association
7 Ridgemount Street
London WC1E 7AE
Tel: 0171-636-7543
Fax: 0171-436-7218

Library of Congress (National
   Library Service for the Blind
   and Physically Handicapped)
1291 Taylor Street North West
Washington, DC 20542
USA
Tel: +1-202-707-5104

Living Paintings Trust
Unit 8
Kingsclere Park
Kingsclere
Newbury
Berkshire RG20 4SW
Tel: 01635-299771

London Regional Transport
Unit for Disabled Passengers
55 Broadway
London, SW1H 0BD
Tel: 0171-226-5600

LOOK (National Federation of
   Families with Visually Impaired
   Children)
Queen Alexandra College
49 Court Oak Road
Harborne
Birmingham B17 9TG
Tel: 0121-428-5038
Fax: 0121-428-5048

LOOK (London office)
LOOK, London
Clapham Park School
127 Park Hill
Clapham
London SW4 9PA
Tel: 0181-678-0555

Lupus UK
PO Box 999
Romford
Essex RM1 1DW
Tel: 01708-731251
Fax: 01708-731252

Macular Disease Society
Mrs Marion Davies
PO Box 247
Heywards Heath
West Sussex RH17 5FF
Tel: 0181-363-7707

Magazine for Graduates with
 Disabilities
Arberry Pink Ltd
Chelsea Wharf
London SW10 0QJ
Tel: 0171-362-5100

Magna Large Print
 Books
Magna House
Long Preston
Near Skipton
North Yorkshire BD23 4ND
Tel: 01729-840225/840526
Fax: 01729-840683

Marfan Association UK
Mrs Diane Rust
6 Queens Road
Farnborough
Hampshire GU14 6DH
Tel: 01252-547441
Fax: 01252-523585

Metropolitan Sports Club for the
 Visually Handicapped
80 Elms Farm Road
Hornchurch
Essex RM12 5RD
Tel: 01708-456832

Micro and Anophthalmic
 Children's Society (MACS)
Mrs Maggie Bourne, Secretary
1 Skymans Fee
Frinton on Sea
Essex CO13 0RN
Tel: 01255-677511

Middlesex Association for the
 Blind (MAB)
Northolt Road Clinic
322 Northolt Road
South Harrow
Middlesex HA2 8EQ
Tel: 0181-423-5141
Fax: 0181-423-9503

'Mobility Aids'
50 Springfield Road
Moseley
Birmingham B13 9NP
Tel: 0121-777-7419

Monument Tape Services (MTS)
20 Laburnum Road
Wellington
Somerset TA21 8EL
Tel: 01823-662104

Moorfields Eye Hospital
City Road
London EC1V 2PD
Tel: 0171-253-3411

Motherwell College
Dalzell Drive
Motherwell
Strathclyde ML1 2DD
Tel: 01698-232323

Multiple Sclerosis Society
25 Effie Road
Fulham
London SW6 1EE
Tel: 0171-736-6267
Fax: 0171-376-9861

National Association for Special
 Educational Needs
NASEN House
Units 4 and 5
Amber Business Village
Amber Close
Amington
Tamworth B77 4RP
Tel: 01827-311500

National Association of
 Industries for the Blind and
 Disabled

Triton House
43a High Street South
Dunstable
Bedfordshire LU6 3RZ
Tel: 01582-606796

National Association of Local
 Societies for the Visually
 Impaired (NALSVI)
Sue Ferguson, Secretary
21 Greencliffe Drive
York YO3 6NA
Tel: 01904-671921

National Association of
 Orientation and Mobility
 Officers
Miss Jean Hollis, Hon. Secretary
107 Cowper Street
Hove
East Sussex BN3 5BL
Tel: 01273-735609

National Association of Toy and
 Leisure Libraries / Play Matters
68 Churchway
London NW1 1LT
Tel: 0171-387-9592
Fax: 0171-383-2714

National Childbirth Trust and
 Parent Ability
Alexandra House
Oldham Terrace
London W3 6NH
Tel: 0181-992-8637
Fax: 0181-992-5929

National Council for Educational
Technology (NCET)
Milburn Hill Road
Science Park
Coventry
Warwickshire CV4 7JJ
Tel: 01203-416994

National Council for Voluntary
Organisations (NCVO)
Regent's Wharf
8 All Saint's Street
London N1 9RL
Tel: 0171-713-6161

National Deafblind League
81 Rainbow Court
Paston Ridings
Peterborough PE4 7UP
Tel: 01733-573511
Fax: 01733-325353

National Diabetic Retinopathy
Network
Jude Andrews
7 Shore Close
Hampton
Middlesex TW12 3XS
Tel: 0181-941-5821

National Disability Council
6th Floor
The Adelphi
1–11 John Adam Street
London WC2N 6HT
Tel: 0171-712-2099
Fax: 0171-712-2075

National Federation of Access
Centres
The ACCESS Centre
Hereward College of Further
Education
Bramston Crescent
Tile Hill Lane
Coventry
Warwickshire CV4 9SW
Tel: 01203-461231
Fax: 01203-694305

National Federation of the Blind
of the United Kingdom
(NFBUK)
Unity House
Smyth Street
Westgate
Wakefield
West Yorkshire WF1 1ER
Tel: 01924-291313
Fax: 01924-200244

National Federation of the Blind
(Scotland)
Miss J. Watt
31/36 Pilrig Street
Edinburgh
Lothian EH6 5AR

National Foundation
for Educational
Research
The Mere
Upton Park
Slough
Berkshire SL1 2DQ

Tel: 01753-574123
Fax: 01753-691632

National Health Service Health
  Advisory Service
Sutherland House
29/37 Brighton Road
Sutton
Surrey SM2 5AM
Tel: 0845 1888 (calls charged at
  local rate)

National League of the Blind
  and Disabled (NLBD)
2 Tenterden Road
Tottenham
London N17 8BE
Tel: 0181-808-6030
Fax: 0181-885-3235

National Library for the Blind
Cromwell Road
Bredbury
Stockport
Greater Manchester SK6 2SG
Tel: 0161-494-0217
Fax: 0161-406-6278

National Mobility Centre
Faculty of Health & Social
  Science
Cox Building
Perry Barr
Birmingham B42 2SU
Tel: 0121-331-6465

National Trust
Valerie Wenham, Adviser

Facilities for Disabled Visitors
36 Queen Anne's Gate
London SW1H 9AS
Tel: 0171-222-9251
Fax: 0171-222-5097

New College Worcester Former
  Pupils Association
Colin Fisher, Secretary
The Gables
90 Barton Road
Lancaster LA1 4EL
Tel: 01524-64706

Nicholls & Clarke Ltd
3–10 Shoreditch High Street
London E1 6PE
Tel: 0171-247-5432
Fax: 0171-247-7738

North Herts Talking Newspaper
  Association
163 Valley Way
Stevenage
Hertfordshire SG2 9DD
Tel: 01438-746700

North London Homes for the
  Blind (NLHB)
Mr G. Geoghegan, Secretary
Honeywood House
Station Road
East Preston
West Sussex BN16 3AL
Tel: 01903-770339

NW SEMERC
1 Broadbent Road

Watersheddings
Oldham OL1 4HU
Tel: 0161-628-0919

Nystagmus Action Group
John Saunders
43 Gordonbrock Road
London SE4 1JA
Tel: 01392-272573

Off The Page
188 Wellfield Road
London SW16 2BU
Tel: 0181-769-9682

Open University
Milton Keynes MK7 6AA
Derek Child, Adviser on the
    Education of Students with
    Disabilities,
Tel: 01908-653442
Dave Jones, Electronics
Tel: 01908-653356
Dr. Tom Vincent, Institute of
    Educational Technology,
Tel: 01908-274066

Opportunities for People with
    Disabilities
74 Great Portland Street
London W1N 5AL
Tel: 0171-580-7545

Opportunities for the Disabled
1 Bank Building
Princes Street
London, EC2R 8EU
Tel: 0171-726-4961

OPSIS: National Association for
    the Education, Training and
    Support of Blind and Partially
    Sighted People
Gretton House
43 Hatton Garden
London EC1N 8EE
Tel: 0171-405-6697
Fax: 0171-405-6698

Optical Information Council
Temple Chambers
Temple Avenue
London EC4Y 0DT
Tel: 0171-353-3556

Organisation of Blind
    Afro-Caribbeans (OBAC)
Gloucester House
Camberwell New Road
London SE5 0RZ
Tel: 0171-735-3400
Fax: 0171-582-8334

Papworth Ability Services Ltd
Unit 11
Langley Business Court
Beedon
Newbury RB20 8RY
Tel: 01635-247724
Fax: 01635-243300

Partially Sighted Society (PSS)
(general administration,
    printing, enlarging, mail
    order, membership,
    publications)

PO Box 322
Queens Road
Doncaster
West Yorkshire DN1 2NX
Tel: 01302-323132
Fax: 01302-365998

Partially Sighted Society
Greater London Office (general
    enquiries, low vision adviser)
9 Plato Place
72–74 St Dionis Road
London SW6 4TU
Tel: 0171-371-0289

Sight Centres (low vision advice
    and training, information and
    counselling)
At Doncaster, London and also
    at:

(1) Dean Clarke House
     Southernhay East
     Exeter
     Devon EX1 1PE
     Tel: 01392-210656

(2) Salisbury District Hospital
     Salisbury
     Wiltshire SP2 8BJ
     Tel: 01722-336262 ext. 2175

Pathway Communications Ltd
Berrows House
Bath Street
Hereford HR1 2HF
Tel: 01432-273311

Pia
102 Bute Street
Cardiff Bay
Cardiff CF1 6AD
Tel: 01222-301000

Playback Service for the Blind
Strathclyde House
India Street
Glasgow G2 4PF
Tel: 0141-248-5811
Fax: 0141-287-8880

Portset Systems Ltd
Shield House
Brook Street
Bishop's Waltham
Southampton SO32 1AX
Tel: 01489-896837

Pre-school Playgroups Association
61/63 King's Cross Road
London WC1X 9LL
Tel: 0171-833-0991

Prince of Wales' Advisory Group
    on Disability
Nutmeg House
60 Gainsford Street
London SE1 2NY
Tel: 0171-403-9433

Professional Vision Services Ltd
Welbury House
90 Walsworth Road
Hitchin
Hertfordshire SG4 9SX

Tel: 01462-420751
Fax: 01462-420185

Projects by the Blind
10–12 Yukon Road
London SW12 9PU
Tel: 0181-675-3900
Fax: 0181-675-3537

PULSEDATA International UK Ltd
Blotts Barn Business Centre
Brooks Road
Rounds
Wellingborough NN9 6NS
Tel: 01933-626000
Fax: 01933-626204

Queen Alexandra College (BRIB)
49 Court Oak Road
Harborne
Birmingham B17 9TG
Tel: 0121-428-5050
Fax: 0121-428-2282

Recording for the Blind Inc.
Headquarters
20 Roszel Road
Princeton NJ 08540
USA
Tel: +1-609-452-0606

Rehabilitation Engineering
  Movement Advisory Panels
  (REMAP)
Technical Equipment for
  Disabled People
Mr J. Wright
Hazeldene

Ightham
Sevenoaks
Kent TN15 9AD
Tel: 01732-883818

Relate
Herbert Gray College
Little Church Street
Rugby CV21 3AP
Tel: 01788-573241

Research Centre for the
  Education of the Visually
  Handicapped (RECEVH)
School of Education
University of Birmingham
PO Box 363
Birmingham B15 2TT
Tel: 0121-414-6733
Fax: 0121-414-4865

Research Institute for Consumer
  Affairs (RICA)
2 Marylebone Road
London NW1 4DF
Tel: 0171-935-2460

Retinoblastoma Society
Jenny Coates
c/o Academic Department of
  Paediatric Oncology
St Bartholomew's Hospital
West Smithfield
London EC1A 7BE
Tel: 0171-600-3309

Royal Association for Disability
  and Rehabilitation (RADAR)

12 City Forum
250 City Road
London EC1V 8AF
Tel: 0171-250-3222
Fax: 0171-259-0212

Royal College of
  Ophthalmologists
17 Cornwall Terrace
London NW1 4QW
Tel: 0171-935-0702

Royal Commonwealth Society for
  the Blind
Commonwealth House
Heath Road
Haywards Heath
West Sussex RH16 73AZ
Tel: 01444-412424

Royal London Society for the
  Blind
Dorton House
Seal
Nr Sevenoaks
Kent TN15 0ED
Tel: 01732-592650

Royal National College for the
  Blind
College Road
Hereford HR1 1EB
Tel: 01432-265725
Fax: 01432-353478

Royal National Institute for the
  Blind (RNIB)

For the following services:
  Community Education
  Education Information
  Employment Development
    Technology Unit (EDTU)
  Employment and Student
  Support Network
  Ethnic Minorities
  Eye Health Unit (Tel:
    0345-669999)
  Grants
  Health
  Hotels, Holidays, Leisure
  New Beacon Magazine
  Ophthalmic advice
  Physiotherapy Support Service
  Reference Library (Website
    Editor: 0171-391-2191,
    j.howell@rnib.org.uk)
  Resource Centre, London
  RNIB/GDBA Mobility Unit
  Voluntary Agencies Link Unit
    (VALU) (Tel: 0345-669999)
    (Directory of Agencies for the
    Blind is obtainable from RNIB)
  Welfare Rights and
    Community Care Advocacy
    Service
224 Great Portland Street
London W1A 6AA
Tel: 0171-388-1266
Fax: 0171-388-2034

*RNIB Accommodation with Care
  Support Service*
RNIB Tate House
28 Wetherby Road

Harrogate
North Yorkshire HG2 7SA
Tel: 01423-881140
Fax: 01423-885192

RNIB Advocacy Service for Parents
C/O RNIB New College
Whittington Road
Worcester WR5 2JX
Tel: 01905-357635

RNIB Book Sales Service
Education Centre (London and
   South East)
Garrow House
190 Kensal Road
North Kensington
London W10 5BT
Tel: 0181-968-8600
Fax: 0181-969-2380

RNIB Customer Services
PO Box 173
Peterborough PE2 6WS
Tel: 01733-370777
Tel: 0345-023153 (for the price
   of a local call)
Tel: 0345-456457 (direct order
   line; for the price of a local call)
Fax: 01733-371555
For the following services:
Braille Library
Cassette Library
Games and equipment
Sales of publications in large
   print, Braille, Moon and on
   cassette tape

Transcription service and advice
*RNIB Education Centre (London
   and South East)*
Garrow House
190 Kensal Road
North Kensington
London W10 5BT
Tel: 0181-968-8600
Fax: 0181-960-3593

*RNIB Employment, Assessment
   and Rehabilitation
   Centres*
Alwyn House
3 Wemysshall Road
Ceres
Cupar
Fife KY15 5LX
Tel: 01334-828894/5/6
Fax: 01334-828911

Manor House
Middle Lincombe Road
Torquay
Devon TQ1 2NG
Tel: 01803-214523
Fax: 01803-214143

*RNIB Employment and Student
   Support Network*
Andy Buchan, Administrative
   Officer
PO Box 49
Loughborough
Leicestershire LE11 3DG
Tel: 01509-211995
Fax: 01509-232013

RNIB Housing Service
Garrow House
190 Kensal Road
North Kensington
London W10 5BT
Tel: 0181-969-2380
Fax: 0181-960-3593

*RNIB Multiple Disability Training
   Services*
7 The Square
111 Broad Street
Edgbaston
Birmingham B15 1AS
Tel: 0121-643-9912
Fax: 0121-643-1738

RNIB New College
Helen Williams,
   Headteacher
Whittington Road
Worcester WR5 2JX
Tel: 01905-357635

*RNIB Northern Ireland Service
   Bureau*
Unit B
40 Linenhall Street
Belfast BT2 8BG
Tel: 01232-329373
Fax: 01232-439228

RNIB Redhill College
Joyce Deere, Principal
Philanthropic Road
Redhill
Surrey RH1 4DG

Tel: 01731-768935

RNIB Resource Centres:

(1) London
     RNIB Headquarters
     Tel: 0171-388-1266

(2) Londonderry
     Sensory Support Service
     16 Bishop Street
     Londonderry BT48 6PN
     Tel: 01504-374619
     Fax: 01504-374810

(3) Scotland
     9 Viewfield Place
     Stirling FK8 1NL
     Tel: 01786-541752
     Fax: 01786-462336

*School of Social Work and RNIB
   Rehabilitation Studies*
University of Central England
Faculty of Health and
   Community Care
Cox Building
Perry Barr
Birmingham BA2 2SU
Tel: 0121-331-6405

RNIB Scotland
10 Magdala Crescent
Edinburgh EH12 5BE
Tel: 0131-313-1498
Fax: 0131-313-1875

RNIB Self Employment Development Unit
Tudor House
RNIB Redhill College
Philanthropic Road
Redhill
Surrey RH1 4DG
Tel: 01731-768935

RNIB Social Service Development Unit (SSDU)
7 The Square
111 Broad Street
Edgbaston
Birmingham B15 1AS
Tel: 0121-643-9912
Fax: 0121-643-1738

RNIB Talking Book Service
Mount Pleasant
Alperton
Wembley
Middlesex HA0 1RR
Tel: 0345-626843 (calls charged at local rate)
Fax: 0181-903-6916

RNIB Transcription Centre North West
67 High Street
Tarporley
Cheshire CW6 0DP
Tel: 01829-732115
Fax: 01829-732408

RNIB Vocational College
Kevin Connell, Principal

Radmoor Road
Loughborough
Leicestershire LE11 3BS
Tel: 01509-611077
Fax: 01509-232013

Royal National Institute
for Deaf People
(RNID)
19–23 Featherstone
Street
London EC1V 8SL
Tel: 0171-296-8000
Fax: 0171-296-8199

Royal School for the Blind (RSB
Leatherhead)
Highlands Road
Leatherhead
Surrey KT22 8NR
Tel: 01372-373086
Fax: 01372-370143

Scottish Braille Press
Craigmillar Park
Edinburgh
Lothian EH16 5NB
Tel: 0131-662-4445
Fax: 0131-662-1968

Scottish Further Education Unit
(SFEU)
Argyll Court
Castle Business Park
Stirling FK9 4TY
Tel: 01786-892000
Fax: 01786-892001

Scottish Higher Education
  Funding Council
  (SHEFC)
Donaldson House
97 Haymarket Terrace
Edinburgh EH12 5HD
Tel: 0131-313-6500

Scottish National Federation for
  the Welfare of the Blind
PO Box 500
Gillespie Crescent
Edinburgh EH10 4HZ
Tel: 0131-229-1456
Fax: 0131-229-4060

Scottish Office (Education and
  Industry)
Victoria Quay
Edinburgh EH6 6QQ
Tel: 0131-556-8400

Scottish Sensory Centre
Moray House Institute of
  Education
Holyrood Road
Edinburgh EH8 8AQ
Tel: 0131-558-6501

SENSE (National Deafblind and
  Rubella Association)
Sense Usher Services
11–13 Clifton Terrace
London N4 3SR
Tel: 0171-272-7774
Fax: 0171-272-6012

SENSE Northern Ireland
Resource Centre
Graham House
Knockbracken
Healthcare Park
Saintfield Road
Belfast BT8 8BH
Tel: 01232-705858

SENSE Scotland
Outreach Advisory Service
15 Newark Drive
Pollockshields
Glasgow G41 4QB
Tel: 0141-424-3222

Sensory Support Services
Cannon Park School
  Annexe
Cannon Hill Road
Coventry CV4 7DE
Tel: 01203-417415

Sensory Systems Ltd
1 Watling Gate
297–303 Edgware Road
London NW9 6NB
Tel: 0181-205-3002
Fax: 0181-205-1192

Share The Vision
Peter Craddock, Director
36 Circular Road
Castle Rock
County Londonderry BT51 4XA
Tel: 01265-848303
Fax: 01265-848003

Shaw Trust
Shaw House
White House Business Park
Trowbridge
Wiltshire BA14 0XG
Tel: 01225-716300

Sight & Sound Technology Ltd
Quantel House
Anglia Way
Moulton Park
Northampton NN3 6JA
Tel: 01604-798070
Fax: 01604-798090

Skill: National Bureau for
    Students with Disabilities
336 Brixton Road
London SW9 7AA
Tel: 0171-274-0565
Fax: 0171-274-7840
Information Service
    Monday–Friday 1.30–4.30 p.m.:
    0171-978-9890

Social Policy Research Unit
    (SPRU)
Professor Sally Baldwin,
    Director
University of York
Heslington
York YO1 5DD
Tel: 01904-433608
Fax: 01904-433618

Society of Blind Lawyers
Jeremy R. Browne, Chairman

82 Cresswell Road
Chesham HP5 1TA
Tel: 01494-772788
Fax: 01494-791581

St Dunstan's Organisation for
    Men and Women Blinded on
    War Service
PO Box 4XB
12–14 Harcourt Street
London W1A 4XB
Tel: 0171-723-5021
Fax: 0171-262-6199

Standing Conference of
    Principals (SCOP)
Woburn House
20 Tavistock Square
London WC1H 9HB
Tel: 0171-419-5550
Fax: 0171-388-7327

Star Housing Association
    Ltd
Mrs D. McLoughlin
c/o 5 Watford Way
Hendon
London NW4 3JN
Tel: 0181-202-3858
Fax: 0181-202-9513

Stroke Association
CHSA House
Whitecross Street
London EC1Y 8JJ
Tel: 0171-490-7999
Fax: 0171-490-2666

Stroke Information Centre
(North Wales)
HM Stanley Hospital
St Asaph
Wales LL30 2PT
Tel: 01745-582368

Support Into Work (SIW)
The Disability Employment
Centre
4 Osmaston Road
The Spot
Derby DE1 1SB
Tel: 01332-292915

Tactile Audio Braille Services Ltd
(TABS)
Tony Feetam
YP1 Building
83-93 George Street
Hull
Yorkshire HU1 3EN
Tel: 01482-595383

Talking Newspaper Association
of the United Kingdom
(TNAUK)
National Recording Centre
10 Browning Road
Heathfield
East Sussex TN21 8DB
Tel: 01435-866102
Fax: 01435-865422

Tandy
Bilston Road
Wednesbury

West Midlands WS10 7JN
Tel: 0121-556-6429
Fax: 0121-556-0786

Tape Recording Service for the
Blind
48 Fairfax Road
Farnborough
Hampshire GU14 8JF
Tel: 01252-547943

Dr. A.F. Tatham
The Map Room
Chesham Building
King's College
University of London
The Strand
London WC2R 2LS

Teaching and Learning
Technology Support Network
University of Wales at Bangor
Information Services:
Sackville Road
Bangor
Gwynedd LL57 1LD
Tel: 01248-382425

Techno-Vision Systems Ltd
76 Bunting Road
Industrial Estate
Northampton NN2 6EE
Tel: 01604-792777

Telephones for the Blind Fund
7 Huntersfield Close
Reigate

Surrey RH2 0PX
Tel: 01737-248032

The Advisory Committee on
   Telecommunications for
   Disabled and Elderly People
(DIEL)
Terry Walker and Barbara Powell
DIEL Secretariat
50 Ludgate Hill
London EC4M 7JJ
Tel: 0171-634-8773/4
Fax: 0171-634-8845

The Albino Fellowship
Mr Mark Sanderson, Hon.
   Secretary
9 Burnley Road
Hapton
Near Burnley
Lancashire BB11 5QR
Tel: 01282-776145

The Chartered Society of
   Physiotherapy
14 Bedford Row
London WC1R 4ED
Tel: 0171-306-6666
Fax: 0171-306-6611

The Computability Centre
PO Box 94
Warwick CV34 5WS
Tel: 01926-312847
Fax: 01926-311345
Freephone Helpline: 0800-269545

The Leadership Consortium
Nutmeg House
60 Gainsford Street
London SE1 2NY
Tel: 0171-403-9433
Fax: 0171-403-6404

The London Voluntary Resource
   Centre
356 Holloway Road
London N7 6PA
Tel: 0171-700-0100

The Prince's Youth Business
   Trust
18 Park Square East
London NW1 4LH
Tel: 0171-543-1234

The Stationery Office
Publication Centre
PO Box 276
London SW8 5DT
Tel: 0171-873-9090 (telephone
   orders)
      0171-873-0011 (general
   enquiries)
Fax: 0171-873-0011

The Toxoplasmosis
   Trust
Room 26
61–71 Collier Street
London N1 9BE
Tel: 0171-713-0663
      0171-713-0599-(Helpline)
Fax: 0171-713-0611

The Prince of Wales' Advisory
 Group on Disability
Nutmeg House
60 Gainsford Street
London SE1 2NY
Tel: 0171-403-9433

Torch Trust for the Blind
Torch House
Hallaton
Market Harborough
Leicestershire LE16 8UJ
Tel: 01858-555301
Fax: 01858-555371

Toys for the Handicapped
76 Barracks Road
Sandy Lane
Industrial Estate
Stourport-on-Severn
Worcestershire DY13 9QB
Tel: 01299-827-820
Fax: 01299-827-035

Tripscope
The Courtyard
Evelyn Road
London W4 5JL
Tel: 0181-994-9294

Ulverscroft Large Print Books
 Ltd
The Green
Bradgate Road
Anstey
Leicester LE7 7FU
Tel: 01533-364325

University and College
 Admission Service (UCAS)
Fulton House
Jessop Avenue
Cheltenham
Glos GL50 3SH
Tel: 01242-222444

UKCOSA: The Council for
 International Education
9–17 St Albans Place
London N1 0NX
Tel: 0171-226-3762
Fax: 0171-226-3373

VIEW: Association for the
 Education and Welfare of the
 Visually Handicapped
Mrs C. Arter, Hon. Secretary
York House Annexe
Exhall Grange School
Wheelwright Lane
Coventry CV7 9HP
Tel: 01203-361127
Fax: 01203-645074

Viewpoint Technology
PO Box 66
Hereford HR1 1YZ
Tel: 01432-343623

VISability
5 Burnham Gardens
Cranford
Hounslow
Middlesex TW4 6LS
Tel: 0181-897-8587

Vision Aid
22a Chorley New Road
Bolton BL1 4AP
Tel: 01204-531882
Fax: 01204-394218

Visually Impaired Musicians
    Association (VIMA)
Julie Smethurst, Secretary
76 Duncan Road
Crooks
Sheffield S10 1SN
Tel: 0114-268-5405

Voluntary Council for
    Handicapped Children
National Children's Bureau
8 Wakley Street
London EC1V 7QE
Tel: 0171-843-6000
Fax: 0171-278-9512

Wales Council for the Blind
Shand House
20 Newport Road
Cardiff CF2 1YB
Tel: 01222-473954
Fax: 01222-455710

Ways & Means (Nottingham
    Rehab)
Ludlow Hill Road
West Bridgford
Nottingham NG2 6HD
Tel: 0115-945-2121/936-0319

Women's Royal Voluntary Service
Milton Hill House
Milton Hill
Abingdon
Oxford OX13 6AF
Tel: 01235-441900

Workable
David Bennett, Director
Premier House
10 Greycoat Place
London, SW1P 1SB
Tel: 0171-222-8866
Fax: 0171-222-1903

The Workers' Education
    Association (WEA)
Vaughn College
St Nicholas Circle
Leicester LE1 4LB
Tel: 0116-251-9740
Fax: 0116-251-8731

Index

Page references in bold indicate figures.

Spectacles 120–1
Speech systems 179–80
    for use with personal
        computers 180–3
    for use with portable
        computers/note takers
        183–4
    voice recognition 184–5
SSEN *see* Statement of special
    educational need
Statement of special educational
    need 67, 68, 230, 231
Statistics 6, 35–6, 72, 80, 81, 82,
    83, 112, 291, 294, 295, 297
Stereotyping 29–32
Strategy
    definitions of 95
    institutional 300
        marketing and publicity
            312–13
Stress
    associated with:
        aspects of college life 74
        change in/deterioration
            of/loss of sight 73–4
        concealment of
            impairment 79
        life-cycle 74
        negotiating the
            environment 79
    techniques to reduce 104–7
Students' Union 277–8
Study skills 259–60
    Braille 261
    cassette tape 261
    group work 262
    note taking 107

readers *see* Readers
    screen based 262
Support staff/workers 69, 243
    learning support tutor *see*
        Disability co-ordinator

Tactile code *see* Braille
Tactile diagrams 201–2
    see also Raised diagrams
    methods of production
        202–6
Tactile displays *see* Braille;
    electronic displays
Tactile indicators 128–30
    Bump-ons/Locator Dots
        129–30, **129, 130, 131**
    Hi Marks **128,** 129
Tactile surfaces 147, 151
Taught helplessness *see* Disability
Teaching strategies 252
    before the teaching begins
        252–53
    external lecturers 259
    lectures 253–56
    practical classes 256–58
    verbal instructions 258
Technical support 161–3
Technology training 161, 162,
    297
Terminology xv
Tomlinson Committee Report
    71, 292–93
Transition
    from college to employment
        234–37
    difficulties associated with
        232–33